MANAGING SUICIDAL RISK

MANAGING SUICIDAL RISK

A Collaborative Approach

SECOND EDITION

David A. Jobes

Foreword by Marsha M. Linehan

THE GUILFORD PRESS
New York   London

Library of Congress Cataloging-in-Publication Data

Names: Jobes, David A., author.
Title: Managing suicidal risk : a collaborative approach / David A. Jobes ; foreword by Marsha M.
Linehan.
Description: Second edition. I New York : The Guilford Press, 2016. I Revised edition of the author's
Managing suicidal risk, 2006. I Includes bibliographical references and index.
Identifiers: LCCN 2016001913 I ISBN 9781462526901 (paperback) I ISBN 9781462533657 (hardcover)
Subjects: LCSH: Suicide. I BISAC: PSYCHOLOGY / Suicide. I MEDICAL /
    Psychiatry / General. I SOCIAL SCIENCE / Social Work. I MEDICAL / Nursing / Psychiatric.
Classification: LCC RC569 .J63 2016 I DDC 616.85/8445—dc23
LC record available at *http://lccn.loc.gov/2016001913*

Once again, to Colleen, Connor, and Dillon
and to the memory of
Frank Jobes, Helen Jobes, and Steve Jobes

About the Author

David A. Jobes, PhD, ABPP, is Professor of Psychology and Associate Director of Clinical Training at The Catholic University of America. He is also Adjunct Professor of Psychiatry in the School of Medicine at the Uniformed Services University of the Health Sciences. With research interests in suicidology for over 30 years, he has published extensively in the field and routinely conducts professional training in clinical suicidology, professional ethics, and risk management. Dr. Jobes has served as a consultant to the Department of Defense, the Department of Veterans Affairs, the Centers for Disease Control and Prevention, and the Institute of Medicine of the National Academy of Sciences. A past president of the American Association of Suicidology (AAS), he serves on the Scientific Council and the Public Policy Council of the American Foundation for Suicide Prevention. His work has been recognized with the Marsha Linehan Award for Outstanding Research in the Treatment of Suicidal Behavior and the Louis I. Dublin Award for Career Contribution to Suicide Prevention from the AAS, among other honors. Dr. Jobes is a Fellow of the American Psychological Association and is board certified in clinical psychology. He maintains a private clinical and forensic practice in Washington, DC.

Foreword

When I was asked to write the foreword to the second edition of *Managing Suicidal Risk*, I immediately accepted. I have a long and interesting history with David Jobes. He has spent his professional life at The Catholic University of America, where I began my own academic career as an assistant professor before joining the faculty at the University of Washington. Some 30 years ago, when Dave was a graduate student at American University, his first-year practicum supervisor in psychotherapy was Allen Leventhal, who was a major influence in my life and early career. At that time, Dave wrote me a letter asking questions about my research, and I wrote him back. We met in person a few years later at an American Association of Suicidology conference, and I began encouraging his early assessment research that ultimately led to the development of the Suicide Status Form (SSF), which is described in depth throughout this book.

A critical turning point in our history was when I was invited to present at the Aeschi Conference in Switzerland, a fabulous series of meetings with clinician–researchers who endeavored to find empathic and compassionate ways of working with suicidal patients. At one of these meetings, Dave and I had a series of in-depth discussions about his becoming a suicide treatment researcher. I pushed him to ramp up his scientific work and pursue funding to further investigate the Collaborative Assessment and Management of Suicidality approach (CAMS—the focus of this book). Dave pursued a National Institute of Mental Health R-34 grant, on which I served as a consultant. He did not get the grant, but it cemented our bond, and I was able to mentor him in grant writing and help him develop further as a suicide treatment researcher.

Anyone who knows me is aware of my passion for science and data and the obvious need to develop effective treatments through randomized controlled trials (RCTs). A decade ago, there was very little RCT research on suicide under way outside of my own work on dialectical behavior therapy. I made a commitment to change the field when I initiated and convened a series of research meetings in Seattle with some senior colleagues and a number of more junior investigators to support the writing of grants that would lead to funded RCT research in suicide. I am pleased to report that these meetings were very effective in helping a generation of researchers to obtain funding for a series of RCT investigations that are now transforming the field of suicide prevention. As a member of this cohort, Dave was one of those investigators who went on to seek and obtain multiple RCT grants and publish data about the effectiveness of CAMS. Through this work we know that CAMS dramatically decreases suicidal ideation and overall symptom distress while increasing hope, patient satisfaction, and retention to clinical care. In addition, there are now *four* RCTs of CAMS under way around the world seeking to replicate and extend earlier clinical trial findings and to better understand the impact of CAMS on suicidal behaviors.

Many people assume that I am a borderline personality disorder treatment researcher. In truth, I have always in my heart been a suicide treatment researcher first. Suicides are the fatalities within mental health care, and frankly we should know much more about suicide treatment than we do. Dave shares my lifelong passion for helping people find their way out of suicidal despair. With its emphasis on empathy, honesty, and collaboration, there is evidence that CAMS helps stabilize suicidal patients so that their self-defined suicidal "drivers" can be effectively treated with various evidence-based interventions. The SSF provides a useful guide to help suicidal patients stabilize as clinician and patient work collaboratively within the CAMS framework; I believe CAMS is a unique contribution to clinical literature.

It has been a pleasure to support Dave's scientific development of CAMS over the past 20 years, and I am gratified to know that he considers me to be a major influence in his growth as a clinical scientist. It is rewarding to see that RCT research in clinical suicide prevention is now robust and thriving, and Dave's research on CAMS is a big part of that. We suicidologists believe that suicidal people must be meaningfully understood, appreciated, and given particular skills to find their way in life. This book is a major contribution in this singular pursuit. The CAMS approach to suicidal risk is a valuable remedy for a pervasive "shame-and-blame" culture that is too commonly seen in contemporary mental health care when mental health providers encounter a suicidal patient. I believe this text will help both clinicians and patients find a way to cope with the suicidal struggle, overcoming those forces that lead to self-inflicted death, to one day find their way out of hell and then truly realize a life that is worth living.

MARSHA M. LINEHAN, PhD, ABPP
Professor and Director
Behavioral Research and Therapy Clinics
University of Washington

Preface

My professional identity has always been that of a *clinician–researcher*. In my mind, this is an entirely different worldview from that of *research clinician*. Over the years of developing the Collaborative Assessment and Management of Suicidality (CAMS), I have consistently heard from clinicians that CAMS tends to "make sense" to many providers in the trenches of mental health care. CAMS is decidedly not an "ivory-tower" approach to clinical work with suicidal people. My feeling has always been that the best clinical research should directly inform clinical practices and make good clinical sense. But I also strongly believe in science and the importance of proving through empirical validation that something that makes intuitive clinical sense actually does work (and does not cause harm).

Beyond these reflections, as a clinician and as a clinical researcher I have been deeply engrossed in the study of the suicidal mind for more than 30 years. What this in-depth study has revealed to me is described throughout this book. Perhaps most important, I have grown to believe firmly that most suicidal patients who are talking to a mental health professional in actuality *do not want to die*. Instead, they are fundamentally struggling in a psychological space and time in which they just do not know what else to do. If we understand this simple notion—and the patient sees and feels that we do indeed "get it"—we are well on our way to a potentially life-saving clinical endeavor.

In the first edition of this book, I felt driven to make a persuasive case for the use of the CAMS approach; I wanted to convince readers that this approach, while novel, was valuable and worthy of their consideration. But to make the case, I had to make the argument for some key (and controversial) points, including (1) seeing *suicide* as a proper focus of treatment (vs. necessarily focusing on a mental disorder), (2) the virtue of working to keep a suicidal person *out* of an inpatient setting, (3) the superiority of various forms of stabilization planning to no-harm contracting or commitments to safety, (4) the critical importance of empathy for suicidality and collaboration to successful treatment, and (5) the role of the *patient* as a key partner in therapy through the treatment of *patient-defined* problems that make the patient suicidal. In the decade since the first edition, many of these ideas have gained some traction in the field. But I nevertheless still routinely encounter clinicians who remain surprised by these ideas, somewhat wary, or downright resistant to them. I have thus come to appreciate that changing familiar clinical practices is extremely hard.

CAMS is fundamentally designed to empower clinicians by empowering their patients. Throughout my career, I have been determined to develop an effective approach to help my suicidal patients fight for their lives, before they felt inexorably compelled to take them. To realize this goal, I knew I had to find a way to build the best possible clinical alliance and also inspire motivation within my patients. Every major component of CAMS is intended to maximize the power of the clinical alliance while simultaneously enhancing patient motivation and autonomy.

While use of CAMS (and the Suicide Status Form [SSF]) has helped change practice behaviors with suicidal patients over the past 25 years, there is still a long way to go if we really intend to save more lives by using CAMS or any other replicated evidence-based approach (such as dialectical behavior therapy or cognitive therapy for suicide prevention, which are both discussed throughout this book). It remains alarming to me how rarely clinical practices that are suicide-specific and proven to work from scientific investigation are actually used. In the business of clinical life-saving, the status quo is not acceptable. We need agents of change who use practices that are proven to work in treating the causes of suicidality, thereby decreasing suicidal suffering.

Merely understanding the nature of a patient's suicidal struggle may not be enough to clinically prevent suicide, but it is an excellent starting point for life-saving work. Beyond understanding, there is a fundamental requirement to effectively *manage* suicidal risk both clinically with the patient and within ourselves as providers of care. Suicide is simultaneously complex, contentious, mysterious, terrifying, compelling, seductive, and horrifying—across all cultures and around the world. No socioeconomic group, no religion, no demographic is immune or "safe" from suicide. Moreover, no suffering soul can guarantee that suicidal thoughts will not arise if life circumstances get bad enough. As clinicians, we cannot ultimately ensure that we will never encounter or be compelled to treat suicidal risk in the course of our professional work. Suicide is ubiquitous; it is in our news, culture, movies, and literature, and in many of our personal and professional lives. Suicide appears to be a part of the human condition and it simply cannot be denied or avoided.

The ubiquity of the suicide option invariably breeds fear, anxiety, and dread not only among the suicidal and their loved ones, but also among clinicians. In the face of this fear, I have learned that we must focus on what we *need*. In relation to clinically working with suicidal risk, that need boils down to providing the best possible care that may not save everyone, but will make a major difference with most. We must therefore remain steadfast in our resolve to focus on the need to competently assess, understand, track, and treat what makes someone aspire to one of the most profound things a human being can do—terminating one's own existence.

I hope this book, and the approach it describes, can help clinicians effectively manage this anxiety-producing clinical concern. Our suicidal patients are typically desperate people enduring terrible circumstances fraught with uncertainty, fear, pain, and hopelessness. Yet if they are sitting with us, there is hope. How we fan the embers of that hope is what this book is about and lies at the heart of clinically saving a life from suicide.

Acknowledgments

No single author can ever take sole credit for writing a book; there are so many contributors and developments that make it happen. In the first edition, I acknowledged all the "first-generation" contributors to that book, many of whom were my students at The Catholic University of America, and their work is just as relevant to this second edition. But in the years since, there is now a new generation of students and protégés who have made this second edition possible.

I experience a tremendous happiness and pride from the mentoring work I get to do with undergraduate and graduate students who make up The Catholic University of America Suicide Prevention Laboratory (CUA-SPL). There are countless moments when I go into the lab and find students coding forms, working as a study team, and entering endless data into the computer. I love these moments because I get to witness the purity of scientific discovery and learning. Without these students, much of what you are reading would simply not exist, and I am grateful to them for their energy and passion. This next generation of SPL alums and current students include Gary Stone, Elicia Nademin, Ellen Kahn-Greene, Mira Brancu, Melinda Moore, Stephen O'Connor, Matt Fitzgerald, M. K. Yeargin, Vivian Rodriguez, Tara Kraft, Elizabeth Ballard, Andrea Kulish, Julian Lantry, Keith Jennings, Kevin Crowley, Rachel Martin, Liz Hirschhorn, Emma Cardeli, Katie Brazaitis, Rene Lento, Blaire Schembari, Chris Corona, Molly Bowers, Abby Anderson, Asher Siegelman, Josephine Au, Margaret Baer, Maureen Monahan, Brian Clark, Ryan Horgan, Josh Holmes, Sami Saghafi, Samantha Chalker, Brian Piehl, Jorge Ponce, Paul El-Meouchy, Chris Willard, Nikki Caulfield, Tara Casey, Kaitlyn Schuler, Lisa Peterson, and Mariam Gregorian. Special thanks goes to SPL alums John Drozd, Aaron Jacoby, Jason Luoma, Rachel Mann, Steve Wong, and Amy Conrad, who were all key players in the early development of the SSF and the birth of CAMS.

Countless professional colleagues and collaborators deserving acknowledgment include Peter Cimbolic, Barry Wagner, Diane Arnkoff, George Bonanno, Carol Glass, Sandra Barreuco, Brendan Rich, Claire Spears, Marcie Goeke-Morey, Marc Sebrechts, Ralph Albano, Rick Campise, Michael Mond, Larry David, Steve Stein, Bruce Crow, Debra Archuleta, Lynette Pujol, Julie Landry Poole, John Bradley, Aaron Werbel, Brett Schneider, Reggie Russell, Russ Carr, Lisa Horowitz, Liz Marshall, Jon Allen, Katrina Rufino, Roar Fosse, Elaine Franks, Kelly Keorner, Linda Dimeff, J. J. Rasimus, Leticia Duvivier, Jeff Sung, David Huh, Sara Landes, Karin Hendricks, Jan Kemp, Marc DeSantis, Eve Carlson, Caitlin Thompson, Gretchen Ruhe, Grace Keyes, Denise Pazur, and Empathos Resources. I am also indebted to the members of the CAMS-care team, which includes my wife, Colleen Kelly, Andrew Evans, and Devon Evans, as well as our consultants Jennifer Crumlish, Keith Jennings, Stephen O'Connor, Melinda Moore, Amy Brausch, Jan York, Brad Singer, Amber Miracle, Eoin Galavan, Christian Pedersen, Kevin Crowley, Natalie Burns, Steve Wong, and Tom Ellis.

Within the field of suicide prevention, I owe a significant debt of gratitude to Israel Orbach, Konrad Michel, Michael Bostwick, Tim Lineberry, Rory O'Connor, Keith Hawton, Mark Williams, Bent Rosenbaum, Thomas Joiner, Craig Bryan, Marjan Holloway, Matt Nock, Mort Silverman, Jim Overholser, Greg Carter, David Klonsky, Skip Simpson, Susan Stefan, Amy Kulp, Lars Mehlum, Merete Nordentoft, Kate Andreasson, Ellen Townsend, Diego DeLeo, Marianne Goodman, Maria Oquendo, Shawn Shea, Jacque Pistorello, Jane Pearson, Barbara Stanley, Cheryl King, Keith Harris, John Draper, Julie Goldstein-Grumet, Mike Hogan, David Covington, Ursula Whiteside, Steve Vannoy, Peter Britton, Jerry Reid, Dan Reidenberg, Richard McKeon, Maddy Gould, Barry Walsh, Christine Moutier, Bob Gebbia, John Madigan, Anja Gysin-Maillart, Dave Adkins, and Amanda Kerbrat. A special thanks goes out to the guiding professional influences of my graduate mentor Lanny Berman, as well as Bob Litman, Norman Farberow, Jerome Motto, Terry Maltsberger, Aaron Beck, and of course the late Ed Shneidman, who remains one of the most influential voices in my career (and who graciously penned the foreword to the first edition of this book). My colleagues David Rudd, Greg Brown, Tom Ellis, and the "CAMS Brain Trust" of Kate Comtois, Stephen O'Connor, Lisa Brenner, and Peter Gutierrez deserve special recognition and are the best collaborators imaginable. Jennifer Crumlish, Assistant Director of the CUA-SPL, and Keith Jennings, CUA Research Assistant Professor, are valued friends and key CAMS collaborators who "have my back" and keep all our research and projects on track. Heartfelt thanks goes to Marsha Linehan for her thoughtful foreword and for "shaming" me into becoming a treatment researcher! Marsha has truly been an inspiration, a guiding force, and a dear friend.

I am grateful to The Guilford Press and the ongoing support of Editor-in-Chief Seymour Weingarten. My Senior Editor at Guilford, Jim Nageotte, has been a particularly valuable influence in shaping both editions of this book. I appreciate Jim's steady and guiding hand, professional wisdom, and friendship. Thanks also to Jane Keislar, Kathy Kuehl, and Laura Patchkofsky at Guilford for their valuable contributions over the years. This edition was wonderfully edited and supported by my superb doctoral student René Lento, who helped craft my language and did exhaustive research to fully update the research literature that is cited throughout this edition.

I have been blessed all my life with a loving and supportive family; my brothers, Steve and Bill, and my parents, Frank and Helen, have always believed in me and celebrated my successes. I was fortunate to "marry up," and my wife, Colleen, is an endless source of love, support, humor, good judgment, and tolerance. Colleen has been intimately involved in the development of CAMS over our 25 years of marriage, and she has been an unwavering source of perspective and wisdom. Our boys, Connor and Dillon, have grown up in a household where the topic of suicide prevention has been omnipresent, and they have shared our home on countless occasions with my students, colleagues from abroad, and various research collaborators. The boys have also worked for the cause of suicide prevention and have always been understanding and supportive of my passion for this topic as my life's work. While I have many blessings in my personal journey, my family is the center of my happiness and gives my life both purpose and meaning.

Finally, there are the patients (and I would note that there are references to many cases throughout this book that are based on well-disguised actual cases to preserve the anonymity of the individuals). I have likely sat with hundreds of suicidal people over 30 years, and *they* are the ones who have taught me the most about this topic. I am humbled by their courage in the face of despair and inspired by their ability to rally and overcome in the face of seemingly insurmountable odds. While I am sobered that we may not save every life, the pursuit of this noble cause should nevertheless remain the unwavering focus in our work.

Contents

CHAPTER 1

Collaborative Assessment and Management of Suicidality

A Suicide-Specific Clinical Intervention within Contemporary Health Care

Bill is a middle-aged white male who arrives for the first therapy session at a private-practice outpatient setting. He is a highly successful architect who runs a large firm. For 30 years Bill has been married to his wife, Kathy, and they have four successful young-adult children. Despite his many successes in life, Bill reports an extensive history of depression, anxiety, intermittent bouts of insomnia, and periods of binge drinking. He further describes recent marital distress and reports that his life is "generally adrift." Bill has sought mental health care on two previous occasions, dropping out each time after a handful of sessions. Bill endorsed various symptoms related to stress, depression, and anxiety on a screening tool that he completed in the waiting room prior to his appointment. On a screening item related to suicidal thoughts, Bill checked that he "frequently" has thoughts of ending his life. While it is unbeknownst to the clinician, Bill is an avid gun owner with many firearms in his home, and he has selected his "favorite" handgun to use for his suicide. In addition, Bill has put his affairs in order and he has written drafts of suicide notes to his wife and children.

Bill's case poses many challenges to a mental health clinician in contemporary clinical practice. Both demographically and diagnostically, Bill presents as the modal suicide completer in the United States (Centers for Disease Control and Prevention [CDC], 2014). Given his cluster of psychiatric symptoms, his poor history of mental health treatment compliance, and his chosen method of a readily accessible handgun, Bill's potential objective risk is alarmingly high. In addition, Bill's wife Kathy is a trial lawyer, and any clinician treating the spouse of an attorney might have anxiety about a malpractice lawsuit if the patient ends his or her life.[1]

Given all these considerations, it is fair to say that most mental health providers (across disciplines and theoretical orientations) encountering a patient like Bill would experience some worry. For some clinicians, such a clinically challenging case may actually be a terrifying prospect because they feel ill equipped to care for someone as potentially lethal as Bill. Sitting with Bill in our first session, I was worried and anxious about him. As a career suicidologist, I quickly appreciated the serious objective risk for suicide that he presented. But my worry and anxiety were lessened because I knew that I had a therapeutic approach that could be the exact life-saving remedy for him.

*   *   *

When I first worked in the field of mental health more than 30 years ago, a clinical presentation like Bill's would have prompted an immediate hospitalization to a psychiatric unit, even if he was not necessarily deemed to be in "clear and imminent" danger. Back in the early 1980s, such an inpatient psychiatric stay would likely last many weeks; with especially good insurance, such a stay might last for months. (In those days with some cases, inpatient stays sometimes lasted for years!) However, these days, a patient like Bill (while undoubtedly worrisome) might not be "suicidal enough" to earn a precertification from an insurer for an inpatient admission. Some insurance companies require *both* "clear and imminent" danger *and* an actual suicide attempt to have occurred before they will approve an inpatient psychiatric admission. In any case, in the event of such an admission, a typical contemporary length of an inpatient psychiatric stay is 7–8 days (Stranges, Levit, Stocks, & Santora, 2011); many stays are brief as 24–48 hours. Moreover, in most contemporary inpatient settings, typical "treatment" may consist only of prescribing some psychotropic medications, and perhaps some brief psychoeducationally oriented groups (National Alliance on Mental Illness, 2014). It is a far cry from the days when psychiatric inpatient care routinely included individual psychotherapy, group therapy, various activity therapies, psychological testing, and a full psychiatric work-up as the standard of care.

So how does one best proceed with a case as daunting as Bill's? Upon reflection, there are two noteworthy factors in his case. First, despite his considerable suffering and objective suicide risk factors, Bill is nevertheless still *alive*. Second, despite his poor history of seeking mental health care, Bill is nonetheless apparently seeking treatment from yet another mental health professional. In fact, Bill

---

[1]Survey data confirm that suicide-related malpractice litigation is a commonly considered by surviving family when a suicide occurs while a loved one is engaged in mental health care (Peterson, Luoma, & Dunne, 2002).

is sitting with a clinical psychologist who is skilled in the use of a suicide-specific innovation called the Collaborative Assessment and Management of Suicidality (CAMS) approach—the evidence-based intervention described throughout this book.

In this first chapter, we begin our consideration of CAMS in relation to three important organizing concepts that directly bear on using it effectively. We will first explore the CAMS philosophy and then examine it as a clinical framework. The chapter ends by situating the use and application of CAMS within the context of contemporary mental health care.

CAMS PHILOSOPHY

As I have described elsewhere in depth with some of my key research collaborators (Jobes, Comtois, Brenner, & Gutierrez, 2011; Jobes, Comtois, Brenner, Gutierrez, & O'Connor, 2016), CAMS is first a clinical *philosophy* of care. The success of CAMS rests firmly on a foundation of a particular philosophical orientation to clinically working with suicidal risk. In many ways, this approach to suicidal risk proposes some significant departures from conventional clinical practices about how best to understand and clinically assess and treat a person with suicidal risk. What follows are key features of the CAMS philosophical approach to caring for suicidal patients.

Empathy for Suicidal States

In 2001, the late Israel Orbach published an influential article in the field of suicidology that focused on *empathy with the suicidal wish*. Orbach and I were charter members of the Aeschi Group, a cadre of clinician-researchers who were fed up with conventional clinical approaches to working with suicidal risk involving diagnostic reductionism that emphasizes the primacy of mental disorders over the phenomenology of suicidal states (Michel et al., 2002). In an intentional effort to chart a new course, the members of the Aeschi Group championed an empathic, narrative, and noncoercive approach to working with suicidal patients. At the heart of this orientation is a core tenet that clinicians must truly *listen* to the patient's suicidal story in an empathic and nonjudgmental fashion. As I have written about for years (Jobes, 1995a, 2000, 2012), the nature of clinical work with suicidal patients often unravels into a patient versus clinician adversarial relational dynamic. We in the Aeschi Group felt compelled to propose a range of alternative ways of forming a therapeutic alliance in the presence of suicidal risk; an entire book is dedicated to this particular approach (Michel & Jobes, 2010). Marsha Linehan once told me that the default professional response to a suicidal patient throughout mental health settings was to *shame and blame* such patients. In my experience, particularly in

4 MANAGING SUICIDAL RISK

emergency departments, this has been all too true. I once sat in a hospital emergency department (ED) into the wee hours of the morning with a patient of mine who had overdosed. She was shackled to a gurney and awaited a charcoal treatment. We were both shocked to overhear her ED nurse say to a colleague, "Yeah, we have another overdoser. I wish we could work with *real* patients!" Within CAMS we never shame or blame; we endeavor to enter the mind of the suicidal person respectfully, and to understand the phenomenology of suicidal suffering from an empathic, nonjudgmental, and intrasubjective perspective.

Collaboration

Collaboration is perhaps the most important ingredient to successful CAMS-guided clinical care. Through collaboration we engage in a highly interactive assessment process and we directly solicit patient input to their treatment plan. Moreover, every session of CAMS actively considers the patient's feedback and sense about what is and is not working within their treatment. All CAMS assessment work is collaborative; all treatment-related aspects of CAMS are collaborative. When conducting assessments, we never interrupt or talk over the patient; instead we endeavor to draw them out and seek their input at every opportunity. In terms of treatment planning, the patient is actively engaged and is said to be a "coauthor" of their suicide-specific treatment plan. From the treatment research literature, all good clinical outcomes are defined by the quality of the therapeutic alliance (Horvath & Symonds, 1991). In CAMS we foster that alliance through a consistent emphasis on collaboration and interactivity over the course of care. From beginning, to middle, to end—collaboration is the key.

Honesty

Finally, in terms of CAMS philosophy, honesty and forthrightness are essential. For any patient teetering between life and death, there can be no more important component of care than direct and respectful honesty about the entire situation created when suicidal risk is present. Clinical honesty related to suicidal risk begins with thoughtful and thorough informed consent (Jobes, Rudd, Overholser, & Joiner, 2008; Rudd et al., 2009). Suicidal patients usually struggle with issues pertaining to control, trust, betrayal, coercion, civil liberties, shame and blame, and abject paternalism. I therefore present some version of informed consent to a suicidal person that goes as follows:

"Let's begin our discussion about suicide with something plain: you can of course kill yourself, and in the grand scheme of things there is remarkably little I or anyone else can do about it. To be frank, it is your life and ultimately up to you whether you choose to live it. However, from a clinical standpoint, we have a dilemma because state laws and the clinical standard of care require me to not permit you to take your life if you pose a 'clear and imminent' danger to yourself. This duty can create a serious strain between your personal autonomy and my professional obligation, which could mean that I might have to commit you to an inpatient hospital setting, even against your will. While I do not want any of my patients to die by suicide, I nevertheless understand that for some people there is no other way to cope with their situation. By the end of the day on average 100-plus Americans will die by their own hand, and about 30% of them will be in concurrent mental health care. I therefore have no illusions that mental health care will necessarily save your life. That said, I would rather not debate with you whether you can kill yourself; instead I would propose an evidence-based treatment designed to save your life. The research shows that most suicidal people respond to this treatment within 3 months. So why not give it a try? You have everything to gain and really nothing to lose. You can of course kill yourself later, when you are no longer in treatment. It is your life to live or not as you see fit. But then, what is the hurry? One day we all die. Finally, if suicide is the best way to do to deal with your situation, then what are you doing here with me? Perhaps it is not yet your time to die?"

Perhaps this is too provocative? Some mental health professionals think so. When I present some version of this suicide-specific informed consent to mental health professionals, I routinely see some raised eyebrows and sometimes even overt objections among certain audience members. Some believe I am baiting the patient to take his or her life. Others are uncomfortable by my frank admission about the limits of my influence and control. Still others object to my acknowledgment that a patient can kill him- or herself later when he or she is no longer in treatment. When such objections are raised, I encourage audience members to pause and reflect, and place themselves into the mindset of a truly suicidal person. Then I repeat this line of informed consent. Usually most clinicians "get it"—we cannot make people not take their lives through coercion, intimidation, or inpatient commitment. In my experience, this kind of informed consent actually *comforts* and *reassures* the suicidal person, making the patient less inclined to see me as a potential adversary and more likely to see me as an ally. By giving up any illusion of control and power *over* the patient, I have actually gained more credibility and influence *with* the patient. While I am clear about my professional duty I still propose a viable path to avoid an adversarial dynamic. Moreover, this line of thinking has the noble virtue of being the absolute *truth* about contemporary clinical demands related to suicidal risk. When I was in graduate school one of my favorite professors once told me, "The truth is highly underrated in psychotherapy." All these years later, I could not agree with her more. In fact, this kind of clinical truth-telling and transparency has become fundamental to CAMS philosophy of clinical care and is indispensable to ethical and effective clinical practice (Jobes, 2011).

CAMS AS A SUICIDE-FOCUSED THERAPEUTIC FRAMEWORK

CAMS is emphatically *not* a new psychotherapy. Rather, it is a suicide-focused therapeutic framework—a clinical platform—guided by a unique multipurpose clinical tool called the Suicide Status Form (SSF). The SSF functions as a clinical roadmap within CAMS, guiding all assessments, treatment planning, tracking of ongoing risk, and, ultimately, clinical outcomes. As is discussed at length in this book, the SSF has been extensively studied for over 25 years in a broad range of clinical settings around the world. It has excellent psychometrics and extensive clinical utility (see Jobes, 2012, for a review). The SSF is in part an assessment tool that provides a unique blend of quantitative and qualitative assessment data. Collaboratively completing the assessment portions of the SSF is often a therapeutic experience for the patient in itself. Indeed, Poston and Hanson (2010) have empirically demonstrated that the CAMS-based SSF assessment functions as a "therapeutic assessment" in their meta-analysis of 17 published studies of psychological assessments that have positive and clinically meaningful effects on treatment, including treatment processes. Other portions of the SSF focus on the development of a suicide-specific treatment plan that features a stabilization plan and targeting and treatment of *patient-defined* suicidal "drivers"—those issues or problems that make suicide compelling to the patient (Jobes et al., 2016). Successful stabilization work in CAMS and ongoing treatment of suicidal drivers is further guided by the use of interim and then outcomes versions of the SSF. As discussed in Chapter 8, the use of the SSF can help to significantly decrease the risk of malpractice liability by creating an extensive documentation trail. Let us now further consider some of the key features of this therapeutic framework for suicidal risk.

Focus on Suicide

CAMS clinicians are singularly focused on preventing their patient's suicide. Within CAMS the inherent clinical bias is that there is nothing more important to consider in mental health treatment than the prospect of the patient's suicidal death. To this end, there is persistence—sometimes even doggedness—in our primary focus on saving the patient's life. In other words, we continually work together to eliminate suicide as a coping option as we endeavor to treat, ameliorate, or eliminate the suicidal drivers that imperil the patient's life. We therefore make no apologies for this emphatic focus: We are trying to save a life. For example, over the course of a session a patient may want to talk about her kids or the economy. While the CAMS clinician may find these topics interesting, we still resist the temptation to focus on unrelated topics; unless these topics are relevant to the patient's suicide risk the CAMS clinician must gently redirect the discussion back to those issues that threaten the patient's life. If the patient is frustrated with the singular emphasis on suicide, we will comment on how we would love to talk about the kids or economy *after* suicide has been eliminated from the patient's coping repertoire. As noted earlier, when using CAMS we should remain unwaveringly focused on helping to save the patient's life and assisting in the development of purpose and meaning.

Outpatient Oriented

In the first edition of this book, I asserted that CAMS as a clinical approach to suicidal risk is fundamentally oriented toward keeping a suicidal person *out* of an inpatient psychiatric hospital setting, if at all possible. Ten years ago this approach was a somewhat novel idea. But based on my experiences training thousands of clinicians, I still get a strong impression that many (if not most) mental health clinicians continue to harbor a strong inpatient focus to care. In other words, when a typical clinician encounters suicidal risk their approach often *begins* with an a priori hospitalization bias: "Uh-oh, where can I get a bed?" Using CAMS as a therapeutic framework, we earnestly endeavor to find ways to keep a suicidal patient *out* of the hospital. We achieve this through our collaborative development of a suicide-specific outpatient treatment plan that includes a carefully developed stabilization plan and a problem-focused treatment of the patient's idiosyncratically defined suicidal drivers. Consequently an inpatient psychiatric hospitalization is the ultimate *last* resort in CAMS-guided care. The need for inpatient care naturally emerges only when the dyad is not able to collaboratively develop a satisfactory outpatient plan that includes stabilization and driver-focused treatment options. A notable exception to this general outpatient bias of CAMS-guided care is when CAMS is used as an *inpatient* intervention. In this case the proper course of inpatient CAMS care still focuses on stabilization planning and driver-oriented treatment that becomes central to effective discharge planning and successful post-hospital disposition (cf. Ellis, Green, Allen, Jobes, & Nadorff, 2012; Ellis, Rufino, Allen, Fowler, & Jobes, 2015).

Flexible and Nondenominational

As a therapeutic framework, CAMS is designed for flexibility and adaptation; we think of CAMS as theoretically "nondenominational." While there are not many replicated evidence-based treatments for suicidal risk, two excellent exceptions clearly do stand out: dialectical behavior therapy (DBT) and cognitive-behavioral therapy (CBT). As Marsha Linehan has shown in rigorous clinical trials, DBT effectively treats both suicide attempt behaviors as well as self-harm behaviors (Linehan et al., 1999, 2006, 2015). In addition, Brown and colleagues (2005) have shown that 10 sessions of a suicide-focused cognitive therapy for suicide prevention (CT-SP) can significantly reduce repeat suicide attempts by *half* in their randomized controlled trial. Using a similar brief cognitive-behavioral therapy (B-CBT) approach for suicide risk, Rudd and colleagues (2015) found a 60% decrease in suicide attempt behaviors for those receiving B-CBT in comparison to usual treatment.

Across these effective and replicated treatments, there is a clear expectation of close adherence to highly structured treatment manuals in order to effectively deliver these interventions faithfully. In the case of DBT one must be able and willing to practice behavior therapy, and in the case of the CBT approaches one must practice cognitive therapy to effectively deliver the intervention. As adherence to an evidence-based approach is a critical component of effective delivery of that care, the training necessary to achieve reliable adherence to a manualized treatment is an important consideration. For both of these excellent approaches to treating suicidal risk, the amount and duration of both didactic and experiential training can be considerable. Moreover, as noted by one of my CBT colleagues, "If you don't take the time to learn to carefully and faithfully follow the recipe, it's really not a cake."

In contrast, CAMS is designed to be highly flexible and can be adapted to a range of theoretical approaches and the spectrum of clinical treatments. As a suicide-specific clinical framework, clinicians across the gamut of theories can equally and effectively use CAMS when working with suicidal patients. Whenever I train providers in CAMS, I emphasize that I want clinicians to retain their own clinical skills, their own clinical judgment, and their own treatment approaches; we do want a clinician to transform into a different provider, someone he or she does not recognize. Consequently, CAMS has been successfully used by mental health clinicians of all theoretical orientations (psychoanalytic, humanistic, interpersonal, cognitive-behavioral, etc.) and professional disciplines (psychologists, psychiatrists, social workers, counselors, nurses, marriage and family therapists, case-managers, substance-abuse clinicians, etc.). We thus encourage providers to practice as they typically do, but to do so *within* the flexible and highly adaptive CAMS therapeutic framework. As discussed in depth in Chapter 9, CAMS has been extensively adapted for brief use in emergency departments and crisis settings, as a post-inpatient discharge group therapy (Johnson, O'Connor, Kaminer, Jobes, & Gutierrez, 2014), and modified for different populations (e.g., military, college students, suicidal youth). While there is undoubtedly a need for effective and highly structured manualized evidence-based treatments, there is an obvious need for highly flexible and adaptive interventions like CAMS as well.

Unlike other replicated evidence-based approaches, CAMS is relatively easy to learn, and achieving adherence can be quick and enduring. Training research has shown that CAMS can be learned in live-didactic forums (Pisani, Cross, & Gould, 2011) as well as within an e-learning training approach (Jobes, 2015, 2016; Marshall et al., 2014). Interestingly, in an online study of 120 providers whose training in CAMS ranged from merely reading the first edition of this book to a daylong live training plus role playing, Crowley, Arnkoff, Glass, and Jobes (2014) found moderate to high self-report adherence to the CAMS framework across the range of learning experiences. Within our large randomized controlled trial of using CAMS with suicidal U.S. Army Soldiers, it is noteworthy that all CAMS clinicians in the study achieved adherence to CAMS within *four sessions* of their first use with a suicidal patient. Generally speaking, by their third CAMS case, these providers were relatively expert at using the intervention and they did not later fall out of adherence in follow-up fidelity and adherence reviews of their work (Corona, 2015).

CONTEMPORARY MENTAL HEALTH CARE

As I have previously noted, within my 30-year professional lifetime there have been extraordinary changes in the delivery of mental health care in relation to suicide risk. In the United States, even more change is currently under way as a result of the passage and enactment of the Affordable Care Act (Patient Protection and Affordable Care Act; Public Law No. 111–148, March 23, 2010). Among all the challenges of the highly politicized issues associated with American health care reform, there is a rather blunt truism that has the power to meaningfully shape and influence the treatment of suicidal risk for years to come. The sheer costs of mental health care related to suicide risk and behaviors are extremely high. For example, inpatient psychiatric care has become quite expensive (Stranges et al., 2011) with an average cost of $5,700 per inpatient stay (ranging from $2,900 to $13,300). Yang and Lester (2007) estimate a typical inpatient stay for suicide risk averages $13,690, with a range from $1,997 to $68,150. Moreover, the use of emergency departments by suicidal people, more specifically attempters, has become costly as well (Owens, Mutter, & Stocks, 2010; Stensland, Zhu, Ascher-Svanum, & Ball, 2010; Valenstein et al., 2009). The collective expense of suicide-related medical procedures such as sewing up "cutters," surgeries related to self-inflicted gunshot wounds, and lavaging stomachs following intentional drug overdoses is considerable (Bennett, Vaslef, Shapiro, Brooks, & Scarborough, 2009). Add costly attorney's fees to defend against suicide wrongful death malpractice lawsuits, and the overall expensive of suicide-related care and management is plain. While it is perhaps a tactless consideration in a discussion of life or death, within a "fee-for-service" approach to health care, one can understand why insurers are struggling to shoulder mounting expenses created by mental health patients in general, and patients with suicide-related morbidity and mortality in particular.

As a member of the National Action Alliance Clinical Care and Intervention Task Force, I had the opportunity to explore in depth the many and various challenges connected to contemporary suicide-related health care. As part of our charge, we were directed to pay particular attention to these suicide-related cost issues as it would pertain to the Affordable Care Act. The task force report entitled "Suicide Care in Systems Framework" (National Action Alliance, 2011) thus strongly emphasized a *systems* approach to clinical suicide prevention. Key health care systems-related phrases such as "evidence-based approaches" and "least-restrictive treatments" and "cost-effective care" were frequently mentioned during our deliberations and ultimately within our report focusing on systems-level issues.

Inspired by the work of the task force, I presented a model at an international suicide prevention conference of a potential spectrum of care for suicidal risk (Jobes, 2013a). I argued in this presentation that potential changes in suicide-related care (largely driven by purely economic forces) do not necessarily have to have a negative impact if we can pursue the goal of reliably differentiating (i.e., "stratifying") suicidal states and then matching our best evidence-based interventions in a least-restrictive manner to each level of risk. I also talked about exciting innovations in suicide interventions that are increasingly focused on brief (one to four sessions of contact) interventions (e.g., Gysin-Maillart, Schwab, Soravia, & Michel, 2016). We also know the potential therapeutic power of follow-up letters, postcards, phone calls, and other means of caring outreach such as texting and e-mails are being studied as well (see Luxton, June, & Comtois, 2013). Follow-up contacts are often referred to as "nondemand" or "caring-contacts," and the data that support their use are impressive. Moreover the potential value of crisis center suicide hotlines has been proven (Gould, Kalafat, Harris-Munfakh, & Kleinman, 2007), and crisis center workers can also provide caring-contact follow-up calls that are typically well received by suicidal people (Gould, 2013).

Figure 1.1 shows the model I am describing of an array of suicide-specific interventions that are both least restrictive and cost effective. Along the x-axis there are graduated steps of interventions that reflect different types and intensities of care. For example, a relatively "low-risk" suicidal person with ideation might be effectively supported and managed purely through a crisis hotline level of intervention. For someone who needs more intensive contact, a brief suicide-specific intervention with follow-up may be sufficient. Persons with more serious risk may require

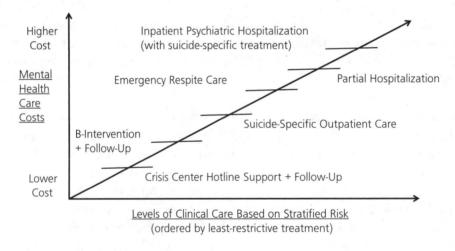

FIGURE 1.1. Stepped model for suicide interventions.

suicide-specific outpatient care, respite crisis care, or partial hospitalization. For someone who is imminently at high risk, an inpatient admission may be necessary (with suicide-specific care provided during the stay). As you follow the arrow that transects the figure, you can see a full continuum of care with increasing steps of intensity and focus. Note that on the *y*-axis there is the corresponding consideration of mental health care costs.

Within this model of stratified risk and stepped care, evidence-based and suicide-specific interventions can be provided at each level of intervention. CAMS itself can be adapted and used at almost every level of stratified clinical care model—from brief crisis intervention, to standard outpatient CAMS, to adapted brief versions of CAMS used in respite care, partial hospitalization, and within inpatient settings (see Chapter 9). CAMS is thus well positioned for use in our evolving health care environment (Jobes & Bowers, 2015).

Another major consideration alluded to earlier pertains to anxieties that many providers have about the risk of malpractice lawsuits should a suicide occur. As I discuss in depth in Chapter 8, using CAMS may actually significantly *decrease* such risk because of the central use of the SSF that creates an extensive clinical documentation trail. Risk of liability is further reduced because CAMS is evidence based and suicide specific; any potential ongoing suicidal risk is monitored and treated until optimal clinical outcomes are ultimately realized.

Having said all this, it would be naïve to suggest that there is a "one-size-fits-all" evidence-based intervention that will work in every clinical environment, with every suicidal patient, for every type and kind of mental health provider. CAMS has nevertheless proven to be an effective and adaptive approach in range of clinical environments, with a diverse spectrum of suicidal patients around the world. Providers across professional disciplines and theoretical orientations have been able to effectively use CAMS as a suicide-specific therapeutic framework that can make a meaningful difference in their clinical practice with suicidal patients.

If we truly aspire to clinically save lives we must use practices that have been proven to be effective for working specifically with suicidal risk. But as a trainer of mental health providers for decades, I have the strong impression that evidence-based practices are often not reliably used in the "trenches" of mental health care (these impressions are further confirmed by literature on the topic; e.g., McHugh & Barlow, 2010; Shafran et al., 2009). As I have reflected on this elsewhere (Jobes, 2015), there are various reasons why any clinician might be willing to change practice behaviors to embrace a proven treatment for suicidal risk. While these are in no particular order, some of these considerations may include:

- A genuine desire to help patients do better.
- Empirical support for the treatment.
- Directives or mandates by leadership (i.e., being forced to do it).
- Fear of losing a patient to suicide and then being blamed.

- Fear of litigation for malpractice wrongful death.
- Different incentives to change practices (e.g., money or comp time).
- Everyone else is doing it and feeling left behind.
- Seeing is believing (being convinced that a treatment could actually work).

Even with all these potential motivators, I am still circumspect about the willingness of many clinicians to change their practice behaviors to use an intervention that works. As you read these words, where do you stand in terms of *your* willingness to change your practice behaviors? It is my hope that by the end of this book you will be convinced that CAMS is both a sensible and compelling approach for effectively working with any suicidal patient you may encounter.

In closing this chapter I would hasten to add that as this book was going into production, a landmark document was released by The Joint Commission (2016), which is *the* accrediting body within U.S. health care. On February 24, 2016, The Joint Commission released a "Sentinel Event Alert" titled "Detecting and Treating Suicide Ideation in All Settings." This extraordinary document has the power to shape and influence mental health assessment and treatment of suicide risk for decades to come within medical institutions accredited by The Joint Commission. And to this end, DBT, CT-SP, and CAMS were specifically mentioned as evidence-based clinical approaches that help reduce suicidal thoughts and behaviors for at-risk patients. This is indeed a most noteworthy development for the cause of clinical suicide prevention.

*   *   *

Within the first 10 minutes of my initial session with Bill, I proposed the use of CAMS. In the true spirit of informed consent, I talked plainly about suicide and my duties as a licensed mental health professional. We discussed the DC Mental Health Act and what the law says about "clear and imminent danger" to self. This discussion both raised Bill's anxiety but also intrigued him about the possibilities of doing a suicide-specific intervention, and with some wariness Bill agreed to proceed with CAMS. But our potentially life-saving treatment began in earnest when I asked for permission to take a seat next to Bill. I did so and handed Bill a copy of the SSF, saying, "Here is an assessment tool that will help me understand in depth the nature of your pain and suffering so I can see how things are going for you right now. The first page here is for you to complete with my help. But you are the expert of your own struggle—please help me understand what it is like to be you so we can pursue a treatment together that may just help save your life."

CHAPTER 2

The SSF
and the Evolution of CAMS

In the fall of 1987, I began my career at The Catholic University of America (CUA) Counseling Center with a part-time appointment as an assistant professor in the Department of Psychology. I had just finished my clinical internship and I was in the final throes of completing my doctoral dissertation, directed by a suicidologist, Lanny Berman, who was my major professor. Around this time I was charged by the director of the counseling center to scour the suicide literature to identify a psychometrically sound suicide risk assessment tool and some sort of systematic methodology for reliably assessing such risk and making sure that our suicidal students did not "fall through the cracks." This simple directive was the genesis of what was to become the SSF and what later led to the development of the CAMS approach described throughout this text. In spite of suicide being a leading cause of death, surprisingly no such clinical tool existed, and there were no reliable evidence-based systemic approaches for reliably dealing with suicidal risk in a mental health care environment. My early search of a markedly limited literature led to a survey study of suicide risk assessment practices (Jobes, Eyman, & Yufit, 1995) that was pivotal to the ongoing development of the SSF and CAMS.

OVERVIEW OF THE SSF

Simply stated, the SSF is a multipurpose engagement, assessment, treatment-planning, tracking, updating, and outcome/disposition clinical tool that serves as the indispensable roadmap for CAMS-guided care. Over 25 years, it has gone through four major revisions based on rigorous clinical research, as well as patient and clinician feedback. As shown in Appendix A, the most recent version—the SSF-4—is made up of eight pages (or eight screens in electronic versions) that are divided into three distinct phases of clinical care: (1) index assessment and treatment planning in the first session (SSF pages 1–4), (2) tracking the risk and updating the treatment plan in interim sessions (SSF pages 5–6), and (3) clinical outcomes and disposition (SSF pages 7–8) used in the final CAMS session.

CAMS is typically initiated with a *currently* suicidal patient, although I have occasionally seen clinicians productively use CAMS *preemptively* with patients they thought might become suicidal. In turn I have also seen CAMS used with patients who have been suicidal in the past, with the goal of exploring this history *retrospectively*. But in most cases of currently suicidal patients, CAMS requires the completion of SSF Sections A–D in the initial session (note that the CAMS "Stabilization Plan" is subsumed under the Section C "Treatment Plan"). After the initial session, there are additional tracking and treatment plan updates that occur in all interim CAMS-guided sessions leading up to clinical outcomes. For the interim phase of care, the same version of the SSF "Tracking/Update" document is repeatedly used. The third and final phase of CAMS involves the clinical "Outcome/ Disposition" version of the SSF that is administered in the final session of CAMS. Given the central importance of the SSF within CAMS, the following discussion will navigate the entire SSF in more detail to further elucidate its use and the three distinct treatment phases of CAMS-guided care.

SSF ASSESSMENT AND TREATMENT PLANNING
(INITIAL SESSION)

The current multipurpose SSF was originally a simple one-page document that we used at the CUA Counseling Center back in 1987. It had some open-ended spaces for entering limited identifying information, some description about any suicide-related matter, and a space for describing disposition. In the subsequent 25 years, the simple version of the form significantly evolved to present-day SSF-4, having been used with thousands of suicidal patients around the world and used in dozens of SSF-related studies (Jobes, 2012).

SSF Section A—The SSF Core Assessment

As shown in Figure 2.1, the SSF Core Assessment includes six variables. The first three assessment variables (psychological pain, stress, and agitation) are based on the seminal theoretical work of Edwin Shneidman (1988); these items make up Shneidman's "cubic model of suicide." The fourth variable—hopelessness—is based on Aaron Beck's work and refers to expectations that things will not get

Rate and fill out each item according to how you feel <u>right now</u>. Then rank in order of importance 1 to 5
Rank   (1 = most important to 5 = least important)

Rank	
	1) RATE PSYCHOLOGICAL PAIN (*hurt, anguish, or misery in your mind, **not** stress, **not** physical pain*): **Low pain:** 1 2 3 4 5 :**High pain** What I find most painful is: _____
	2) RATE STRESS (*your general feeling of being pressured or overwhelmed*): **Low stress:** 1 2 3 4 5 :**High stress** What I find most stressful is: _____
	3) RATE AGITATION (*emotional urgency; feeling that you need to take action; **not** irritation; **not** annoyance*): **Low agitation:** 1 2 3 4 5 :**High agitation** I most need to take action when: _____
	4) RATE HOPELESSNESS (*your expectation that things will not get better no matter what you do*): **Low hopelessness:** 1 2 3 4 5 :**High hopelessness** I am most hopeless about: _____
	5) RATE SELF-HATE (*your general feeling of disliking yourself; having no self-esteem; having no self-respect*): **Low self-hate:** 1 2 3 4 5 :**High self-hate** What I hate most about myself is: _____
N/A	6) RATE OVERALL RISK OF SUICIDE: **Extremely low risk:** (will **not** kill self) 1 2 3 4 5 :**Extremely high risk** (will kill self)

FIGURE 2.1. The SSF Core Assessment.

better no matter what one does (Beck et al., 1979). The fifth variable, self-hate, is derived from the work of Roy Baumeister (1990), who links intolerable perceptions of self (i.e., self-hate) to a need for suicidal escape. The sixth SSF variable is overall risk rating, or the behavioral bottom line: Are you going to kill yourself or not? Let us now consider each of the SSF Core Assessment constructs in more depth.

Psychological Pain

The influential contributions of the field's "founding father"—the late Edwin Shneidman—were both far-reaching and multilayered. As I have discussed elsewhere (Jobes & Nelson, 2006), Shneidman's groundbreaking theoretical work, his innovative empirical research, and especially his clinical wisdom have been central to the development of the SSF and the clinical spirit of CAMS. Arguably one of Shneidman's most enduring contributions to the field of suicidology was an entire theoretical metapsychology (a distinctly mentalistic approach) of suicide organized around the construct of "psychache"—a profound and seemingly unbearable suffering that exists at the heart of every suicidal drama (Shneidman, 1993). From this perspective, if we mean to help any suicidal person, we must fundamentally understand the person's idiosyncratic psychological suffering. Shneidman further argued that *every* suicide invariably occurs when the person's individually defined psychological pain threshold is exceeded. Reducing suicidal risk thus requires finding a way of raising the threshold or tolerance to their suicidal pain. Of course it is also critical to remove or ameliorate the root of the psychological pain itself. Many contemporary clinical researchers have imported Shneidman's ideas into their treatment approaches (e.g., Chiles & Strosahl, 1995; Ellis & Newman, 1996; Joiner, 2005; Linehan, 1993a; Rudd et al., 2015; Rudd, Joiner, Jobes, & King, 1999; Rudd, Joiner, & Rajab, 2001; Wenzel, Brown, & Beck, 2009).

Press (Stress)

Beyond the primary emphasis on psychological pain, Shneidman (1993) further highlighted the construct "press," which he took from his intellectual mentor Henry Murray (1938). Fundamental to Murray's classic personality theory of *personology* was an interactive matrix of various psychological needs and presses. For our purposes, this term refers to those largely external (occasionally internal) psychological pressures, stressors, or demands that impinge on, move, touch, or otherwise affect the individual. These typically include external things like relational conflicts, job loss, events that occur in life that create significant distress; alternatively, however, internal stressors like command hallucinations can obviously be pressing too. Presses are closely linked to feeling overwhelmed; that is, perceptions that one is overrun by psychological demands. I should note that I have used the more standard term s*tress* on the SSF itself because that word is more familiar to the typical patient (but I will continue to use the term *press* within the text to stay true to Shneidman's conceptual language).

Perturbation (Agitation)

Shneidman's (1993) construct of "perturbation" is sometimes unclear, as it can be confused with psychological pain and stress. Yet Shneidman insisted that perturbation is a unique and pivotal suicide construct. He asserted that perturbation captures the state of being emotionally upset, disturbed, and disquieted. For Shneidman, perturbation includes both cognitive constriction *and* a penchant for self-harm or ill-advised action. Perturbation can be described as the patient's impulsive desire to do *something* to change or alter his or her current unbearable situation. It is an essential psychological *energy* that is the vital driving force behind all suicidal behaviors. In clinical practice it is not uncommon to see patients in a great deal of psychological pain, with little to no perturbation. But completed suicides rarely occur without the psychological "oomph" that is necessary to overcome our natural thresholds to avoid pain and death. While it is not synonymous, I have used the term *agitation* on the SSF in place of *perturbation* because it is more familiar to the typical patient (for clarity in this text, I use the conceptual term *perturbation*). In recent years, anxiety, agitation, and activated psychological states have become a major empirical preoccupation in suicidology (Capron et al., 2012; Ribeiro, Bender, Selby, Hames, & Joiner, 2011; Selaman, Chartrand, Bolton, & Sareen, 2014; Sublette et al., 2011; Winsper & Tang, 2014). The recent emphasis on suicidal "warning signs" (Rudd et al., 2006; Tucker, Crowley, Davidson, & Gutierrez, 2015) further underscores the significance of Shneidman's original perturbation construct.

The Cubic Model

Shneidman (1985) used the three preceding constructs to form the cubic model of suicide. While there are some compelling theoretical models of suicide in the field (e.g., Joiner, 2005; Klonsky & May, 2015; O'Connor, 2011), the elegant simplicity of Shneidman's suicidal cube has stood the test of time. One reason that I have particularly liked this model over the years is that it was the first "perfect storm" approach to understanding suicidal risk. In a field that has been remarkably obsessed with delineating countless suicide "risk factors" (that do little for clinically understanding acute risk), Shneidman's suicidal cube provides a useful window into the nature of the suicidal mind and can directly inform the assessment of suicide risk particularly in relation to "clear and imminent" danger.

Moreover, the suicidal cube usefully accentuates an important point strongly argued in the first edition of this book. CAMS assessment and treatment is strongly focused on *suicide* versus mental disorders. While we know that mental disorders are present in well over 90% of people who die by suicide, the mere presence of a mental disorder does remarkably little to help us understand proximate suicidal behavior. For example, depression is widespread throughout the world (Bromet et al., 2011), yet depression *does not equal* suicide—by a lot! Indeed, we know that in the course of a typical day, 100 Americans on average will die by suicide; of those, only 60% will have a clinical depression (CDC, 2014; U.S. Department of Health and Human Services, n.d.). Moreover, such a mental disorder bias does not begin to account for thousands of people with depression who have neither suicidal thoughts nor have made attempts. This line of discussion highlights the singular virtue of Shneidman's cubic model because it gets us thinking about the suicide risk assessment problem in *three dimensions*. Actually, the cubic model helps us think about situation specificity—how do at-risk people find themselves in circumstances that spark a suicidal behavior? As shown in Figure 2.2, the cubic model of suicide conceptualizes suicidal behaviors as occurring from a synergy of the three psychological forces that we have just discussed. Each of Shneidman's constructs of pain, press, and perturbaion exists on one of three axes in the model and can be rated from low (1) to high (5). Within this model, Shneidman has asserted that *every* suicidal act occurs when maximum levels of psychological pain, press, and perturbation psychologically co-occur.

The lethal 5-5-5 corner cubelet of the model is particularly noteworthy as a dangerous intersection and interaction of these psychological constructs and provides an excellent operational definition of "clear and imminent" danger. The

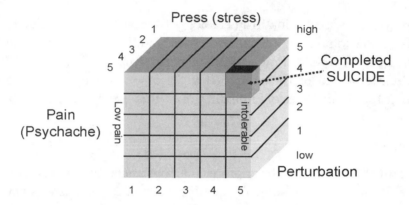

FIGURE 2.2. Shneidman's cubic model of suicide. From Shneidman (1987). Copyright 1987 by the American Psychological Association. Reprinted by permission.

model can thus be used to directly inform the assessment of suicide risk as well as inform useful treatment targets for clinical intervention. Any clinical intervention that effectively treats any of the three axes has the potential to meaningfully move a high-risk suicidal patient into a fundamentally less dangerous psychological space.

Hopelessness

Aaron Beck's concept of hopelessness refers to an expectation that your negative situation will not get better no matter what you do change the situation. The construct of hopelessness is intimately linked to future thinking and represents a third leg of Beck's larger theory of depression that emphasizes the "cognitive triad": hopelessness about self, others, and the future. Future thinking as it relates to suicide is an increasingly important construct that is being more widely discussed in the suicidology literature (e.g., O'Connor et al., 2004; Williams, 2001). As the founder of cognitive therapy, Beck has led the way in our appreciation of the critical role of *thinking* within psychological and psychiatric problems.

Within my own research group we have unpublished data that show distinctly different cognitive content among college students (*n* = 201) who are suicidal versus college students (*n* = 201) who are not suicidal (Nademin, Jobes, Downing, & Mann, 2005). In this study, we found that the nonsuicidal sample had more than *twice* as many self-reported coding themes of "plans and goals" and "hopes for the future" than the suicidal sample. In addition, the nonsuicidal sample had significantly more frequent *belief*-based reasons for living. It is clear that the capacity to think about the future with a sense of hope is protective against suicide. It follows that a sense of hopefulness in our future thinking and related beliefs may help us weather the rough spots that invariably occur in life. Alternatively, the absence of hopefulness—particularly in terms of abject hopelessness—is an extremely pernicious risk factor for suicide. In terms of prospective research there is perhaps no single risk-factor construct that has been more highly correlated with completed suicide than hopelessness (Beck, Steer, Kovacs, & Garrison, 1985; Brown, Beck, Steer, & Grisham, 2000).

Given these considerations, I felt it was imperative to include hopelessness as a key SSF construct. It has the virtues of theoretical and empirical support but there is also a clinically relevant aspect related to actively working with the construct of *hope*. While the relative presence or absence of hope is extremely important to note from an assessment standpoint, it also provides an important organizing focus for successful treatment. Developing treatments that specifically target future thinking and endeavor to actively build a sense of hope is a clinical imperative. I recall one of my first supervisors insisting that we must be "hope vendors" to our patients. This notion strikes me as being uniformly true to successful mental health treatment in general and is particularly true when working with a suicidal person.

Self-Regard (Self-Hate)

Roy Baumeister's 1990 paper conceptualizing suicide as an escape from self is a suicidology classic; in his view, suicidal people are fundamentally driven to psychologically escape unacceptable perceptions of self. According to Baumeister's theory, one's negative views of the self can become so unbearable (i.e., one's self-hatred is so extreme) that suicide becomes a compelling option for escaping intolerable self-perceptions. In fact, within our own SSF research the construct of self-hate and psychological need for escape has proven to be one of our most reliable and persistent findings (Jobes, 2005; Jobes, Kahn-Greene, Greene, & Goeke-Morey, 2009; Jobes & Mann, 1999). In one study with suicidal active-duty Air Force personnel, we found that 60% of our Reasons for Dying responses were variations on themes of escape (Jobes, 2004b). In another related study of suicidal inpatients we found that the majority perceived suicide as the "easy way out" (Kraft, Jobes, Lineberry, & Conrad, 2010).

Beyond escape, Baumeister's approach emphasizes issues related to the self. From Carl Jung to Heinz Kohut, the notion of self is a central construct within psychodynamicallyoriented metapsychology. Intuitively we know that people who think about suicide are fundamentally preoccupied with their unhappiness, and in most cases that misery is often psychologically rooted close to home—in the person's subjective sense of self. Simply stated, most suicidal people do not feel self-love, and their need to escape from their suffering can be profound. The beauty of Baumeister's conceptual approach is that it captures these two essential components of the suicidal struggle—the need for escape and the malignant role of suicidal self-loathing.

Overall Risk

Finally, there was a need to capture the overall *behavioral* possibility of suicide on the SSF (i.e., is this person going to actually take his or her life?). This final SSF Core Assessment construct does not reference any particular theorist, but obviously captures a generic behavioral perspective on suicide risk. In this regard, the sixth rating scale simply asks whether patients will or will not kill themselves. This question is not only significant because of the obvious implications for life and death but also because it goes to one of the most essential and elusive struggles in clinical suicidology—namely, the medical–legal challenge to determine whether there is a "clear and imminent" risk for suicidal behavior. Consider for a moment the issue of risk from a legal standpoint. What exactly does "clear and imminent" danger to self actually mean? In truth, suicidal states are hardly ever "clear"— invariably suicidal states are much more shades of gray rather than black or white. And "imminent?" Does it mean right this second, later today, sometime this week, or perhaps later in the month? While exact definitions of these terms remain elusive both within mental health and the law, these terms are nevertheless important for purposes of clinical care and disposition and have significant implications for malpractice related to wrongful death if a suicide does occur. For these reasons an overall behavioral assessment of risk was included as a final SSF Core Assessment variable.

Psychometrics of the SSF Core Assessment

Within the tradition of psychological test construction research, we have conducted two rigorous psychometric studies of the SSF Core Assessment. The first study was conducted with an outpatient sample of treatment-seeking suicidal college students at CUA (Jobes, Jacoby, Cimbolic, & Hustead, 1997). The second study was conducted with suicidal inpatients at the Mayo Clinic and sought to replicate and extend the findings of our earlier study using a higher-risk and more diverse sample (Conrad et al., 2009). In the counseling center study we were able to demonstrate that the six SSF Core Assessment variables functioned quasi-independently and that the variables were both valid (good to excellent convergent and criteria-prediction validity) and reliable (significant test–retest reliability). Following the publication of this study, legitimate concerns were raised about the generalizability of our findings because the sample was made up of lower-risk, upper-socioeconomic, white Catholic college students, which markedly limited the external validity of our findings. To address this concern, the second study was conducted to investigate a more diverse sample of more seriously suicidal inpatients. The second study robustly replicated the psychometric validity and reliability findings of the first study and further showed that the SSF was markedly more effective when used with high-risk suicidal inpatients. Specifically in terms of factor analyses, the SSF Core Assessment in the first study of college students accounted for 36% of the total variance, whereas in the second study of suicidal inpatients 72% of the total variance was described by the SSF Core Assessment (Conrad et al., 2009; Jobes et al., 1997).

While establishing the validity and reliability of the Core SSF Assessment was essential, we have also learned a great deal about the SSF Core Assessment through other quantitative studies. For example, one early study (Eddins & Jobes, 1994) investigated the similarities and differences in how suicidal patients and their clinicians independently view and rate these constructs. I should note that these data later prompted the *collaborative* completion of these rating scales when CAMS was developed. Other early studies used the first session (index) ratings of the SSF Core Assessment constructs to describe and predict categorical treatment outcomes (Jobes, 1995a; Jobes et al., 1997). Similarly, one-time first session ratings of the SSF Core Assessment variables were used to significantly predict different reductions in suicidal ideation over the course of treatment as well as the moderating effects of certain SSF variables using hierarchical linear modeling (HLM) analyses (Jobes, Kahn-Greene, et al., 2009). In terms of specific findings, this study showed that suicidal patients' one-time first session SSF ratings of Overall Risk of Suicide differentially predicted four distinct linear reductions in suicidal thinking over the course of care. In a second level of HLM analysis of the remaining SSF variables, we found that first session ratings of SSF constructs of Hopelessness and Self-Hate significantly moderated the effect of the Overall Risk of Suicide rating. The SSF Core Assessment has also been used as an outcome assessment in various correlational studies of CAMS as a clinical intervention (e.g., Ellis, Green, Allen, Jobes, & Nadorff, 2012).

SSF Core Assessment Qualitative Responses

Perhaps one of the more novel aspects of the SSF has been the integration of *both* quantitative and qualitative assessments. Within the field of mental health assessment it is rare that the two major assessment traditions are integrated into a single assessment approach. Generally those who embrace quantitative assessment approaches typically publish in quantitatively oriented journals and present at quantitatively oriented conferences. Similarly, those who embrace qualitative (narrative) approaches to assessment publish in qualitative journals and present at qualitatively oriented conferences. In contrast, we have seen the distinct virtue of an integrated approach on the first page of the SSF.

To this end, the SSF Core Assessment variables are followed by qualitative prompts that allow patients to respond to sentence stem prompts *in their own written words*. This particular SSF assessment is akin to Rotter's (Rotter & Rafferty, 1950) projective assessment called the "incomplete sentence blank" (ISB). Figure 2.3 is an example of an SSF completed by a suicidal combat veteran. Note that each

Rank

Rank	
_1_	1) RATE PSYCHOLOGICAL PAIN (*hurt, anguish, or misery in your mind, **not** stress, **not** physical pain*): **Low pain:** 1 2 3 4 ⑤ :**High pain** What I find most painful is: _guilt over firefight/causing my wife pain_
_5_	2) RATE STRESS (*your general feeling of being pressured or overwhelmed*): **Low stress:** 1 2 3 4 ⑤ :**High stress** What I find most stressful is: _getting over it and everything else in my life_
_4_	3) RATE AGITATION (*emotional urgency; feeling that you need to take action; **not** irritation; **not** annoyance*): **Low agitation:** 1 2 3 ④ 5 :**High agitation** I most need to take action when: _after a fight with my wife_
_3_	4) RATE HOPELESSNESS (*your expectation that things will not get better no matter what you do*): **Low hopelessness:** 1 2 3 4 ⑤ :**High hopelessness** I am most hopeless about: _ever being over what happened here_
_2_	5) RATE SELF-HATE (*your general feeling of disliking yourself; having no self-esteem; having no self-respect*): **Low self-hate:** 1 2 3 4 ⑤ :**High self-hate** What I hate most about myself is: _how I make my wife feel_
N/A	6) RATE OVERALL RISK **Extremely low risk:** 1 2 ③ 4 5 :**Extremely high risk** OF SUICIDE: **(will *not* kill self)** **(will kill self)**

FIGURE 2.3. Example of a suicidal veteran's SSF Core Assessment.

of the five initial SSF qualitative stems are followed by a line of space for patients to write their own personal responses. For example, in relation to the psychological pain question, suicidal patients who are completing the SSF provide a response to "What I find most painful is: _____." As I discuss in Chapter 4, the clinician encourages the patient to respond to each of the SSF sentence stems, as the patient writes or types whatever comes to mind in reaction to each incomplete sentence.

Perhaps one of the more interesting findings out of our lab is qualitative research about what suicidal people write when prompted by the SSF, particularly in relation to what they are *not* writing about. In one study (Jobes et al., 2004), we observed two samples of suicidal SSF-responding patients (*n* = 119 college students and *n* = 33 active-duty Air Force personnel) who were notably *not* preoccupied with symptoms of mental disorders (e.g., depression, anxiety, or voices). In this study, four reliably coded themes captured 67% of the 636 total prompted responses across the combined sample. Specifically, these four themes described "relational" (22%), "vocational" (20%), "self-oriented" (15%), and "unpleasant internal states" (10%) patient-written responses. In other words, these patients revealed that their suicidal struggles were dominated by relational, vocational, and self-oriented issues. Considering that the suicide prevention literature tends to be fixated on psychopathology, mental disorders, and symptoms of mental illness (what we coded as "unpleasant internal states"), these SSF-based qualitative findings were both unanticipated and intriguing, with distinct implications for clinical care. Refer to Appendix B for a more detailed discussion of coding these responses.

Self versus Relational Suicide Risk

Some years ago I argued that suicidal states might exist on a spectrum anchored by "intrapsychic" versus "interpsychic" poles (Jobes, 1995a). More simply stated, we have long observed that some suicidal people are preoccupied with their internal thoughts and feelings, whereas for other suicidal people there is a distinctly relational preoccupation. Within this model I argued that those with self-focused suicidality may be more at risk of dying by suicide, while those who are relationally focused in their suicidality may be more at risk of making a nonfatal suicide attempt. In accordance with this theory, the SSF has two separate 5-point rating scales pertaining to a patient's perception that his/her suicidal risk is self- versus other-focused. In one unpublished study of suicidal inpatients, Lento, Ellis, and Jobes (2013) found that overall suicide risk assessment might be meaningfully enhanced when the patient rates high on *both* constructs. That is, the relationship between a patient's *self*-focus rating and the intensity of his or her suicidal ideation significantly depended on the patient's *other*-focus rating. Among those who attributed their suicidality highly to self-focused reasons, a simultaneously high attribution to other-focused reasons appeared to serve a protective function and was associated with less suicidal ideation compared to those with a *high* self-focus and *low* other-focus combination. In a variation of this research, Brancu, Jobes, Wanger, Greene, and Fratto (2015), using a software program to analyze SSF written responses of suicidal college students, found that patients with self-oriented SSF responses were significantly associated with longer durations of clinical care.

SSF Reasons for Living versus Reasons for Dying

In my experience of talking to suicidal patients over the past 30 years, I have been struck by the internal debate endemic to the suicidal struggle. On the one hand, most of these patients have clear thoughts about why they want to die; on the other hand, these same patients invariably also have at least some reasons for wanting to live. Interestingly, many of the things that patients list regarding reasons for living can simultaneously be listed as reasons for dying as well—such is the nature of the suicidal mind. For example, a patient may write "my wife and kids" as a reason for living, and yet also write "to stop being a burden to my family" as a reason for dying. Such apparent contradictions raise the critical construct of *ambivalence,* which is psychologically fundamental to most suicidal states. Let me clear, if some-one is in a clinician's office talking about suicide, he or she is ambivalent. Suicidal people who are not ambivalent about living or dying are not talking to clinicians; they are dead.

As shown in Figure 2.4, the SSF Reasons for Living (RFL) versus Reasons for Dying (RFD) assessment prompts the suicidal patient list up to five RFLs and RFDs, respectively, in spaces provided (the respective psychological importance of each response is rank-ordered from 1 to 5).

Our research team has developed a highly reliable coding system to orga-nize these responses into response themes (Jobes & Mann, 1999). The RFL themes include "Family," "Friends," "Responsibility to Others," "Burdening Others," "Plans and Goals," "Hopefulness for the Future," "Enjoyable Things," "Beliefs," and "Self." The RFD themes include "Relationships," "Unburdening Others," "Loneliness," "Hopelessness," "General Descriptors of Self," "Escape in General," "Escape the Past," "Escape the Pain," and "Escape Responsibilities." Generally this assessment has shown both the pervasiveness of RFLs among suicidal patients and the marked need for *escape* as a common reason for dying (Jobes & Mann, 1999). The RFL/RFD assessment approach has been applied to additional studies within our lab (e.g., Corona et al., 2013) and elsewhere in the field (e.g., Harris, McLean, Sheffield, & Jobes, 2010) as a means of further examining the ambivalent nature of the suicidal mind. I would note, however, that recent research investigating a large sample of suicide *attempters* showed RFLs dominated by family-oriented responses, whereas RFD responses focused almost entirely on issues of the self with virtually no escape-oriented responses (Jennings, 2015). It would thus appear that the psychology of RFL and RFD may be markedly different among those who are "upstream" with suicidal ideation prior to attempting versus those people who are "downstream," having recently made a suicide attempt yet survived.

As mentioned earlier, there are interesting unpublished data focusing only on SSF Reasons for Living (Nademin et al., 2005). In this study, SSF RFLs for 201 suicidal college students were compared to RFLs provided by a sample of 201 non-suicidal undergraduate students in introductory psychology courses at CUA. Two

Rank	REASONS FOR LIVING	Rank	REASONS FOR DYING
1	wife	1	my wife
2	family	2	I'm a scumbag
		3	what I did over there

FIGURE 2.4. Suicidal veteran's reasons for living versus reasons for dying.

distinct findings emerged. First, the psychology student sample had more total RFL responses than the clinical sample (1,004 compared to 598). Second, the suicidal clinical sample endorsed RFLs focusing on coding themes of "Family," "Burdening Others," and "Enjoyable Things." In contrast, the subject pool students' RFL responses were significantly more focused on the coding themes of "Hopefulness for the Future," "Plans and Goals," and "Beliefs." In other words, the nonsuicidal sample had markedly more total RFL responses that were focused on *aspirational* and *inspirational* themes of hope, future, plans, goals, and beliefs when compared to the RFLs of the suicidal sample. While there are obvious limitations to this kind of research, it does perhaps reflect an inability of suicidal people to protectively think about the future and harbor hope that might help them weather the difficult times in their life (see O'Connor et al., 2004). Refer to Appendix C for information about coding these responses.

SSF Wish to Live versus Wish to Die Assessment

One of my favorite articles in the field of suicidology was authored by Maria Kovacs and Aaron Beck (1977), who wrote an important paper about what they called the "internal struggle hypothesis," which posited that suicidal people struggle with competing wishes for living versus dying. Brown, Steer, Henriques, and Beck (2005) later used this methodology to assess suicidal risk among psychiatric outpatients. They combined ratings of two items (the Wish to Live and the Wish to Die) to create an interval-scale index score for each patient, and found that this index score was significantly associated with prospective suicidal risk. More specifically, those with a higher index score (indicating a stronger wish to die) were at significantly higher risk for completing suicide. Our research group at CUA has further validated this WTL/WTD methodology in a range of additional studies (Corona at al., 2013; Jennings, 2015; Lento et al., 2013; O'Connor et al., 2012a; O'Connor, Jobes, Yeargin, et al., 2012).

The SSF One-Thing Response

As shown in Figure 2.5 the SSF "One-Thing Response" is used to gather useful information from the patient about the one thing that would make them no longer suicidal.

In our research we have seen a remarkable range of responses to this question (Jobes, 2004b). For example, one suicidal Air Force patient wrote, "five million dollars and a ticket home." Frankly, this response is rather flip and not particularly useful clinically. In contrast, however, I had another patient write, "to get my medications right—I have been having mood swings related to mixing an oral contraceptive with my antidepressant medicine." Such a response is much more

The one thing that would help me no longer feel suicidal would be: _getting rid of guilt_

FIGURE 2.5. Suicidal veteran's One-Thing Response.

clinically helpful, prompting an immediate referral to a consulting psychiatrist. In comparing these two examples I do not mean to be pejorative about the first example; it is just that the second example provides the clinician with useful information that leads directly to a treatment intervention. The original SSF One-Thing Response coding system reliably organized responses into "Self" versus "Relational," "Realistic" versus "Unrealistic," and "Clinically Useful" versus "Not Clinically Useful." In an unpublished study of 191 suicidal college students we saw that those who most quickly resolved their suicidal risk had SSF One-Thing Responses that were reliably coded as "self," "realistic," and "clinically useful" (Fratto, Jobes, Pentiuc, Rice, & Tendick, 2004; see Appendix D). An additional reliable coding system for the SSF One-Thing Response was developed by Kulish, Jobes, and Lineberry (2012) to organize these responses into the following categories: "Specific Intimate Relationships," "General Social Relationships," "Economic/Professional/ Academic Stability," "External Intervention," "Internal Intervention," "No Desire to Live," "Not Suicidal," and "No Answer." This newer system provides more coding content complexity and generally more detailed information to further inform clinical assessment and treatment.

SSF Macro-Coding

Finally, we developed a "macro-coding" methodology to consider SSF qualitative responses from a larger overview—a "gestalt" perspective (Jobes, Stone, Wagner, Conrad, & Lineberry, 2010). To achieve this, our research team reliably coded the entire first page of *all* SSF qualitative responses taken together into two major "Suicidal Orientations": Self versus Relational (refer to Figure 2.6).

Similarly, we have reliably coded only the RFL/RFD assessment into three different "Suicidal Motivations": Life Motivation (frequencies of RFL > RFD) versus Ambivalent Motivation (frequencies of RFL = RFD) versus Death Motivation (frequencies of RFL < RFD). Organizing the SSF qualitative responses into these broader coding superordinate themes of suicidal motivation has enabled us to reliably differentiate a cross-sectional sample of suicidal inpatients showing significant between-group differences on standardized assessment tools and in relation to attempt history (Jobes et al., 2010). Macro-coding a sample of suicidal outpatients into life, ambivalent, and death motivated groups using first RFL/RFD responses was also able to differentially predict longitudinal outcomes related to outpatient mental health treatment (Jennings, Jobes, O'Connor, & Comtois, 2012).

Rate and fill out each item according to how you feel right now. Then rank in order of importance 1 to 5 (1 = most important to 5 = least important):

Rank	
_4_	1) RATE PSYCHOLOGICAL PAIN (hurt, anguish, or misery in your mind, **not** stress, **not** physical pain): Low pain: 1 2 3 (4) 5 :High pain What I find most painful is: _when my wife says she doesn't like me_
_3_	2) RATE STRESS (your general feeling of being pressured or overwhelmed): Low stress: 1 2 3 (4) 5 :High stress What I find most stressful is: _relationships, work_
_4_	3) RATE AGITATION (emotional urgency; feeling that you need to take action; **not** irritation; **not** annoyance): Low agitation: 1 2 (3) 4 5 :High agitation I most need to take action when: _when people belittle me_
_4_	4) RATE HOPELESSNESS (your expectation that things will not get better no matter what you do): Low hopelessness: 1 2 (3) 4 5 :High hopelessness I am most hopeless about: _relations, work, being a father_
_3_	5) RATE SELF-HATE (your general feeling of disliking yourself; having no self-esteem; having no self-respect): Low self-hate: 1 2 3 4 (5) :High self-hate What I hate most about myself is: _drinking, me and wife don't get along_
N/A	6) RATE OVERALL RISK OF SUICIDE: Extremely low risk (1) 2 3 4 5 :Extremely high risk (will not kill self) (will kill self)

1) How much is being suicidal related to thoughts and feelings about yourself? Not at all: 1 2 (3) 4 5 : completely
2) How much is being suicidal related to thoughts and feelings about others? Not at all: 1 2 3 (4) 5 : completely

Rank	REASONS FOR LIVING
_4_	son
_1_	wife
_1_	brother
_1_	support family

Rank	REASONS FOR DYING
_4_	not good enough father
_5_	I'm a bad husband
_3_	not a good mentor
_3_	failing at providing

I wish to live to the following extent: Not at all: 0 1 2 3 4 5 (6) 7 8 : Very much
I wish to die to the following extent: Not at all: 0 1 2 3 (4) 5 6 7 8 : Very much
The one thing that would help me no longer feel suicidal would be: _wife saying negative things_

RELATIONALLY ORIENTED

Rate and fill out each item according to how you feel right now. Then rank in order of importance 1 to 5 (1 = most important to 5 = least important)

Rank	
_1_	1) RATE PSYCHOLOGICAL PAIN (hurt, anguish, or misery in your mind, **not** stress, **not** physical pain): Low pain: 1 2 3 4 (5) :High pain What I find most painful is: _nihilistic thinking_
_5_	2) RATE STRESS (your general feeling of being pressured or overwhelmed): Low stress: 1 2 (3) 4 5 :High stress What I find most stressful is: _philosophizing_
_4_	3) RATE AGITATION (emotional urgency; feeling that you need to take action; **not** irritation; **not** annoyance): Low agitation: 1 (2) 3 4 5 :High agitation I most need to take action when: _I "determine" I need to die_
_2_	4) RATE HOPELESSNESS (your expectation that things will not get better no matter what you do): Low hopelessness: 1 2 3 (4) 5 :High hopelessness I am most hopeless about: _meaning of life_
_3_	5) RATE SELF-HATE (your general feeling of disliking yourself; having no self-esteem; having no self-respect): Low self-hate: 1 2 3 (4) 5 :High self-hate What I hate most about myself is: _I "realize" there is no such thing as love_
N/A	6) RATE OVERALL RISK OF SUICIDE: Extremely low risk 1 2 3 (4) 5 :Extremely high risk (will not kill self) (will kill self)

1) How much is being suicidal related to thoughts and feelings about yourself? Not at all: 1 2 3 (4) 5 : completely
2) How much is being suicidal related to thoughts and feelings about others? Not at all: 1 (2) 3 4 5 : completely

Rank	REASONS FOR LIVING
_1_	life is meaningful
_2_	so many things to do
_3_	family/friends
_4_	"voice" is wrong
_5_	I will get better

Rank	REASONS FOR DYING
_1_	me life is meaningless
_5_	I am stupid
_3_	internal voice
_2_	no one loves me
_4_	so many questions

I wish to live to the following extent: Not at all: 0 1 2 (3) 4 5 6 7 8 : Very much
I wish to die to the following extent: Not at all: 0 1 2 3 4 5 (6) 7 8 : Very much
The one thing that would help me no longer feel suicidal would be: _to disprove all statements of nihilistic_
inner voice

SELF-ORIENTED

FIGURE 2.6. SSF Macro-coding of "Suicidal Orientation" (self vs. relational).

27

SSF Section B: Risk-Factor Assessment

Section B of the SSF includes 14 well-researched empirically based risk factors (and warning signs) that are among the best variables for assessing suicidal states. The original list of variables was developed by a work group of experts convened by the U.S. Air Force Suicide Prevention Program (Oordt et al., 2005). These variables were used in early SSF versions and have proven to be a valuable short list of suicide-risk and warning-sign variables with good empirical support (Jobes & Berman, 1993; Jobes et al., 1997).

SSF Section C: Treatment Planning

Section C of the SSF is the Treatment Plan section and is discussed in depth in Chapter 5. The treatment plan section flows directly from the collaborative assessment performed by the patient and clinician in Sections A and B. For now, there are a few points I would like to emphasize about the treatment planning section of the SSF. First, unlike traditional treatment planning, where the clinician alone writes up the patient's plan (and may or may not share that plan with the patient), the CAMS approach emphasizes collaborative treatment planning wherein the patient functions as a *coauthor* of the plan (Jobes & Drozd, 2004). The CAMS premise is that the clinician is uniquely positioned to consider various interventions *with* the patient, having completed SSF assessment sections A and B with the patient's active involvement. Within CAMS, a central and overt goal is to consider what interventions will be necessary to pursue and justify *outpatient* care. Collaboratively developing an outpatient treatment plan is thus an expressed overarching goal of CAMS. Accordingly, it is important to note that within the SSF treatment plan section there a "Problem Description" section, and Problem 1 is "Self-Harm Potential." Next there is a "Goals and Objectives" section that initially emphasizes "Safety and Stability." Theses sections are then followed by spaces for "Interventions" and "Duration." This sequence of treatment planning is by design because the number-one clinical problem is not negotiable—self-harm potential must be appropriately addressed within the treatment planning section. If the clinician and patient are not able to sufficiently address the clinical problem of self-harm potential through their collaborative treatment planning and the development of an outpatient stabilization plan, an inpatient hospitalization may be necessary as the only means of ensuring the patient's immediate physical safety in accordance with state law. Fortunately, a great deal of work has been done on different versions of outpatient stabilization planning over the past decade. Otherwise known as "safety planning" (Stanley & Brown, 2012) or "crisis response planning" (Rudd et al., 2001), these approaches are the clear remedy for the ill-advised use of "no-suicide" contracts or the notion of "contracting for safety," which is still used too much in contemporary mental health care.

When I first worked on an inpatient psychiatric unit as a member of the nursing staff more than 30 years ago, prior to discharge the attending doctors would instruct us to "get the patient to commit to their safety prior to discharge." We would dutifully carry out the order and the patients typically eagerly agreed, knowing this was needed to get out of the hospital. The problem is that there was little to no discussion about what they would do in a dark moment if they became suicidal again! The worst part about traditional no-harm contracting is that it often can become a game in which both parties know how ineffective this intervention actually is. In many cases, our patients know what they must say, or not say, to be hospitalized or discharged. Worse yet, we know that they know that we know. It simply makes no sense. This is particularly true because of the emphasis on what the patient *won't* do versus what they *will* do should they become suicidal. In contrast, various versions of stabilization planning go into great depth about what the patient will endeavor to do should he or she become suicidal, which is much more helpful and practical. More will be said of this in Chapter 4, particularly in reference to the CAMS version of stabilization planning that is now embedded within the SSF-4. In that chapter we will also explore "driver-oriented" treatment that is first broached in the initial CAMS session with the identification of Problems 2 and 3, respectively, on the treatment plan section of the SSF. Driver-oriented treatment is unique to CAMS; it is a signature feature setting it apart from other evidence-based practices for suicide.

SSF Section D: Supplemental Clinical Documentation

During the 1990s the U.S. Congress passed a significant piece of legislation with major implications for health care delivery. The Health Insurance Portability and Accountability Act (HIPAA) was passed (in part) as a means of ensuring the privacy and security of medical health records as well as standardizing practices related to personal health information (e.g., rules related to electronic transmission). The legislation required full compliance of providers across health care disciplines as of April 13, 2003. The implications of HIPAA have been far-reaching for all health care providers, including mental health professionals. Consequently, key elements of HIPAA have been incorporated into various aspects of SSF documentation.

At each phase within CAMS—the initial session, all interim sessions, and the final session—there are specific pages of documentation that we loosely refer to as the "HIPAA pages" of the SSF (pages 4, 6, and 8 of the SSF-4 shown in Appendix A). The inclusion of these pages is meant to provide an efficient way of maintaining a comprehensive medical record that complies with HIPAA. As is discussed in Chapter 8, the protective aspect of careful documentation in relation to malpractice litigation is important. In relation to these various considerations, the SSF has been specifically constructed to both decrease potential malpractice liability *and* function as a fully HIPAA-compliant and comprehensive medical record. I generally recommend using the SSF as *the* medical record for any suicidal patients while they remain suicidal, displacing the documentation one would ordinarily maintain. In other words, while CAMS patients are being assessed, tracked, and treated using the SSF, there is no particular need for additional documentation (unless the clinician so chooses). When the risk of suicide has been successfully addressed by CAMS, clinicians can then transition back to their normal medical record documentation that they routinely use.

CAMS is used in a range of clinical settings (e.g., outpatient clinics, counseling centers, hospitals, crisis centers); consequently, there may be a need to adapt CAMS and the SSF depending on the setting. For example, certain university counseling centers have opted not to use the HIPAA pages of the SSF, arguing that the nature of work in these centers does not meet the criteria for having to be HIPAA compliant. Generally, I have been supportive of modified uses of CAMS and the SSF depending on the setting and the nature of the practice.

SSF TRACKING/UPDATE (INTERIM SESSIONS)

Another critical and unique element of CAMS-guided care is the expectation that patients will be clinically "tracked" until their suicidal risk is either eliminated through treatment or other outcomes occur (e.g., referral or treatment dropout). To this end, the CAMS Tracking/Update portion of the SSF is used for every interim session until outcomes are realized. As is discussed in much greater detail in Chapters 4 and 5, every interim session begins with a relatively quick patient rating of the six SSF Core Assessment variables (Section A) to get a sense of current suicidal risk and ends with a collaborative update of the patient's suicide-specific treatment plan (Section B). After every interim CAMS session the clinician fills in the related interim HIPAA page to complete the comprehensive medical record (Section C).

SSF CLINICAL OUTCOME/DISPOSITION (FINAL SESSION)

As a clinical intervention, CAMS comes to a close when criteria for "resolution" are met or other outcomes arise. As discussed in Chapter 7, when three consecutive sessions of low overall risk and the successful management of suicide thoughts, feelings, and behaviors are realized, then the final SSF outcome/disposition documentation is administered with a final check of the SSF Core Assessment and verification of the resolution criteria (Section A). The session ends with the completion of the patient's treatment outcome and disposition (Section B).

Importantly, the SSF Outcome/Disposition should be used to document the full range of possible outcomes. For example, a patient's CAMS-guided care might end with an incarceration for serious domestic violence. Other patients may drop out of treatment or be hospitalized—all of which can be documented on SSF Outcome/Disposition sections to ensure that the medical record is complete no matter the outcome. As with every phase of CAMS, there is a final posttreatment HIPAA-specific page of documentation that completes a comprehensive medical record of the case (Section C) and marks the end of using clinically using CAMS.

THE EVOLUTION OF CAMS

In 1996, I was sitting in the cramped office of the Executive Director of the American Association of Suicidology with two graduate students in tow. At that time, Lanny Berman had a psychiatrist colleague who led a large managed-care mental health system. This colleague was interested in engaging a team of clinician-researchers to find a better way to assess and treat the ubiquitous suicidal patients in this system of care. There was some budding interest in the field at this time about the unique assessment aspects of the SSF following some early SSF-related publications (e.g. Jobes, 1995a; Jobes & Berman, 1993). It was an exciting opportunity to be invited to adapt the use of the SSF to fit across a relatively large mental health care system. A central challenge within this effort was to find a way to decrease hospitalizations (thereby saving money) while still effectively managing the risk of suicide. Notably, an early SSF study had just been published showing some intriguing differences between patient and clinician independent ratings of the SSF variables (Eddins & Jobes, 1994). In this study, we found a tendency for clinicians to overrate some SSF variables (in comparison to patient ratings) but significantly underrate the potentially lethal variable of suicidal perturbation (agitation). In our meeting I was asked how I wanted to reconcile these differences between clinician and patient ratings as we considered the use of the SSF across this large mental health system. It then occurred to me that we should have the patient and clinician complete the assessment *collaboratively*. This idea was in part inspired by the data but was also influenced by my teaching the Rorschach inkblot test, which routinely uses a side-by-side seating arrangement. An essential aspect of administering the Rorschach is the notion that the *patient's* responses to the inkblot stimuli are what matters. Thus, the clinician-administrator of the Rorschach has a singular assessment mission: to see what the patient sees in the inkblots. In other words, we endeavor to see the stimuli *through the eyes of the patient*. What would become the heart of CAMS was born in that moment. I would also note that this simple notion of directly understanding and empathically appreciating the suicidal patient's perspective has since evolved into a major focus within the larger field of clinical suicide prevention (refer to Michel & Gysin-Maillart, 2015; Michel & Jobes, 2010; Michel et al., 2002; Orbach, 2001; Tucker et al., 2015).

The early development of CAMS was therefore organized around a particular way of administering the SSF as an assessment approach to suicidal risk. But in a relatively short time the approach evolved into a suicide-specific clinical framework and intervention. As CAMS developed, the assessment-heavy early versions of the SSF evolved into the more multidimensional clinical tool. Today, the SSF-4 is a multipurpose assessment, treatment-planning, risk tracking, and outcome clinical tool and functions as the "roadmap" of CAMS-guided care (Jobes, 2006, 2012). Hence, CAMS has evolved in direct response to fundamental clinical needs related to:

1. Establishing a strong clinical alliance and increasing patient motivation.
2. Thoroughly and comprehensively assessing suicidal risk.
3. Developing and maintaining a problem-focused treatment plan that is suicide specific.
4. Having a way to track the ongoing suicidal risk until it is reduced and/or eliminated.
5. Having clinical documentation that reflects excellent practice, thereby decreasing liability.
6. Flexibility and adaptability across theoretical orientation, discipline, and clinical setting.
7. Having an approach that is relatively easy to learn, leading to quick adherence/mastery.
8. Having a relatively cost-effective approach to caring for suicidal risk.
9. Having a least-restrictive clinical approach to working with suicidal risk.
10. Having an evidence-based approach that effectively treats suicidal risk.

While there were various fits and starts in our initial efforts to clinically roll out CAMS and conduct clinical research in "real-world" treatment environments (refer to Jobes, Bryan, & Neal-Walden, 2009), the use of CAMS, and our related clinical research, evolved and matured over time. The effectiveness-oriented research foundation of CAMS (both successes and failures) helped to meaningfully evolve CAMS as an intervention (Jobes, Comtois, Brenner, & Gutierrez, 2011). In the course of our ongoing effectiveness research we have discovered and consolidated some important points. Seeing CAMS as a *philosophy* of care and as a suicide-specific *therapeutic framework* is paramount. In addition, the development of driver-oriented treatment marks an exciting innovation in suicidal care and, our research is continuing to refine this aspect of the approach (Jobes, Comtois, Brenner, Gutierrez, & O'Connor, 2016). What follows is a brief review of the evidence base in support of CAMS to date.

Open Trials and Correlational Studies of CAMS

As shown in Table 2.1, there are seven published nonrandomized clinical investigations on the effectiveness of CAMS (and the embedded use of the SSF) used in a variety of clinical settings with varying samples of suicidal patients.

Two studies using different research methods with suicidal college students show significant pre–post within-group treatment results using the SSF (Jobes et al., 1997), as well as significant CAMS-related reductions in overall symptom distress and suicidal ideation using repeated measures linear analyses (Jobes, Kahn-Greene, et al., 2009). Two other studies show the cross-cultural impact of CAMS when it was used in two within-group pre–post investigations of suicidal outpatients in Danish community mental health care (Arkov, Rosenbaum, Christiansen, Jonsson, & Munchowm, 2008; Nielsen, Alberdi, & Rosenbaum, 2011). Even though CAMS was originally developed as an outpatient intervention, it was first effectively adapted and used in an unpublished study with an inpatient sample in Switzerland (Schilling, Harbauer, Andreae, & Haas, 2006). Research collaborators at the Menninger Clinic have published a series of articles (Ellis, Allen, Woodson, Frueh, & Jobes, 2009; Ellis, Daza, & Allen, 2012; Ellis et al., 2015) about an adapted inpatient use of CAMS in that inpatient setting (referred to as "CAMS-M"). This team published both a within-subjects and an open trial investigation of the effectiveness of CAMS within this longer-term inpatient psychiatric setting (Ellis et al., 2012). Another Menninger study has shown significant between-group changes (using "propensity score matching" to create a matched comparison control group) in overall suicide ideation and suicide-related cognitions (Ellis et al., 2015).

CAMS was used naturalistically in two U.S. Air Force outpatient mental health settings in a nonrandomized case–control study of 55 suicidal Air Force personnel

TABLE 2.1. Correlational and Open-Trial Support for SSF/CAMS

Authors	Sample/setting	$n =$	Significant results
Jobes et al. (1997)	College students, university counseling center	106	Pre–post distress; pre–post SSF core ratings
Jobes et al. (2005)	Air Force personnel, outpatient clinic	56	Between-group suicidal ideation; ED/PC appointments
Arkov et al. (2008)	Danish outpatients, CMH clinic	27	Pre–post SSF core ratings
Jobes et al. (2009)	College students, university counseling center	55	Linear reductions in distress/ideation
Nielsen et al. (2011)	Danish outpatients, CMH clinic	42	Pre–post SSF core ratings
Ellis et al. (2012)	Psychiatric inpatients	20	Pre–post SSF core ratings; suicidal ideation, depression, hopelessness
Ellis et al. (2015)	Psychiatric inpatients	52	Suicidal ideation and cognitions

(Jobes, Wong, Conrad, Drozd, & Neal-Walden, 2005). Within this correlational ex-post-facto design, suicidal ideation was reduced significantly more quickly for patients treated by providers using an early version of CAMS in comparison to a control group of patients treated by providers using "treatment as usual" (TAU) care. Moreover, using an interrupted time-series analysis, CAMS was significantly correlated with comparative reductings in primary care appointments and emergency department visits. While these correlational data were promising, we could not infer a *causal* impact of CAMS because there was neither randomization nor any formal check of adherence and fidelity, which obviously affected the internal validity of the study. That said, this archival study was conducted *after* care was already rendered, which meant that the external validity of our findings was high; these patients were seen naturalistically and were not engaged as research participants. In addition, a series of post-hoc statistical analyses were performed to account for possible "third variables" that may have affected the study's significant findings (e.g., medication or provider). These analyses did not demonstrate any changes in the overall pattern of results showing the uniform superiority of CAMS care.

Randomized Controlled Trials of CAMS

Because *causality* is a central goal of science, our current CAMS research is focused on randomized controlled trial (RCT) designs (Jobes et al., 2016). Our first published RCT was a small feasibility study comparing CAMS to "enhanced care as usual" (ECAU) with a community-based sample of suicidal outpatients (Comtois et al., 2011). In this study, 32 suicidal outpatients were randomly assigned to the respective treatment arms in an outpatient mental health treatment clinic housed within a large urban medical center. Despite limited statistical power given the small sample, there were statistically significant experimental findings on all of the primary and secondary measures, including between-group differences in suicidal ideation, overall symptom distress, reasons for living, and optimism/hope (see Figure 2.7).

Prominently, the between-group differences were *most* robust at the most distal assessment time point (12 months after the start of care) showing the possible enduring impact of CAMS long after the treatment ended (on average around eight sessions). Finally, CAMS patient satisfaction ratings were significantly higher than control patient ratings, and the patients receiving CAMS demonstrated superior treatment retention in comparison to control patients.

A second RCT investigation has been conducted by colleagues in Copenhagen, Denmark. The "DiaS" trial was a parallel-group superiority design in which 108 suicide attempters with borderline features were randomly assigned to either 16 weeks of DBT or up to 16 weeks of CAMS (Andreasson et al., 2014). With an extensive (and replicated) empirical literature on the effectiveness of DBT for self-harm and suicide-attempt behaviors, this investigation surprisingly found *no* statistically

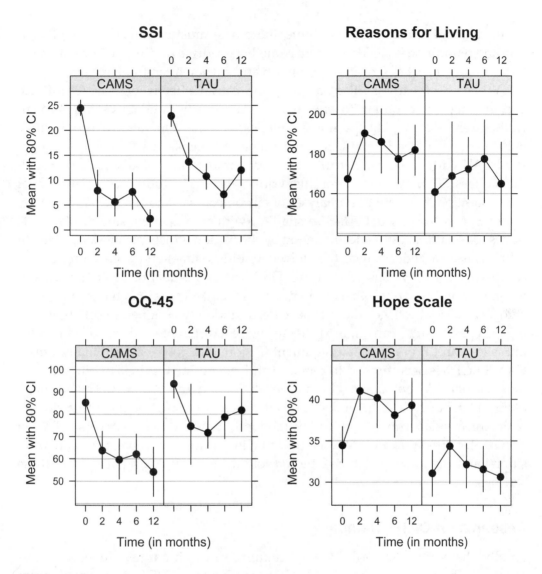

FIGURE 2.7. Results of the Harborview randomized controlled trial (Comtois et al., 2011).

significant between-group differences between DBT and CAMS for self-harm and suicide attempts (Andreasson et al., 2016). Specifically, at the 28-week follow-up, DBT patients had 21 self-harm episodes (36.8%) and CAMS patients had 12 episodes (23.5%); DBT patients made 12 attempts (19.3%) and CAMS patients made 5 attempts (9.8%). While this ambitious study had some methodological constraints and was statistically underpowered, these nonsignificant findings are nevertheless important as the CAMS patients received markedly less direct care (typically fewer than 16 weeks of once/week sessions) in comparison to DBT patients who received 16 weeks of individual therapy, skills training in groups, access to telephone coaching with therapists, and supervision and consultations for the team of therapists.

As the authors of the DiaS study note, these data must be interpreted with caution and replication is clearly needed. Nonetheless, these findings are promising in terms of the impact of CAMS on self-harm and suicide-attempt behaviors.

While these early RCT data about the causal effectiveness of CAMS are encouraging, we continue to endeavor to empirically validate CAMS through well-powered RCTs and experimental replication. The "Operation Worth Living" (OWL) study funded by the U.S. Department of Defense is a RCT of CAMS versus ECAU with an outpatient intent-to-treat sample of $n = 148$ suicidal U.S. Soldiers (Jobes, 2014). At the time of this writing, the OWL study is completing final data collection and statistical analyses of our outcomes. Another RCT is currently under way in Norway of CAMS versus TAU with an outpatient sample of $n = 100$ (Jobes, 2014, 2015). A small RCT funded by the National Institute of Mental Health (NIMH) is also under way at the University of Nevada–Reno Counseling Center comparing CAMS versus TAU versus DBT within a sequential, multiple assignment, randomized trial (otherwise known as "SMART") research design. In this study, 62 suicidal college students have been randomly assigned to different dosing of types of care in an effort to effectively treat different kinds of suicidal states in Stages I and II of random assignment (Pistorello & Jobes, 2014). Finally, a new CAMS RCT has been funded to replicate and extend the findings of our previous RCT with suicidal outpatients (Comtois et al., 2011). In the "Aftercare Focus Study" (AFS), a total of 200 discharged suicide attempters from inpatient psychiatric care or emergency department care will be randomly assigned to CAMS versus TAU in a "next-day appointment" (NDA) model of clinical care that centers on "care transition" and the known high-risk period following clinical discharge from these settings.

Research on CAMS Training

Finally, there are noteworthy CAMS training research studies. Indeed, as discussed by Pisani, Cross, and Gould (2011), training in CAMS has been recognized as one of only a handful of suicide-specific professional training approaches at the national level. There is interesting unpublished evidence that CAMS training can be effective in changing clinicians' knowledge and attitudes about working with suicidal risk. In a study conducted by Schuberg and colleagues (2009) of 165 CAMS-trained Veterans Affairs mental health providers, we found significant (p < .05) pre–post training differences related to decreasing clinician anxiety about working with suicidal risk in general, while specifically increasing clinician confidence in assessing and treating suicidal risk. There were other significant pre–post positive training findings related to clinicians' perceptions about forming an alliance with a suicidal patient, increasing patient motivation, and conducting safety planning. Most of these significant CAMS-training pre–post effects were sustained in a 3-month follow-up assessment with a subset of the original sample ($n = 36$).

In an online survey of 120 mental health practitioners, Crowley, Arnkoff, Glass, and Jobes (2014) found moderate to high self-reported adherence to the CAMS therapeutic philosophy, which was comparable to other studies gauging the impact of suicide-focused training. Participants further reported relatively high adherence to CAMS practice, which was higher than findings on adherence to interventions for other psychiatric issues. Overall adherence to CAMS philosophy and practice did not vary as a function of contextual variable (e.g., clinician discipline, type of practice setting, or different CAMS training modalities).

We have also seen the positive impact of CAMS training delivered within an e-learning training modality (Marshall et al., 2014). In this study, 215 Veterans Affairs mental health providers across five sites were randomized to three conditions: 69 to CAMS e-learning, 70 to in-person CAMS training, and 76 to a control no-training group. We found in this study that both CAMS live training and e-learning training were favorably received, with no significant differences between clinician ratings of the two training methods. This study showed the potential value of providing an accessible broad-based e-learning CAMS training to a wide range of mental health providers.

While these training studies have some limitations (e.g., their self-report nature), we nevertheless know that clinicians can quickly learn key CAMS concepts, and with support and guidance can become CAMS adherent often with their first case. Ongoing training research is now under way to further investigate training that leads to actual clinician *behavior change* to become competent CAMS-adherent clinical providers (Jobes, 2015).

SUMMARY AND CONCLUSIONS

The SSF has evolved significantly over 25 years of clinical practice and research. As part of this evolution, a novel suicide-specific evidence-based clinical intervention has emerged. CAMS is now best understood as a philosophy of care and as a therapeutic framework. CAMS has been purposely designed to enhance the therapeutic alliance and inspire motivation within the patient *to want to live*. CAMS is clinically used to both stabilize suicidal patients and fully engage them in a problem-focused course of care that systematically targets and treats the patient's self-defined suicidal drivers. At its best, CAMS effectively treats the patient's suicidal drivers and helps provide a new coping repertoire as the clinical dyad pursues a "post-suicidal" life for the patient—a life with purpose and meaning as well as plans, goals, and hope for the future.

CHAPTER 3

Systems of Clinical Care and Optimizing the Use of CAMS

Successful clinical assessment and treatment of suicidal risk requires *both* a system of care that is reliably attuned to the prospect of encountering patients with suicidal risk *and* a clinician who is equally prepared to engage that risk in a reliable and competent fashion. To achieve this, CAMS-guided care thrives within a clinical environment where there is an expectation that suicidal presentations will be identified early and that potential risk will be effectively engaged as far "upstream" as possible. Over the past decade, I have conducted a number of process improvement (PI) initiatives in both public and private sector clinical treatment settings and large health care systems. Such initiatives are often pursued when there has been a particularly significant suicide, a series of suicides, or a malpractice wrongful-death lawsuit prompting a thorough examination of existing practices (with the goal of improving those practices). Within any effective PI initiative there are various ways to improve how suicidal risk is identified, clinically assessed, treated, documented, and administratively tracked over the course of care for optimal outcomes. Implementing such improvements will not only help save lives but also decrease the risk of malpractice liability.

Whether large or small—within a single clinic or across a network of hospitals—the PI model developed and used by the CUA Suicide Prevention Lab (and our close collaborators) involves three distinct phases: (1) evaluation and needs assessment of the existing system of care for suicidal patients, (2) the delivery of a tailored training and any adaptations of CAMS to providers within that system, and (3) follow-up consultation and further evaluation of the impact of the intervention for quality assurance purposes (Archuleta et al., 2014). Having conducted many PIs within private medical centers, university counseling centers, psychiatric inpatient facilities, community mental health systems, a large network of Veterans Affairs medical centers, and military treatment facilities, we have learned a great deal about clinical care for suicidal patients in a range of clinical settings. In my experience of conducting PIs, providing consultation, training countless mental health professionals, and serving as a forensic expert in cases of suicide-related malpractice tort litigation, I have seen both excellent systems of care for suicidal risk as well as shockingly naïve and utterly inept approaches to effectively caring for suicidal patients (and everything in between). As a general matter, a system of care can markedly improve clinical practice for suicidal patients by following the four basic steps discussed in this chapter. Notably, these four steps are as pertinent to private practitioners working out of a modest home office as they are to a statewide suicide prevention program working across the full gamut of mental health care services. Moreover, these steps will greatly enhance the success of CAMS-guided care.

STEP 1: DEVELOP POLICIES AND PROCEDURES

Written policies and procedures related to suicide risk are critical to have in place. Depending on the size and scope of the practice and/or system of care, such policy and procedures can be modest to exhaustive and detailed. In any case, a plaintiff's attorney will routinely subpoena any and all policies and procedures statements related to suicide risk when considering pursuing a malpractice lawsuit against a provider or a larger system of care. The absence of suicide-specific policies and procedures can therefore increase the potential of litigation after a completed suicide because it creates the appearance of neither anticipating the prospect of suicidal presentations nor establishing a "usual and customary" approach for systematically dealing with such cases. A caveat to this line of thinking is that previously established suicide-specific policies and procedures only reflect good practice when providers actually follow their suicide policy and procedures! At a minimum, an effective suicide-specific policy and procedure statement will acknowledge the anticipated prospect of seeing suicidal patients and will then outline usual and customary practice procedures related to routine assessment, tracking, and treatment of these patients. Most mental health professional trade associations can provide general guidance about developing practice policy and procedures; review and approval by an attorney who is knowledgeable in state mental health laws and professional standards is also an important additional step to take.

STEP 2: DEVELOP A RELIABLE WAY
TO IDENTIFY SUICIDAL RISK EARLY ON

It is self-evident that it is impossible to effectively treat suicide risk if that risk remains unknown to the clinician. Fundamental to clinical suicide prevention is the importance of having a way to reliably and effectively identify suicide risk as early as possible. In this realm both traditional and innovative approaches can be used to help identify suicide risk in a routine and timely manner, thereby opening the door to potentially effective life-saving treatment.

Direct Interview-Based Identification of Suicidal Risk

As noted in Chapter 2, I was involved in a survey study of suicide-specific assessment practices among a range of practicing clinicians (Jobes et al., 1995). Beyond these data, a few general impressions from this study are worth noting. First, I was impressed by the clinicians' confidence in their own clinical judgment—a confidence that bordered on hubris. Particularly in their open-ended responses, there was a critical attitude toward the known psychometric limits of suicide assessment tools and the application of psychological tests to assessing suicide risk, which sharply contrasted their own obvious confidence in their clinical judgments based on interview-format assessment questions and clinical observations. In this regard, I have been fascinated by a line of important (and underappreciated) research by the late Paul Meehl about the distinct limits of clinical judgment in sharp contrast to actuarial assessments (Dawes, Faust, & Meehl, 1989; Meehl, 1997). Across this line of research, the use of assessment tools was *always* superior to clinical judgments, yet in my experience clinicians do not appear to believe these data and remain remarkably overconfident in their "gut" judgments based solely on their interview skills.

Given that many clinicians eschew the use of suicide assessment tools or symptom-based screeners, it is imperative to be sensitive and clinically attuned to the ever-present prospect that any patient may harbor suicidal thoughts. It is thus vital to listen for statements of despair or allusions to their situation being hopeless or feeling trapped. A clinician's ears should certainly prick up when a patient says things like "I'm so tired; I feel like giving up," or "I feel trapped—I really don't have any options," or "Things never work out for me, what's the point?" Such vague insinuations should be followed by a direct question from the clinician about the prospect of suicidal thinking. In an empathic and nonshaming manner the clinician should say something like "Things sound really desperate for you right now and pretty hopeless. Have you thought about suicide as a way to deal with this situation?" Along these lines, the more forthright and direct the questioning, the better. But make no mistake—no potentially life-saving clinical work can follow unless one is willing to ask the patient directly about his or her suicide risk. If you are unwilling to use a screener or an assessment tool to routinely assess for suicide risk, it is incumbent on you to read between the lines for clues and vague references to suicide and then do not hesitate to ask about the possibility in an empathic and earnest manner. Remember, when it comes to suicide risk identification, there should be no leading or shaming questions: "You're not thinking of suicide, are you? How could you do that to your wife?"

While the evidence supports the use of an actuarial assessment approach, I still believe that interview-based assessment through an informed approach can be both effective and even therapeutic. Indeed, as a charter member of the Aeschi Group, I have coedited an entire book on clinical interviewing and how such interview assessments can be effective, therapeutic, and even transformative (Michel & Jobes, 2010). The Aeschi Approach to clinically working with suicidal risk emphasizes empathy with the suicidal wish, following the patient's lead, and listening to the patient's "suicidal story" in a nonshaming and never judgmental manner. Over the years the Aeschi conferences held in Switzerland, and now in the United States, have afforded a unique opportunity to showcase the development and maturation of SSF and CAMS, because CAMS-guided care is consistent with the core Aeschi attitude.

Indirect Identification of Suicidal Risk

As mental health professionals know, there is a certain subset of patients who say they have "suicidal ideation" when in truth there may be little to no threat that the patient will actually terminate his or her existence. This issue is one of the most complicated that we face in the field of mental health. Whole systems of public mental health care are plagued by the dilemma of encountering countless chronically mentally ill people who threaten suicide as means to achieve various nonterminal ends (e.g., attention, shelter, or food). The significant challenges of the "instrumental" nature of threatening suicide or behaving in a sublethal manner as a means to an end go far beyond the scope of the present discussion. Suffice it to say that instrumental suicide risk is sometimes rather obvious but other times can be difficult to discern from "genuine" risk for a serious self-inflicted injury or death. Because many of our assessment approaches transparently ask about suicide, such direct queries can prompt affirmative disclosures of instrumental suicidality but may alternatively produce a denial from those who are genuinely suicidal but wish to hide it. Given this tricky dialectic, there has been increased interest in identifying suicide risk in nontransparent or *indirect* manner such that a patient may not know that his or her suicide risk is being evaluated. The following are examples of indirect suicide risk assessments sometimes referred to as the identification of "occult" or latent suicide risk assessment (e.g., Claassen & Larkin, 2005).

Kessler K-10

As noted earlier, our research team created a large database of suicidal and nonsuicidal psychiatric inpatients in an extensive psychometric study of the SSF (Conrad et al., 2009). From this Mayo Clinic data set, an occult study of indirect suicide risk was performed (O'Connor, Beebe, Lineberry, Jobes, & Conrad, 2012). We investigated the use of the Kessler "K-10" (a brief 10-item symptom checklist that has *no specific question about suicide risk*). A factor analysis of K-10 results was conducted producing a two-factor solution characterizing depression and anxiety, respectively, of 149 inpatients. These factor loadings were found to be highly correlated with psychometrically sound measures of suicidal risk and could effectively discriminate suicidal patients from nonsuicidal patients. Such indirect assessments can therefore be used to conduct follow-up assessments to help lead a patient to seeking and receiving potentially life-saving suicide-specific clinical care.

Technological Assessments of Brain Activation

There is experimental use of technology to study correlations between increased suicidal risk and central nervous system activation. For example, Goodman (2012, 2015) has used electronic sensors placed around the eyes to measure eye-blink startle responses to a range of visual stimuli presented on a computer screen. In this research pleasant, neutral, or unpleasant images (e.g., a person with a gun to his head) are presented to subjects with suicidal ideation, or have made a single attempt, or have made multiple attempts. The eye-blink response data show that multiple attempters were extremely reactive to the unpleasant images. These data may thus reflect an acquired affective sensitivity (or a lack of emotion regulation) among those who have made multiple suicide attempts. While cross-sectional and correlational in nature, such data are intriguing and may reflect Thomas Joiner's (2005) notion of "acquired capability" for suicide through exposure (i.e., their own multiple attempt behaviors).

In another line of research, Familoni and Rasmusson (2012) have conducted research using military thermal imagery technology to measure the opening of sweat pores on the face and thumb as an index to autonomic nervous system activation. In this study, high-resolution thermal imagery was used with active duty military personnel. These investigators found significant correlational effects between embedded questions pertaining to combat-related posttraumatic stress disorder and suicide that corresponded to real-time opening of sweat pores on the face and thumb as measured by thermal imaging. Again, while such correlational data are intriguing, we cannot assume any *causal* prospective suicidal risk from these data. But such methodologies in combination with other assessment approaches may incrementally increase our ability to understand prospective risk.

Implicit Association Test

Along these lines, Matthew Nock at Harvard University has developed an important indirect assessment of prospective suicide risk. Through his use of the Implicit Association Test (IAT), Nock has developed an "objective" or "behavioral" assessment of *prospective* suicide attempts. In one key study, Nock and colleagues (2010) measured implicit associations about death/suicide in 157 people seeking treatment at a psychiatric emergency department. The IAT revealed a significant sixfold increase for prospective suicide attempt behaviors in the 6 months following completion of the IAT assessment. Specifically, on computer-based IAT administrations of paired stimuli, participants who had stronger reaction-time responses to "death" stimuli (vs. "life" stimuli) had higher prospective risk of attempting suicide (i.e., their behavioral reactivity to classifying such semantic stimuli revealed automatic mental associations). This line is of work is one of the most significant breakthroughs in assessment research in the past decade, and numerous IAT studies are now being undertaken to further understand the nature of this objective (and indirect) assessment of prospective risk for suicide-related behaviors (Glashouwer et al., 2010; Harrison, Stritzke, Fay, Ellison, & Hudaib, 2014; Randall, Rowe, Dong, Nock, & Colman, 2013; Tang, Wu, & Miao, 2013).

Symptom-Based Screener Identification of Suicidal Risk

In 2010, The Joint Commission that accredits health care institutions in the United States issued suicide assessment-oriented "National Patient Safety Goals," as suicide deaths have proven to be a leading "sentinel event" within health care facilities nationwide (The Joint Commission, 2010; Mills et al., 2010). Moreover as noted in Chapter 1, The Joint Commission's (2016) landmark sentinel event alert has further emphasized this point as they assert the paramount importance of detecting suicide ideation in nonacute and acute care settings. Health care settings in the United States have thus been challenged to find a short, user-friendly, psychometrically valid and reliable (and free) suicide screening tool that has both high sensitivity and specificity for predicting a suicide. But to the dismay of many in the field, such a tool does *not* exist. What does exist, however, are a number of screening tools with limited predictive validity that are mostly proprietary (and not widely used). Nevertheless interest in enhancing systematic screening for suicide risk across health care settings and useful guidelines for developing and using screening tools is evolving (Boudreaux & Horowitz, 2014). While existing screeners have their limits, they nevertheless have the virtue of actually asking about potential suicide risk in a routine and systematic manner, which consequently can open the door for further in-depth suicide risk assessment and potential life-saving treatment. What follows is only a brief review of some of the existing screening tools that may be effective for identifying risk and triggering the potential use of CAMS.

Symptom Checklist–90/Brief Symptom Inventory

The measure first used in our SSF-based research at the CUA Counseling Center (Jobes et al., 1997) was the Symptom Checklist–90 (SCL-90). The original SCL-90 was a public domain assessment tool that was first developed by Derogatis and colleagues (Derogatis, Lipman, Rickels, Uhlenhuth, & Covi, 1974; Derogatis,

Rickels, & Rock, 1976). The original scale provided a Global Severity Index of general symptom distress and various clinical subscales. Although the 90-item format was long and some patients complained about the overall length of the assessment, it was valuable tool for our pre–post treatment studies. Since the time of our initial research, Derogotis has improved the assessment tool by significantly decreasing the number of items to 53 and improving the structure and psychometrics of the clinical subscales (Derogotis & Savitz, 1999). The measure is now called the Brief Symptom Inventory (BSI) (Tarescavage & Ben-Porath, 2014).

Behavioral Health Measure

The Johns Hopkins University Counseling Center has used the Behavioral Health Measure (BHM) with great clinical and research success. The BHM, developed by Kopta and Lowry (2002), is a 20-item self-report measure of general symptom distress. The BHM has been shown to have good to excellent construct validity, concurrent validity, and test–retest reliability (ranging from .71 to .83; Kopta & Lowry, 2002). A clear merit of the BHM is that it is mercifully short and can be easily administered at every clinical contact. With multiple data points for any given course of treatment, the clinician can closely track the course of care in terms of both process and outcomes. From a research perspective, the routine and repeated use of the BHM at Johns Hopkins has enabled us to perform much more sophisticated linear analyses (e.g., hierarchical linear analyses; HLM) to understand treatment process and outcomes (Jobes, Kahn-Greene, et al., 2009; Kopta et al., 2014). The BHM has a specific question about suicidal thoughts that can be used as a trigger for using CAMS in treatment settings. It is important to note that there are limits to using a shorter assessment tool such as the BHM. For example, the BHM does not capture more severe psychopathology as comprehensively as longer measures. Although not particularly problematic in a higher-functioning university population, it may not be as suitable in other settings, where there is a broader range of psychopathology (Bryan et al., 2014; Bryan, Corso, Rudd, & Cordero, 2008; Kopta et al., 2014).

Outcome Questionnaire–45.2

Another symptom-based tool that is short enough to be administered at every clinical contact is the Outcome Questionnaire–45 developed by Lambert, Hansen, and colleagues (1996). The OQ-45.2 is a 45-item self-report measure that again provides an overall measure of symptom distress as well as three subscales that address (1) subjective discomfort, (2) interpersonal relationships, and (3) social role functioning. The OQ-45 has good internal consistency ($r = .93$; Lambert, Hansen, et al., 1996) and test–retest reliability—at 3 weeks, the test–retest value is $r = .84$ (Lambert, Burlingame, et al., 1996). Lambert and colleagues further report that the OQ has good concurrent validity and sensitivity to treatment change in the course of care. Patients become quite familiar with the measure, especially with repeated administrations, and the OQ can be completed in only 5 minutes or less. In addition, there is also an online version of the OQ, which provides a useful alternative way of administrating the measure. I prefer the OQ for its range to handle the spectrum of psychopathology. The OQ item 8, "I have thoughts of ending my life," has been used with success as a trigger item for CAMS and as a proxy index for suicidal ideation in our Air Force research (Jobes et al., 2005).

AsQ'em

In direct response to an earlier Joint Commission directive, Horowitz and colleagues (2013) have developed a two-question suicide screener called Ask Suicide-Screening Questions to Everyone in Medical Settings (AsQ'em). These authors assert the importance of asking questions that are related to the most critical risk factors for completed suicide, namely present thoughts and past behavior. The AsQ'em questions include: (1) "In the past month, have you had thoughts about suicide?" and (2) "Have you ever made a suicide attempt?" If a patient answers "yes" to either question, a follow-up question is asked: "Are you having thoughts of suicide right now?" This screening approach is based on previous work by members of the National Institute of Health research team, using similar brief suicide screener questions with pediatric and teenage samples (e.g., Ballard et al., 2013; Horowitz, Bridge, Pao, & Boudreaux, 2014). A feasibility study of the AsQ'em screening with 331 adult inpatients showed the following: the screening took approximately 2 minutes; 87% of the patients reported feeling comfortable with the screening; and 75% of nurses and 100% of social workers agreed that all hospitalized patients could benefit from such a simple and direct screening approach.

Patient Health Questionnaire

Simon and colleagues (2013) performed an important study related to the widespread use of the Patient Health Questionnaire (PHQ-9) that is widely used for depression screening. Its pervasive use may in part be due to the PHQ-9 being nonproprietary and readily available on the Internet. Extracting PHQ-9 responses from electronic medical records in a large integrated health care system, these researchers studied whether the PHQ-9 could be used to examine subsequent suicide attempts and deaths. Using a sample of 84,418 outpatient responses to item 9 of the PHQ ("thoughts that you would be better off dead or of hurting yourself in some way") was significantly associated with increased risk of suicide attempts and suicide deaths. While some criticize the compound nature of question 9 (talking about death and self-harm), the data are nonetheless impressive and the PHQ-9 has the great virtue of being free and easily available.

It is beyond the scope of the present chapter to fully explore the dozens of suicide-specific assessment tools that are available for clinical use. Again, while these tools tend not to be widely used (Jobes et al., 1995), there are many (particularly those coming out of Aaron Beck's lab at the University of Pennsylvania) that are well constructed with excellent psychometrics. Two of my favorites are the Scale for Suicide Ideation (Beck & Steer, 1991) and the Beck Hopelessness Scale (Beck & Steer, 1993). I also like Marsha Linehan's Reasons for Living Inventory (Linehan, Goodstein, Nielsen, & Chiles, 1983). Kelly Posner's Columbia Scale for Suicide Severity Rating Scale has a sophisticated online option for completing repeat assessment and is receiving a great deal of attention in clinical practice (Posner et al., 2011). As previously noted, there are simply too many suicide-specific assessment tools to fully discuss (refer to Brown, 2001, for a review of adult scales and Goldston, 2003, for youth-oriented scales). But rigorous research is now under way investigating the predictive validity of some of the most promising scales within the U.S. military that should provide useful data about the utility of some of the leading scales and assessment approaches (Joiner, 2015).

STEP 3: USE CLINICAL CONSULTATION

Routine use of clinical consultation is both an ethical expectation and a professional practice requirement. Particularly in relation to complex cases of clinical decision making, the professional input of a second party is extremely valuable. Routine professional consultations can be relatively brief and somewhat informal with a peer-colleague. For a particularly complex case, seeking an in-depth consultation with an expert in the field is recommended practice and may help decrease the risk of malpractice liability. When you do seek consultation, be sure to note your consultations within the medical record, particularly in relation to your formulation of suicidal risk and your suicide-specific treatment planning.

STEP 4: USE SUICIDE-SPECIFIC DOCUMENTATION

The importance of maintaining suicide-specific documentation in your medical record progress notes cannot be overstated and is discussed in much more depth in Chapter 8. Maintaining contemporaneous, thorough, and suicide-specific documentation is critical to both good clinical practice and is the single most important means for decreasing the prospect of malpractice litigation for "wrongful death" following a patient suicide (Simpson & Stacy, 2004). It follows that your policies and procedure statement should further emphasize the value of contemporaneous clinical documentation of suicide risk assessments and related treatments.

OPTIMIZING THE USE OF CAMS

The preceding discussion of systems of clinical care and the four-step approach to enhancing clinical practices with suicidal patients has now set the stage for the optimal use of CAMS with those patients. As we shift our attention to CAMS-specific care, it is important to underscore some key ideas that designed to make CAMS-guided care unique and compelling to both the mental health provider *and* the suicidal patient.

Countertransference and Suicide

One of the best-known papers in the field of suicidology was written by two groundbreaking psychoanalysts: John Maltsberger and Daniel Buie. Their 1974 *Archives of General Psychiatry* classic paper titled "Countertransference Hate in the Treatment of Suicidal Patients" starkly laid out the case that clinicians typically harbor a unique set of negative feelings toward suicidal patients. It is important to note the word *hate* in the paper's title. Hate—certainly stronger than "dislike" or "unpleasant feelings toward"—was used on purpose to emphasize the intensity of feelings that clinicians may have toward their suicidal patients. Moreover, these authors describe a matrix of countertransferential reactions and behaviors that can lead to deep feelings of *malice* and *aversion* in the clinician. In this important early paper, Maltsberger and Buie spoke clearly and directly to the strong negative feelings that clinicians may have that can undermine their ability to treat suicidal patients effectively.

For many years this theoretical paper was quoted and referenced as virtual clinical fact—the paper is well written and intuitively compelling, but the ideas and the theory itself had never been empirically validated. In an effort to investigate this theory, three of my students at CUA have endeavored to test the central components of Maltsberger and Buie's countertransference theory in their doctoral dissertations. In the end, we found that empirically investigating the theoretical constructs of this psychoanalytic approach was challenging. The more we tried to quantify and empirically investigate the constructs of the theory, the more the constructs tended to lose the richness and utility of their clinical meaning. We nevertheless persevered in our attempts to study countertransference reactions that were unique to suicidal patients through both analogue and survey studies (Crumlish, 1996; Jacoby, 2003). However, neither of these studies was able to demonstrate that clinicians do in fact feel differently toward suicidal patients in comparison to other (nonsuicidal) difficult patients.

Nevertheless, one unpublished dissertation study did find interesting differences in how clinicians actually *talked* about their suicidal patients (Judd, Jobes, Arnkoff, & Fenton, 1999). In this study, we had undergraduate blind raters evaluate

80 verbatim transcripts of clinicians presenting cases of patients within a weekly case conference (conducted during the 1940s and 1950s) at the Chestnut Lodge Hospital in Maryland. We had our blind undergraduate coders evaluate hard copies of initial case presentations by the clinician typed verbatim by court reporters (i.e., when they first talked about their patient to their colleagues within this professional forum). Critically, half of the sample of 40 patients were suicidal and eventually died by suicide, whereas the other half (matched for gender, diagnosis, and age) were neither suicidal nor died by suicide. While the effects were modest, there were statistically significant differences in the ways that clinicians talked negatively (e.g., more critical descriptors and negative comments) about their suicidal patients within the case conference setting, providing at least some support for Maltsberger and Buie's theory.

Beyond theory and research, many clinicians in practice can readily acknowledge having strong negative feelings about working with a range of difficult patients, particularly those who are suicidal. Through my extensive workshop training experiences, I am often struck by the intensity of clinicians' feelings about these patients. As discussed in Chapter 1, the clinical concerns with suicidal patients are fairly obvious and can be formidable—for example, suicidal states are difficult to assess and treat; our hands can be tied by health care insurance limitations; and plaintiffs' attorneys are at the ready to litigate for wrongful death when we fail to prevent suicides. All these considerations contribute to an understandable wariness that many clinicians harbor toward these patients. But given that suicidal presentations are common and the implications are so profound, we must find alternative ways of handling these adverse feelings and negative reactions to these patients so we can provide effective interventions.

Another challenge we face in contemporary care is that many of us were originally trained to immediately hospitalize any patient who mentions suicide. In the face of health insurers increasingly restricting precertifications for admission and lengths of inpatient hospital stays plummeting, I have argued that we must endeavor to find ways to form a deeper *outpatient* clinical engagement and a meaningful interpersonal connection with the suicidal patient (Jobes, 2000; Jobes & Bowers, 2015). As noted, being empathic of suicidal states is extremely difficult, yet if we hope to succeed with any suicidal patient, we must first find a way to be empathic. When we manage to be empathic of suicidal desires, we can potentially open the door to connecting and to collaborating *without* necessarily endorsing suicide as a means of coping with pain and suffering. As I have discussed elsewhere in depth (Jobes & Maltsberger, 1995), the key is to be engaged with the suicidal patient as a "therapist-participant"—one who leads with empathic fortitude. In contrast we should endeavor to not be a "therapist-voyeur," someone who avoids full engagement because of empathic dread.

The continued need to shift our attitudes and approach to suicidal patients (and the related consideration of the limits of contemporary inpatient psychiatric hospitalization) cannot be overemphasized. As noted in Chapter 1, I have gone through a shift in attitude and approach as my own career has evolved, particularly because most of my early training occurred within psychiatric inpatient settings. However, as my professional clinical training progressed as an outpatient psycho-therapist, I became increasingly aware of some strong fears and anxieties—my own countertransferential feelings—toward my suicidal patients (e.g., Jobes, 2011). As I came to understand these complex feelings more fully, I also realized that much of my anxiety was rooted in not being able to ultimately control the poten-tially life-threatening behaviors of my patients and the implications of a patient actually ending his or her life under my care. Of course, such fears and anxieties are not unique to me. Again from my workshop training perspective, clinicians routinely describe similar fears and related concerns. Like many of my colleagues, I had a deep dread that even if I performed an excellent clinical assessment of sui-cide risk and provided outstanding treatment, the patient may *still* die by suicide.

But over the years my perspective has evolved. As I have learned more about suicidal states from my patients, and more about effective clinical assessments and possibilities for treatment, I have come to see things differently. Through years of clinical practice and research I have come to better understand the nature of the sui-cidal mind, which has enabled me to provide better clinical practice with suicidal people. With this knowledge, a certain confidence has taken hold—that with the proper therapeutic attitude and the right clinical tools, we can markedly improve the odds of averting suicide outcomes. The majority of my suicidal patients have not been hopeless cases that I felt compelled to shun or avoid. Rather, most suicidal people whom I have seen have significantly lost track of what makes their lives viable—they feel trapped and that there is no other way to cope. Yet with a proper clinical response, *most* of these patients can respond quite well to suicide-specific care in a matter of weeks (Lento, Ellis, Hinnant, & Jobes, 2013). This gradual shift in perception and attitude led me from a place of fear and worry to a place of rela-tive confidence that was fundamentally built on an acquired clinical competence. Variations of this shift in attitude and approach and this kind of mindset toward suicidal patients has been discussed elsewhere in the clinical and research litera-ture by other like-minded clinical suicidologists—refer to the work of colleagues such as Linehan and colleagues (2015), Brown and Beck (Brown, Have, et al., 2005), Bryan and Rudd (2006, 2010), Ellis (2004), Shea (1999), Michel (Gysin-Maillart et al., 2016; Michel & Gysin-Maillart, 2015; Michel, Valach, & Waeber, 1994), Leen-aars (2004), and the previously mentioned work of Orbach (2001) and Maltsberger (1994). This collective attitude adjustment toward working with suicidal patients is a signature feature of the Aeschi approach (Michel & Jobes, 2010), and you do not have to be an expert suicidologist to embrace this clinical outlook.

What I have come to appreciate most in my three decades in the field is the fact that while I cannot guarantee a nonfatal outcome, I can nevertheless provide *the best possible clinical care* to the suicidal patient. Care based on clinical wisdom and rigorous scientific support is the most that we can ever really aspire to offer suffering patients and their families. In this realization, there is a kind of liberation: We do not need to be paralyzed in the face of suicide risk; we can be confident and competent in doing effective suicide-specific care.

The Traditional "Directive" Approach

With some trepidation, I publically critiqued what I called a "traditional" clinical approach to suicide risk during my presidential address at the 1999 American Association of Suicidology Annual Conference (Jobes, 2000). In that address I criticized clinical approaches to suicidal risk that were highly directive (especially anything coercive). I challenged the overreliance on inpatient psychiatric hospitalization, the singular reliance on medication, and the routine use of "no-suicide" or "no-harm" contracts. Based on the research at that time, I further eschewed a clinical approach to suicide that focuses primarily on treating mental disorders, relegating suicide risk to symptom status. The key points of this critique are depicted in Figure 3.1. The response to this critical analysis of the clinical status quo in 1999 was mostly positive. In the years since, a number of issues that I raised then about clinical suicidology have undoubtedly changed for the better, but other things have not changed all that much.

As previously noted, health care reform and the sheer expense of suicide-related care continues to shape mental health practice (Jobes & Bowers, 2015). Shorter inpatient hospital stays have increasingly made this option less effective. One positive development over the last decade has come from RCTs showing that certain psychotropic medications can positively treat suicidal risk (Gibbons, Brown, Hur, Davis, & Mann, 2012; Mann et al., 2005; Meltzer et al., 2003; Tondo, Hennen, & Baldessarini, 2001; Zisook et al., 2011). However, there are contradictory clinical trial data that fail to show that medications can reliably and effectively treat suicidal ideation and behaviors (Fergusson et al., 2005; Gunnell, Saperia, & Ashby, 2005). Obviously, more research is needed to further clarify these conflicting findings.

On another front, the inherent problems of "no-harm" contracting and "commitment to safety" approaches to suicide are increasingly being recognized in the field. The shift in thinking about dealing with suicidal risk is due in part to the work of Barbara Stanley and Greg Brown (2012), who developed "safety planning" as an alternative clinical intervention to "no-suicide" contracting. The collective wisdom of experts in the field is that "contracting for safety" is not clinically effective (Bryan & Rudd, 2006) and may actually *increase* malpractice liability risk following a suicide (Jobes et al., 2008). Consequently, safety planning and related interventions like "crisis response planning" (Rudd et al., 2001), or "stabilization planning" (Jobes et al., 2016) are increasingly taking center stage within the larger field of mental health. Nevertheless, on occasion I still do encounter ardent defenders of

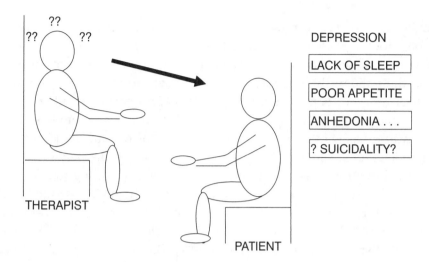

FIGURE 3.1. The reductionistic approach to suicidal risk. According to the reductionist model, suicide = a symptom of psychopathology. Traditional treatment = inpatient hospitalization, treating the psychiatric disorder, and no-suicide contracts.

no-harm contracting despite the noted shifts in expert thinking. In terms of treatment for suicide risk, the data from randomized controlled trials make it abundantly clear that the most effective clinical treatments for suicidal patients are psychosocial interventions that specifically focus on the treating *suicide,* independent of a mental disorder diagnosis (Brown, Have, et al., 2005; Comtois et al., 2011; Jobes, 2012; Gysin-Maillart et al, 2016; Michel & Gysin-Maillart, 2015; Rudd et al., 2015).

As a final consideration of my original critique, I was quite focused on the relational dynamic that is often seen in the traditional directive approach between clinician and patient. What troubled me about this dynamic was that the clinician

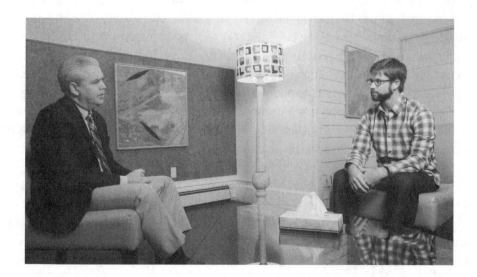

functions as the active expert in a figurative "one-up" position, whereas the patient is in a "one-down" passive position as the naïve recipient of the clinician's treatment. Within this relational dynamic, it is up to the clinician to know and do what is best *for* the patient; the patient's role is relegated to confirming symptoms of mental disorders and then receiving care for a diagnosed mental illness.

Interestingly, my lab has conducted research on the phenomenology of suicidal states that has shown how much symptoms of mental disorders are *not* a particular focus for suicidal patients. We conducted a qualitatively oriented study of 152 suicidal treatment seekers and found four reliable coding themes captured 67% of 636 SSF-based content responses related to their suicidal struggle (Jobes et al., 2004). These themes showed that suicidal patients struggled most with relationship issues (22%), vocational issues (20%), issues of the self (15%), and then symptoms of distress and mental illness (10%). But while only 10% of patients' suicidal responses were related symptoms of mental disorders, the literature on clinical suicide prevention is overwhelmingly focused on mental disorders and psychopathology. Was Sigmund Freud (1961) perhaps right many years ago when he observed that happiness in life tends to focus on the human compulsion to *work* and the power of *love*? In our study, patients confirmed such issues were indeed at the heart of their suicidal struggles.

The CAMS Collaborative Approach

As illustrated in Figure 3.2, CAMS takes a completely different approach to a clinical encounter with a suicidal patient. Within CAMS-guided clinical care, *suicidality* is the bull's-eye of our shared clinical interest; we aim to focus on what it means for patients to be suicidal *through their eyes*. In other words, a CAMS clinician must be singularly preoccupied with the patients' suicidal phenomenology; their intrasubjective understanding of the role that suicide plays in their struggle should be most important to us. I have never talked to a suicidal person who did not have legitimate needs behind his or her suicidal words, thoughts, and behaviors. For example, the need to end seemingly impossible suffering, to silence the voices of psychosis, to make others know how distressed they are, to escape an unbearable feeling of being utterly trapped—all of these are understandable and require meaningful remedies to prevent a potential suicide. Thus the most important clinical question to address is whether suicide is the only solution. To a seriously suicidal person, it often seems so. From our clinical perspective and personal biases we see many alternatives short of a fatal act.

While we do not ignore psychiatric illness, a CAMS provider nonetheless is primarily focused on the patient-defined suicidal drivers—why they want to take their life. Rather than assuming we know the causes of the patient's suicidal thinking and behaviors (e.g., a mood disorder), we endeavor to deconstruct the patient's suicidality through the collaborative use of the SSF. The side-by-side seating

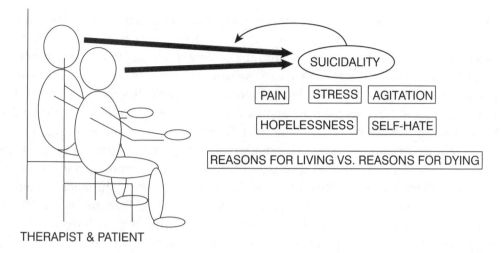

THERAPIST & PATIENT

FIGURE 3.2. The CAMS approach to suicidal risk. CAMS identifies and targets *suicide* as the primary focus of assessment and intervention. CAMS assessment uses the SSF as a means of deconstructing the "functional" utility of suicidality. CAMS as an intervention emphasizes a problem-focused intensive outpatient approach that is suicide-specific and a treatment plan that is "coauthored" with the patient.

arrangement that we use in CAMS is significant on many levels. Perhaps most important, it literally moves us from a face-to-face seating position, which can be a figuratively adversarial position, to a side-by-side collaborative seating arrangement. Working on various assessment and treatment planning sections of the SSF together in this fashion communicates both a shared understanding of the suicidal risk and a treatment planning effort that is defined by *both* members of the clinical dyad. CAMS thus guides a collaborative assessment *deconstruction* of the suicidal

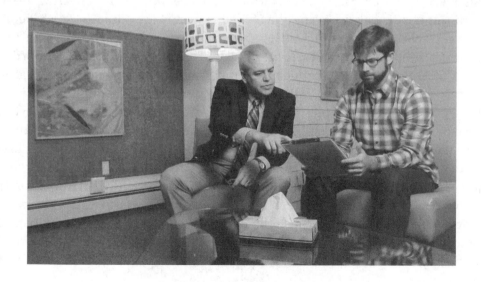

risk that then provides direction for a suicide-specific treatment *reconstruction* of alternative ways of coping that also entails the treatment of patient-defined suicidal drivers. By literally taking a seat next to the patient, the clinician communicates a completely different clinical message to the suicidal patient: "The answers to your struggle exist within you—we will find those answers together as treatment partners, helping you learn to cope differently and endeavoring to help you find a life that you actually want to live, one that is defined by purpose and meaning."

By taking this clinical attitude and approach, the issue of suicidality is *objectified*—it is now an issue that is mutually examined and therapeutically pursued together with the patient. In this sense, rather than approaching the suicidal patient warily—as a potential threat or clinical adversary—CAMS actually facilitates building a therapeutic alliance by focusing on the issue of suicidal risk. Rather than being in a power struggle over whether the patient can take his or her life, CAMS averts the struggle with an alternative proposition: "Let us see if together we can find a viable alternative to suicide to better deal with your pain and suffering." In this manner, the CAMS clinician seeks to form a meaningful therapeutic relationship that ultimately can inspire the most essential ingredient for clinical success—the *patient's* motivation to fight for his or her own life. When you think about it, part of the goal is to help train patients to become "junior suicidologists" who become aware of how suicide functions in their lives so that they may liberate themselves from its seductive grip.

PREPARATIONS FOR USING CAMS

To successfully launch CAMS-guided care, the clinician must be prepared to move seamlessly from the early identification of current suicidal thoughts (via screening or an interview-based query), to the introduction of a more thorough CAMS-based assessment of suicidal risk using the SSF. This means the clinician must literally have a copy of the SSF readily available before any clinical session begins. In addition, the side-by-side seating arrangement that is used during certain portions of CAMS assessment and treatment planning must be anticipated such that the physical arrangement of seating does not prohibit taking a side-by-side or adjacent seating position. In my own office, I do not use the love seat (too close); instead, I move the ottoman to an adjacent position to create the desired CAMS dynamic.

In the course of using CAMS over the years, and based on patient feedback, we have come to see that the mere act of moving from the clinician's chair to an adjacent seat is meaningful to the patient and can have a significant impact on the clinical relationship. For example, in our Air Force work we saw that this seating arrangement was effective because the clinician was an officer and the patients were usually enlisted—a literal authority dynamic based on rank was suddenly modified by the shared sense that the patient and the provider were now on the same team. Such kinesthetic aspects are not trivial; consider the classic Freudian psychoanalytic placement of the analyst sitting *behind* the analysand, who lies on the proverbial couch. Taking a seat next to a patient is never to be done lightly; the request to do so must be sincere, with exquisite sensitivity to personal space, perceived status, trauma history, gender, and cultural dynamics.

SUMMARY AND CONCLUSIONS

In this chapter we have considered systems of care in relation to suicidal risk and how to optimize the use of CAMS-guided care. As discussed early on, one can significantly enhance clinical care for suicidal risk through the development of suicide-specific policies and procedures, the early and reliable identification of potential suicidal risk, the routine use of clinical consultation, and the appropriate use of suicide-specific documentation related to risk assessment and treatment planning. Optimizing the use of CAMS can further be achieved through understanding countertransference issues related to suicidal risk and embracing a collaborative (nondirective) approach to suicidal risk (along with proper preparations for administering the approach). Through enhancing systems of care one can optimize the effective use of CAMS, which invariably means that we will be able to successfully engage a suicidal person through a respectful and empathic attitude in our efforts to understand the how, when, where, and why of suicide within the patient's phenomenology. When we collaboratively understand the true nature of the patient's suicidal struggle, the stage is set for the identification of patient-defined drivers that CAMS-guided care will systematically target and treat in an effort to render suicide—the most dire and extreme of all "coping" options—obsolete over time. But beyond better coping, effective CAMS-guided care also pursues a life with purpose and meaning. When these key elements of CAMS-informed clinical care truly come together, lives can be meaningfully altered and sometimes literally saved from the abyss of suicidal despair.

CHAPTER 4

CAMS Risk Assessment

The Collaborative Use of the SSF

In many ways, this chapter is one of the most important in this book because when the assessment of suicide risk is properly performed, it can be remarkably alliance forming, motivation enhancing, and extraordinarily therapeutic. In this chapter, I discuss both conceptual aspects and concrete procedural steps pertaining to CAMS-based suicide risk assessment. Because *how* this assessment is performed is so important, I provide scripted examples of what one might say at each point in the assessment process. These are merely examples; I do not intend for you to use these scripted examples verbatim. But each example provides insight into the important spirit of the CAMS collaborative assessment approach and perhaps may guide and empower you to say similar things in your words and style.

STEP-BY-STEP INSTRUCTIONS FOR CAMS RISK ASSESSMENT

As noted in Chapter 3, it is important to identify suicidal risk early in the clinical hour, particularly when engaging a new patient. Clinical experience and our research have shown that the initial CAMS assessment and treatment planning phase in the index session takes at least 30 to 40 minutes, but typically a full 50 minutes is used (Archuleta et al., 2014; Comtois et al., 2011). For clinicians who are new to CAMS, the overall pacing of the intervention is one of the biggest challenges early on. People who observe me demonstrating a CAMS assessment remark that I move the assessment along rapidly, even though it does not seem rushed or impatient. The proper pacing of CAMS assessment comes with experience and crafting of technique. I tend to be fairly interactive with the patient and routinely say things like, "Okay, that sounds really important, let's bookmark that and get back to it later." Generally speaking, the pacing goals for the index session of CAMS (Session 1) are as follows: Section A assessment = 20 minutes, Section B assessment = 10 minutes; Section C (including the CAMS Stabilization Plan) treatment planning = 20 minutes. Granted, this is a lot pack into a 50- to 60-minute session, but with practice this becomes quite manageable over time with experience.

This consideration of pacing clearly underscores the importance of addressing the topic of suicide within the first *5 to 10 minutes* of a session (whether one uses a symptom-based screening tool or not). Many clinicians react negatively to "forcing" a focus on suicidal risk so early in a clinical contact, particularly if it is a first encounter with a new patient. Skeptical clinicians may feel that such a direct approach about such a sensitive issue could be off-putting and a distraction to what the patient is prepared to talk about. However, if the topic is broached in a matter-of-fact and empathic manner, most patients for whom it is not relevant will merely dismiss the issue, while others will pause and often seem eager to address this concern. Given the life-or-death implications of suicide, addressing it early on in a forthright manner is an "everything to gain and nothing to lose" proposition. In my experience, putting off the topic with someone who is genuinely suicidal invariably complicates an inherently tricky clinical issue. More than once clinicians at training workshops have said, "I can't imagine doing CAMS with a patient in the first session, before I have formed a clinical alliance." My response is that the opposite is true; we routinely see remarkably strong alliances quickly forged in the crucible of the suicidal crisis by using the SSF to engage the suicidal patient. Both clinical practice and research show that the use of CAMS can actually jump-start the formation of a strong and trusting therapeutic clinical alliance. Moreover, suicidal patients actually *like* being engaged in this manner when compared to usual clinical practices (Comtois et al., 2011). From meta-analysis research we know that CAMS-based assessments function as a *therapeutic assessment,* with its emphasis on a highly personalized, collaborative experience that involves extensive real-time feedback (Poston & Hanson, 2010).

By emphasizing a collaborative clinical effort between the clinician and patient CAMS is fundamentally designed to be alliance enhancing. CAMS facilitates a structured assessment process to delve deeply and empathically into a patient's psychological *pain and suffering,* which is our front-end emphasis. While current suicidal ideation triggers the CAMS administration of the SSF, our initial assessment focus tends to primarily focus on psychological pain and suffering rather than on suicide per se. Questions that are more specific to suicide actually come up later in the assessment process (Section B). No doubt, the topic of suicide can be sensitive for some patients, but the rapid transition into a deep and meaningful discussion of pain and suffering is usually well received, and can actually be quite reassuring and comforting. But *how* the clinician introduces the SSF is crucial for success.

Addressing the Topic of Suicide Risk

A typical question a clinician may ask to start the session could be "What brings you in to see me today?" The patient will then characteristically present initial complaints, concerns, and symptom-related problems. As noted in Chapter 3, it is extremely helpful to have a screening tool or assessment that can tip off the clinician to suicidal risk at the start of the session. Even with a screening tip-off to suicide risk, we still encourage you to allow patients up to 5 minutes to initially describe what they are going through, and then you can transition to the topic of suicide risk in the following manner:

> "It sounds like there is a lot going on for you right now, and I am glad that you came in for help. It seems like you are overwhelmed and that you are in a great deal of pain. It also appears that it is so difficult for you right now that you have actually had thoughts of suicide, based on the assessment form you completed in the waiting room. Because I understand such thoughts as a serious indicator of how bad things are for you, I would like to conduct a deeper and more thorough assessment of your psychological pain and emotional suffering. To that end, I have an assessment tool here that I would like for us to complete together that I think we will find to be helpful. Would it be okay if I move my chair next to you, so that we can work through this assessment together?"

For clinicians who do not use a screener, it especially incumbent that that the provider listens closely for key words of despair, desperation, a desire to escape, or hopelessness. When you pick up a potential latent suicidal "vibe," it is important to broach the topic directly early on. Here is what I might say:

> "Gosh, your situation sounds really overwhelming and emotionally painful— I'm glad you came in for help! But I wonder how bad it gets for you at times? How do you cope? You know it is not uncommon for some people going through what you are going through to consider suicide. Given what you are describing, have such thoughts come up at all for you? If so, there is an assessment process that we can go through together that really helps me understand your situation in much better depth. May I take a seat next to you so that we can work through this assessment together?"

I want to highlight a few key features of each of these passages. First, I want to reassure the patient that it was a good idea to seek help—we must be hopevendors to our patients, affirming them in their decision to seek care. Second, I make it clear that I recognize the patient's sense of being utterly overwhelmed and that I understand that the patient is suffering emotionally. He or she needs to hear that I understand the magnitude of the situation. Third, my direct query about suicide is meant to be interpreted as a proxy of how difficult and painful the patient's situation has become; suicidal thoughts are understandable given the magnitude of their pain. Fourth, I purposely shift our clinical focus by emphasizing the need for a deeper assessment of the patient's *pain and suffering* that will be completed *together,* which will be helpful to us in our efforts to address the patient's presenting concerns. Fifth, I respectfully ask to take a seat adjacent to the patient to complete the SSF. The patient should know that I assume nothing; the patient's willingness to proceed is a paramount concern of mine.

Filling Out Section A of the SSF

At this juncture, it makes sense to return to our case study of "Bill" from Chapter 1. With some trepidation, Bill agreed to my proposal to complete a more thorough assessment, which included my moving the ottoman adjacent to him and presenting him the SSF on a clipboard. As he took the clipboard I said:

> "Okay, Bill, this is an assessment tool called the Suicide Status Form. By completing each part of the tool we're going to get a better understanding of your emotional pain and suffering that may be linked to your feeling suicidal. I'll be helping you complete this first part of the assessment, and I can answer any questions along the way to help clarify some of your responses. Completing this assessment will really help me understand what it's like to be you right now."

The SSF Core Assessment

To begin the assessment process, the *patient* takes pen in hand and proceeds to complete all the rating scales and qualitative responses that make up Section A of the first-session SSF. While there are some exceptions, I actually feel quite strongly that the patient should complete the first page of the SSF—*not the clinician*—because it communicates a completely different and important assessment dynamic. Patients know best about their suicidal pain and suffering; our assessment job is to faithfully follow and support their efforts to respond.

The patient thus begins to rate the initial scales that make up the SSF Core Assessment (i.e., Pain, Stress, Agitation, Hopelessness, Self-Hate, and Overall Risk). After each rating scale, the patient is encouraged to write out his or her qualitative responses to each incomplete sentence prompt. Throughout completion of the SSF Section A assessment, the clinician serves as consultant, coach, and collaborator—clarifying any questions the patient may have and assisting in the patient's efforts to complete the form. It is fine for the patient to leave some of the write-in responses blank (nonresponses can actually yield useful data). The clinician should encourage the patient and help the patient to not get bogged down on any particular item; it is important to move along through the "data collection" (i.e., not tracking off unduly on any one response). After the SSF Core Assessment is completed, the clinician then directs the patient to subjectively rank order the SSF Core Assessment constructs from most (1) to least (5) important.

As shown in Figure 4.1, Bill completed the SSF Core Assessment with no trouble. We see that he is in a great deal of suicidal pain pertaining to life and his marriage. In terms of Shneidman's cubic model of suicide, we see ratings of 5 on Psychological Pain, 4 on Stress, and 3 on Agitation—a 5–4–3 rating. Although not as worrisome as a 5–5–5 rating (i.e., a possible operational definition of clear and imminent danger), we still see a worrisome level of risk. Thankfully, his Agitation rating is somewhat lower, which in my mind is encouraging because agitation is such a lethal psychological force in completed suicides. But Bill's ratings of 5 on Hopelessness and 5 on Self-Hate definitely gets my attention because our research has shown that these two particular variables can significantly moderate the Overall Risk of Suicide rating, which he rates at 3 (Jobes, Kahn-Greene, et al., 2009). As he rank-orders the importance of SSF Core variables (from 1 to 5), his #1 and #2 rankings of Hopelessness and Self-Hate, respectively, are also a cause for concern. Clearly his sense of hopelessness about feeling "trapped" and calling himself "a

Rank

3	1) RATE PSYCHOLOGICAL PAIN (*hurt, anguish, or misery in your mind, **not** stress, **not** physical pain*): **Low pain:** **1 2 3 4 (5)** :**High pain** What I find most painful is: *my life, my marriage*
4	2) RATE STRESS (*your general feeling of being pressured or overwhelmed*): **Low stress:** **1 2 3 (4) 5** :**High stress** What I find most stressful is: *everything*
5	3) RATE AGITATION (*emotional urgency; feeling that you need to take action; **not** irritation; **not** annoyance*): **Low agitation:** **1 2 (3) 4 5** :**High agitation** I most need to take action when: *I fight with my wife*
1	4) RATE HOPELESSNESS (*your expectation that things will not get better no matter what you do*): **Low hopelessness:** **1 2 3 4 (5)** :**High hopelessness** I am most hopeless about: *feeling trapped*
2	5) RATE SELF-HATE (*your general feeling of disliking yourself; having no self-esteem; having no self-respect*): **Low self-hate:** **1 2 3 4 (5)** :**High self-hate** What I hate most about myself is: *I'm a loser*
N/A	6) RATE OVERALL RISK **Extremely low risk:** **1 2 (3) 4 5** :**Extremely high risk** OF SUICIDE: **(will *not* kill self)** **(will kill self)**

FIGURE 4.1. Bill's SSF Core Assessment.

loser" speak to a potentially worrisome combination; he feels hopelessly stuck and is preoccupied with self-loathing.

Self versus Other Orientation to Suicide

The next two questions of Section A of the SSF shift the assessment focus from the SSF Core Assessment to whether the patient's suicidal risk is oriented toward "yourself" or "others" (both or neither). This assessment is relevant to some of my early theoretical work pertaining to *intrapsychic* versus *interpsychic* suicidal states (Jobes, 1995a). An intrapsychic suicidal patient has an internally/self-focused kind of suicidal suffering. In contrast, an interpsychic suicidal patient has a kind of suicidal suffering that is deeply rooted in relational considerations. It is theorized that intrapsychic suicidal patients may be more at risk for *completing* suicide, whereas interpsychic patients may be more at risk for *attempting* suicide. Paradoxically, the theory (and some of our data) suggests that intrapsychic suicidal patients may be less inclined to seek treatment but may be more responsive to care if they do. Conversely, interpsychic suicidal patients may be more likely to seek care but might be more refractory to standard mental health treatments (Jobes, 1995a; Jobes et al., 2005; see also work by Fazaa & Page, 2005). As shown in Figure 4.2, we see that Bill rates both constructs at a 5, which spontaneously prompts a brief discussion about how he "can't take it anymore" and that his family would "be better off without me around." These ratings and this discussion definitely get my attention in that Bill is seeing suicide as a way to both escape from pain and a disturbing "gift" to those who love him (consistent with Joiner's [2005] notion of "perceived burdensomeness"). Moreover, we have research that shows high ratings on both self and other can meaningfully increase the prospect of overall risk (Lento, Ellis, & Jobes, 2013). Specifically, it was found that higher ratings on "self" were associated with higher scores on the Scale for Suicidal Ideation (SSI). However this trend was moderated by the individual's "other" rating in a protective manner. That is, individuals with both high "self" ratings and high "other" ratings scored lower on the SSI than did individuals with a combination of high "self" ratings and low "other" ratings. Other research by O'Connor, Smyth, and Williams (2014) provides further support of these data, as these investigators found that high levels of *intrapersonal* future thinking (i.e., thoughts about the self and no one else) were associated with repeat suicide attempts.

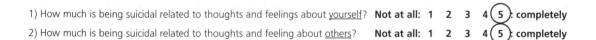

1) How much is being suicidal related to thoughts and feelings about <u>yourself</u>? **Not at all: 1   2   3   4 (5):** completely
2) How much is being suicidal related to thoughts and feeling about <u>others</u>? **Not at all: 1   2   3   4 (5):** completely

FIGURE 4.2. Bill's Self versus Others Ratings.

Reasons for Living versus Reasons for Dying

The next assessment within the CAMS first-session Section A is the RFL versus RFD assessment. This section can be completed in any fashion that suits the patient. For example, some patients begin with RFD and only reluctantly, with the clinician's encouragement, shift their attention to RFL. To complete this section properly, patients should fill in as many spaces as makes sense to them, but they are not required to fill in every space. Following the listing of responses, the patient is then asked to rank-order the items from most to least important (1 to 5 for each side of the assessment—RFL and RFD, respectively). As with all SSF qualitative assessments, it is not crucial for the patient to complete all five RFL/RFD spaces with responses—the relative completeness (or not) is a useful source of information.

For Bill, we see that his only RFL focuses on his family; paradoxically, one of his RFD responses is also focused on his family—such is the nature of the suicidal mind. Similar to his SSF Core Assessment responses, Bill's remaining RFDs are focused on his sense of being trapped, being a loser, and his abject misery. The absence of additional RFLs, particularly in relation to future thinking, is a bit worrisome because we know that *any* expressed future thinking on any part of the SSF may be a protective factor (Jobes, 2004b; Nademin et al., 2005).

Wish to Live versus Wish to Die

Upon completion of the RFL/RFD assessment, the patient is then encouraged to complete the 0–8 ratings pertaining to "wish to live" (WTL) versus "wish to die" (WTD), which is an assessment inspired by the work of Kovacs and Beck (1977) that was mentioned in Chapter 2. When they first introduced their theory of the "internal struggle hypothesis," Kovacs and Beck introduced both a valuable theory about the ambivalent nature of the suicidal mind and an early approach for stratifying suicidal risk. Some years later, Beck and colleagues were able to show that simple self-report ratings of wish to live versus wish to die of a large sample of suicidal patients seen over many years were associated with significant odds ratios

Rank	REASONS FOR LIVING	Rank	REASONS FOR DYING
1	wife	3	wife and kids
2	kids	1	trapped/escape
		2	loser
		4	miserable

FIGURE 4.3. Bill's Reasons for Living versus Reasons for Dying.

I wish to live to the following extent:	Not at all:	0	1	②	3	4	5	6	7	8	: Very much
I wish to die to the following extent:	Not at all:	0	1	2	3	4	5	⑥	7	8	: Very much

The one thing that would help me no longer feel suicidal would be: _to be free—not trapped_

FIGURE 4.4. Bill's Wish to Live versus With to Die and SSF One-Thing Response.

for actual suicidal *behaviors* (Brown, Steer, et al., 2005). In other words, patients' ratings their WTL and their WTD can be used to create an interval scale (called the Suicide Index Score—SIS) that is calculated by merely subtracting a patient's WTD score from their WTL score. In the Brown, Steer, and colleagues (2005) study, the high WTD patients were significantly more likely to engage in suicidal attempt and completion behaviors.

Our team at the CUA Suicide Prevention laboratory has employed this SIS methodology across a range of cross-sectional (Corona et al., 2013; O'Connor, Jobes, Comtois, et al., 2012; O'Connor, Jobes, Yeargin, et al., 2012) and treatment outcome studies (Jennings, 2015; Jennings et al., 2012; Lento, Ellis, Hinnant, & Jobes, 2013). In our lab we examine the 9-point version of WTL versus WTD on the SSF (which is divisible by 3 in accordance with the original approach used by Kovacs and Beck). When WTL and WTD scores are thus converted to 3-point scales, the SIS range can vary from +2 (high WTL) to –2 (high WTD). Similar to the work of Beck's group, we find it useful to "trichotomize" the SIS into three distinct groups: WTL (+2 and +1) versus Ambivalent (where the SIS calculation is 0), vs. WTD (–1 and –2). As shown in Figure 4.4, after converting Bill's 9-point SSF WTL rating of 2 and his 9-point SSF WTD rating of 6 we see that his subsequent SIS score (1–3= –2) places him in the worrisome WTD category of risk—his psychological attachment to suicide is apparently high.

SSF One-Thing Response

The final assessment under Section A of the SSF is the "One-Thing" response, which I sometimes refer to as the "magic wand" assessment. In other words, "If we could somehow magically change just one thing in your life that would eliminate your suicidal risk all together, what would that be?" Patients sometimes respond with unlikely, even fantastic, responses—"bringing my husband back to life" or "if I had a time machine to do everything over," which are not useful for us clinically. Other responses can be quite within our clinical reach—"getting over my guilt of being a bad parent" or "finding a medication that stabilizes my mood." The range and content of one-thing responses can be quite interesting. As with other SSF open-ended responses, patients may respond to this query in any manner they prefer. For example, some patients will give more than one response, while others are utterly stumped. In turn, the CAMS clinician should neither be too directive nor too restrictive in relation to how the patient completes this or any of the SSF qualitative assessments.

Referring back to our case of Bill, we again see in Figure 4.4 yet another cryptic allusion to "to be free—not trapped"—this is now the third mention of a trapped feeling that we have seen across Bill's Section A responses. It is not at all uncommon to see this kind of perseveration of one or two themes reoccurring across the SSF. Importantly, we know from the work of Williams (2001) and O'Connor (2011) that the notion of "entrapment" is a common phenomenological experience that plagues many suicidal people. A recent longitudinal study by these investigators found that entrapment and past frequency of suicide attempts were the only significant predictors of prospective suicidal behaviors in a group of attempt survivors who had filled out the questionnaires 4 years earlier (O'Connor, Smyth, Ferguson, Ryan, & Williams, 2013). Suicide can thus become the mechanism for escape, which is yet another common psychological construct seen in theorizing of suicidal states (Baumeister, 1990) and within our own SSF-based research (Jobes & Mann, 1999, 2000).

Conclusion of Section A

As noted, completion of this first page of the SSF should not be rushed, but neither should the dyad should get bogged down on any one portion of Section A. There is a balance to achieve between pushing too much and getting mired in the details. I do believe that the 15 to 25 minutes spent on completing Section A in the patient's own hand in this collaborative fashion is critical for CAMS success. The process of engaging the patient—coaching, clarifying, and assisting—creates an essential synergy that is the backbone of CAMS. One day when we conduct dismantling studies of the mechanisms of change in CAMS, I believe that the initial collaborative SSF assessment experience will be found to be a fundamental mechanism of therapeutic change. At its best, the initial SSF assessment makes a lasting and important impression: "I am genuinely interested in understanding your pain and suffering by seeing your world as you experience it."

Filling Out Section B of the SSF

After completing Section A, there is an important transition to Section B of the SSF. The clinician remains seated next to the patient and takes the SSF back to complete Section B (the clinician's assessment section). As discussed in Chapter 3, this section contains a listing of key, empirically based risk factors and warning signs for suicide. To make this assessment transition and to further orient the patient to this phase of the SSF assessment process, the clinician may begin this phase by saying something like:

"We have just finished an important part of our assessment, and I feel like I have a much better understanding about the pain and suffering that has led you to feeling suicidal. There is now an additional set of questions that I want to consider together. In combination with the information on the first page, these assess additional suicide-related questions that should help us come up with a workable treatment plan for effectively dealing with your pain and suffering."

It is important to move through the Section B questions with the patient in a matter-of-fact manner. Each question is posed to the patient in a forthright fashion with no hint of judgment or any desired response in the clinician's voice. To complete the Section B assessment, the patient looks on as the clinician completes each item in Section B. Figure 4.5 shows the Section B continuation of Bill's case example.

What follows is a discussion of each of the empirically based assessment items in Section B so that you can become familiar with each question in order to make clarifications and to effectively gather this important and necessary assessment

---

Section B (Clinician):

(Y) N Suicide ideation — Describe: _most nights, before bedtime_
- Frequency — _2–3_ per day _____ per week _____ per month
- Duration — _____ seconds _30_ minutes _2_ hours

(Y) N Suicide plan
When: _evenings, late at night_
Where: _in his study at home_
How: _gunshot to forehead_ Access to means (Y) N
How: _____ Access to means Y N

(Y) N Suicide preparation — Describe: _has drafted suicide notes_

(Y) N Suicide rehearsal — Describe: _has put gun to his head_

Y (N) History of suicidal behaviors
- Single attempt — Describe: _n/a_
- Multiple attempts — Describe: _n/a_

Y (N) Impulsivity — Describe: _"no one would say I'm impulsive"_

(Y) N Substance abuse — Describe: _binge drinking – has been sober before_

Y (N) Significant loss — Describe: _n/a_

(Y) N Relationship problems — Describe: _withdrawing from others/marital problems_

(Y) N Burden to others — Describe: _"they will be better off without me"_

Y (N) Health/pain problems — Describe: _n/a_

(Y) N Sleep problems — Describe: _bouts of insomnia – history of sleep issues_

(Y) N Legal/financial issues — Describe: _no legal – financial stress_

(Y) N Shame — Describe: _loser – "I'm a failure"_

FIGURE 4.5. Bill's responses for Section B of the SSF.

information. I will continue to refer to the Figure 4.5 responses to further illustrate key points in relation to our case example. I should also note that there are literally *hundreds* of potential suicide risk variables that could be in Section B (Maris, Berman, & Silverman, 2000), but for parsimony and effectiveness we have retained a subset of variables that have both robust empirical support and significant clinical utility.

Suicide Ideation

The SSF Section B assessment begins with suicide ideation. By definition, cognitive thinking about suicide is implicated in all suicidal behaviors (Jobes, Casey, Berman, & Wright, 1991; Rosenberg et al., 1988). For our purposes, when a patient has suicidal thoughts, the nature and content of these thoughts are critical. Is it a brief fantasy or something that has been deeply and specifically explored? When we ask about suicide ideation, we are trying to gauge the degree of cognitive engagement on the topic. This is why we ask them to describe their ideation and elaborate on the frequency and duration of their suicide-related thoughts. Implicated in suicidal ideation is the important construct of "intention," which is something suicidologists and clinicians have wrestled with for years (Wagner, Wong, & Jobes, 2002). As clinicians, we are obviously most concerned when a patient's psychological intent is the complete termination of their biological existence. But the vast majority of suicidal patients in clinical practice fall far short of being absolutely determined to die. We must therefore endeavor to understand with the patient the purpose and meaning of their suicidal thoughts. If we can collaboratively understand the goal, the nature of the intent, and the functional utility of suicidal thoughts in the patient's life we are much better positioned to actually help save it.

Suicide Plan

It follows that understanding a patient's suicide plan is a key next step to unraveling some key aspects of psychological intent, particularly as it relates to the construct of *lethality* (i.e., the objective biological danger posed by a particular method of suicide). Sensitively appreciating the significance of a patient's plan is crucial (Stefansson, Nordström, & Jokinen, 2012). Interestingly, Joiner and colleagues (2003) found that "worst point plan" and "worst point preparation" were predictive of future death by suicide (whereas current or "worst point" suicidal ideation/desire was not predictive of subsequent death). For such reasons, while we appreciate the role of suicidal ideation, the magnitude and severity of planning and preparing for suicide is important (which is exactly why these constructs appear on the SSF in Section B).

We thus know that the clarity, specificity, and concreteness of a suicidal plan are a useful window into the seriousness of suicidal intent and lethality. In other words, someone with a vague, inexact, or nonspecific plan is much less serious about dying by suicide. In contrast, a patient who has a specific and detailed plan, including a particular place, time, and date, is much more psychologically invested in their suicide, thereby reflecting a more serious level of psychological intent. Along these lines it is worth noting that among older patients we see more determined and thoroughly planned self-destructive acts, using less violent methods, along with fewer warnings of potential suicidal intent (Conwell et al., 1998). The plan matters a lot.

To further assess the level of suicide intent, the SSF prompts for additional specificity about the "when," "where," and "how" of a suicidal plan with an additional question about whether the patient has access to the means of carrying out the plan (e.g., do they have a stash of lethal pills or access to a firearm?). Identifying components of a suicide plan at this point in the SSF assessment will also provide useful information for effectively formulating "means restriction" strategies as part of the patient's CAMS Stabilization Plan, which occurs during collaborative treatment planning.

Referring back to the case of Bill, this particular Section B SSF query led to a notable elaboration that he had actually picked out his "favorite" handgun and noted in session that "I would shoot myself between the eyes." While he had entertained the idea of putting the muzzle of the gun in his mouth, he was concerned that he might somehow survive and then be a "vegetable." Bill had not really considered any alternative methods, only vaguely considering an overdose, but again noted that there might be some chance of survival. This level of specificity and elaboration of such a lethal plan is quite concerning. Bill has given the topic considerable thought and does not seem to want to leave any wiggle room for surviving an attempt. Consequently, I am now notably concerned about my patient's potential suicide risk. As noted, the SSF suicide plan query can accommodate two separate suicidal plans, which is not unusual to see. While patients sometimes have additional plans, more than two plans are relatively rare, and I usually stop with the two top plans (Florentine & Crane, 2010; Hawton, 2007).

Suicide Preparation

Many suicidal people engage in specific preparation behaviors prior to making an attempt or taking their life (Rudd, 2008; Rudd & Joiner, 1998). In general, preparation behaviors are often related to organizing the suicide attempt itself, such as the procurement of lethal means, doing research on the Internet to determine a lethal dose of drugs, or determining a suitable location where the possibility of interruption or intervention may be reduced. Other preparation behaviors may include putting one's affairs in order, writing a will, writing suicide notes, shooting a good-bye video, posting a cryptic Facebook message, doing a favorite activity one final time, saying a final good-bye to friends and family, or giving away prized possessions. All of these behaviors infer significantly increased risk, as they represent a behavioral "ramping up" to a suicidal act. As noted early on, Bill has in fact drafted suicide notes to his wife and children and says that he has put his affairs in order, both of which again reflect psychological investment and preparatory behavior in the indisputable direction of taking his own life.

Suicide Rehearsal

Separate from suicidal preparation is another related set of relevant behaviors referred to as rehearsal behaviors (Rudd, 2008). Such behaviors typically involve a literal acting out or playing through of the planned suicide attempt. For example, someone may hang a rope, find a beam in the garage, secure the rope at a certain length, position a short stool, and even step up on the stool and place the ligature around the neck without then stepping off the stool to make the attempt. Such rehearsal behavior is serious—sometimes ending just short of an actual attempt. Many completed suicides are known to have held loaded guns to their head, placing the barrel of the gun at different locations or perhaps having put the barrel into their mouth. As noted, Bill has given the location of a self-inflicted gunshot wound some considerable thought —a clear reflection of potential lethal intent. As a general matter, such behaviors are important to identify, as they represent the most dangerous of all preparatory behaviors. Metaphorically, through these rehearsal behaviors, the suicidal person figuratively walks up to the precipice of death and teeters as he or she looks over the edge.

History of Suicidal Behaviors

The history of previous suicide attempts has long been considered a major risk factor for future suicidal behavior (Sveticic & De Leo, 2012). The work of Rudd and Joiner (1998; Joiner et al., 2005) showed distinct differences between people who have only had suicidal thoughts (desire) from those who make a single attempt versus those who have made two or more attempts. The risk of prospective behavior increases significantly with any past attempt behaviors, particularly a multiple-attempt history. In this area, the clinician is assessing for primarily "genuine" attempts, not superficial sublethal acts of scratching or minor overdoses. While attempt history should weigh heavily in our evaluation of risk, a French study of completers versus attempters did find that male suicide completers were less likely than suicide attempters to have a history of previous suicide attempts, so gender effects once again may be relevant in our understanding of suicidal risk (Younes et al., 2015).

Referring back to the case example of Bill, while there is no history of previous suicide attempts, his level of suicidal contemplation and planning is serious. As noted on his SSF, he thinks about suicide two to three times per day in durations lasting from 30 minutes to 2 hours. This is especially worrisome because these situations occur late at night by himself, probably in a state of intoxication, in his study with his favorite handgun sitting conveniently in his desk drawer.

Impulsivity

Because suicide attempts often happen in agitated, dysregulated, and highly impulsive states, it is useful to know about the patient's appraisal of his or her own impulsivity. Generally speaking, impulsivity can be characterized broadly in terms of a range of behaviors and actions that were not well thought through (Anestis, Soreray, Gutierrez, Hernández, & Joiner, 2014). The risk is further increased if such behaviors are inherently self-destructive. For example, suicide attempts are associated with a history of fighting (Bridge, Reynolds, et al., 2015; Simon et al., 2002; Simon & Crosby, 2000), conduct and impulse-control disorders (Nock et al., 2009), and poor premeditation (i.e., diminished ability to think through the consequences of one's actions; Klonsky & May, 2010). In truth, impulsivity is somewhat complex construct with many subcomponents (e.g., issues of state vs. trait impulsivity), which can make it difficult to simply rate as a yes/no question. But in many ways the query about this construct provides an opportunity for patients to reflect on this aspect of their behavioral repertoire—how they see it and how others see it as well which is an important assessment exercise in its self. In the case of Bill he reports being methodical in his behavior—"no one would say I am impulsive."

Substance Abuse

Another risk factor that is often implicated in suicidal behaviors is substance abuse (Esposito-Smythers & Spirito, 2004: Nock et al., 2009). We know that substance abuse contributes significantly to impulsive behaviors by lowering overall impulse control. Moreover, many people complete suicides in a state of intoxication (Borges & Rosovsky, 1996, Hufford, 2001). While the relationship between alcohol and suicide has been well established in the research literature (Wilcox, Conner, & Caine, 2004), many studies show a clear relationship between substance use disorders and suicide both in the near term (Hufford, 2001) and over time (Esposito-Smythers & Spirito, 2004). Bill acknowledges episodes of binge drinking, but does note that there have been periods of considerable sobriety (up to 2 years). His reported drinking behavior of late is a major concern that increases his risk considerably.

Significant Loss

For many years, suicidologists have known that suicides are often precipitated by losses that seem to trigger the suicidal act (Maris, Berman, & Maltsberger, 1992).

Such losses may be big or small; it can be one particularly significant loss or an accumulation of several lesser losses. Examples may include a marital divorce, a romantic breakup, a financial disaster, the death of a loved one or a pet—literally any tangible event that has meaning can be significant (e.g., Ajdacic-Gross et al., 2008; Brent et al., 1993; Joubert, Petrakis, & Cementon, 2012; Stack & Scourfield, 2015). Moreover, suicide-triggering losses can also be symbolic—for example, retirement from a meaningful career. Although losses often contribute to the circumstances that precede the suicide, usually such losses are not singularly causal of a suicide (Maris et al., 1992). In relation to Bill, there are no obvious significant losses that contribute to his risk.

Relationship Problems

Following the work of sociologists, we know that social factors are meaningfully implicated in many suicidal behaviors (Durkheim, 1951). Across the age spectrum, we further know that social relationships and social integration tend to protect a person against suicide (Daniel & Goldston, 2012; Eisenberg & Resnick, 2006; McLaren & Challis, 2009; Rowe, Conwell, Schulberg, & Bruce, 2006). From a clinical intervention standpoint, it is important to endeavor to not let the highly suicidal person be alone. Bill is not as isolated as some, but he does acknowledge withdrawing from family and friends, spending long and miserable evenings alone in his study where he has been veering into suicidal ruminations. In a related but more specific sense, we know that most of the suicidal patients we have studied (Jobes et al., 2004) have relationship isssues as their top suicide-related concern. These suicidogenic relationship problems may be romantically based or focused on friends or family (see also Joiner, 2005). In Bill's case, there are marital difficulties that significantly contribute to his suicidal musings.

Burden to Others

Following the work of Joiner (2005), the construct of "perceived burdensomeness" is yet another relational slant on suicide that is different from isolation or relational problems. The pernicious nature of experiencing oneself as a burden on others can create a dangerous undertow—that suicide becomes a "gift" to caring others who are weighed down with the troubles of the suicidal person. In some cases, I have seen this perception seem almost like a fixed delusion. A 17-year-old boy in my office reassured his pleading and tearful mother that while it would be tough the first year or so, she would be glad he is gone in the long run; they actually argued over the matter while the father looked on in abject horror. While it may not be delusional, Bill clearly does perceive that his family will benefit from his death.

Health/Pain Problems

There are also various data that suggest that general health-related issues, particularly if these issues are chronic, may be implicated in suicidal states (Giner et al., 2013; Maris et al., 2000; Sanna et al., 2014). While many live out their natural lives in the face of chronic physical pain, some find such states utterly unbearable, which may lead to increased suicidal risk fostered by a need to escape (Hooley, Franklin, & Nock, 2014; Smith, Edwards, Robinson, & Dworkin, 2004). In Bill's case, there are no apparent health problems that add to his suicidal misery.

Sleep Problems

Over the past decade, there has been increasing interest in the potential role of sleep disturbances to increased suicidal risk, particularly the pernicious role of insomnia (Pigeon, Pinquart, & Conner, 2012). Sleep problems related to insomnia, hypersomnia, and nightmares have been shown to significantly increase suicidal risk in adolescents (Goldstein, Bridge, & Brent, 2008). Moreover, in a sample 423 veteran suicide decedents, sleep disturbance was temporarily associated with near-term risk for suicide (Pigeon, Britton, Ilgen, Chapman, & Conner, 2012). Notably, Bill has been having recent bouts of insomnia and he has a history of irregular sleep. He further states that his binge drinking helps him "pass out," but he awakens in the middle of the night feeling disoriented and has trouble falling back asleep.

Legal/Financial Issues

We know that legal problems can also contribute significantly to suicidal risk (e.g., Brent et al., 1993). Indeed, suicide attempts and completions among individuals in lockup or holding cells (often picked up for driving under the influence of alcohol) are a notable concern. There is often a window of considerable suicidal risk shortly after a person is first faced with a legal accusation (Oordt et al., 2005). Similarly, financial issues from poverty, unemployment, credit card debt, payday lenders, owing back taxes, and simply not being able to make ends meet can all contribute to increased suicidal risk (Coope et al., 2015; Pompili et al., 2011). There are no apparent legal problems in Bill's situation, but there are some financial stressors.

Shame

Finally, a related but unique risk factor is shame, which can play a key role in the need to escape discovery of past wrongs or experiences that cannot be borne in the eyes of others. For example, I know of cases of priests facing charges of child abuse who have attempted or completed suicide rather than face the misery of prolonged litigation that will be both professionally and personally humiliating. Conversely, being the victim of abuse can play a particularly critical role in suicidal and self-destructive behavior (Linehan, 1993a). In our work with military populations, we see that issues of shame can be an important factor in suicide risk among service members where strength and toughness are central to the culture (refer to Bryan, Jennings, Jobes, & Bradley, 2012; Bryan, Morrow, Etienne, & Ray-Sannerud, 2013; Jobes, 2013c). My patient Bill is ashamed for becoming such a "loser" and a "failure" in life.

Conclusion of Section B

After completing Section B of the SSF, the clinician and patient are ready to transition to Section C of the SSF, which centers on the focused and collaborative development of a suicide-specific stabilization plan and the driver-oriented treatment plan that defines CAMS-guided care. In terms of wrapping up the first session SSF assessment, I might typically say:

> "I appreciate your willingness to complete this assessment with me. I think we now both have a much better sense of what's been going on with you and why suicide has been on your mind. Knowing why you are suicidal is crucial to finding alternative ways of coping with your pain and suffering. Do you have any questions before we start working on your treatment plan?"

CASE EXAMPLE: RISK FORMULATION FOR BILL

Considering all the assessment data gathered in Sections A and B for our case example of Bill, I would consider his potential suicide risk to be quite high. In fact, given his serious risk, I am actually struck that he is still alive and I am almost surprised by his willingness to even meet with me. Given the substantial risk that Bill poses, most clinicians would be eager to immediately hospitalize him, and I seriously considered that option myself. Yet within the CAMS approach to care, we endeavor to do the best we can to *avert* a hospitalization—when possible—and rely on inpatient care only as the *last* resort. Bill's SSF Core Assessment speaks to considerable suffering, and his self-hate and hopelessness are a major source of concern to me. He confirms that his suicidal risk is both connected to his sense of self and his key relationships. Bill's reasons for living are trumped by his reasons for dying, and overall he appears to be more attached to dying than living. Bill's sense of psychological entrapment is particularly worrisome to me as well.

  From Section B of the SSF we see that Bill has invested considerable time and energy into the prospect of taking his life using the most lethal means possible. He has put affairs in order and has actually written drafts of suicide notes. His drinking and poor mental health treatment history does not bode well either.

Thankfully, there is no reported previous attempt history among an otherwise bleak set of suicide risk variables. And yet, Bill is sitting in the office of clinical psychologist who is increasingly drawing out of him critical information related to his suicidal struggle and journey. He is still alive and talking, not dead and silent—this is perhaps the most important (even encouraging) assessment data that we have about Bill at this point.

SUMMARY AND CONCLUSIONS

Completing SSF Sections A and B in the first session with a patient is pivotal to the success of CAMS. Everything about the CAMS approach to assessing suicide risk is designed to enhance the alliance and more deeply engage the patient within his or her own care. The emphasis of Section A is expressly meant to communicate to patients that they are the experts of their own experience. In turn, the clinician's job to see the suicidal risk through the eyes of the patient. The patient's perceptions of the struggle are the assessment gold standard; the clinician's job is to be the proverbial prospector looking for nuggets of suicidal truth so as to empathically appreciate and understand those critical perceptions.

As discussed, Section A heavily emphasizes a focus on pain and suffering more than suicide per se. Having emphasized the patient's pain and suffering, Section B marks a transition to focusing more specifically on empirically based suicide risk factors and warning signs, thereby providing some objective perspective on various suicide-related variables. The intentional backloading of the more suicide-specific focus of Section B makes this assessment section secondary to the primary assessment section that focuses of the patient's phenomenology and intrasubjective suicidal struggle (Section A). By doing suicide risk assessment this way, we underscore an empathic and collaborative approach by working with the patient in a concerted effort to sidestep the suicide-hospitalization/no-hospitalization power struggle. In so doing, we increase the likelihood of forming a collaborative alliance and inspiring patient motivation, which can be embodied and operationalized in the patient-defined, driver-oriented, suicide-specific CAMS treatment plan.

In terms of Bill, the treatment challenges we face are formidable. Across Bill's responses on Section A and B of the SSF, we have many reasons to be concerned about his prospective risk of suicide. Bill should certainly be considered a high-risk suicidal person with ready access to lethal means and a significant psychological attachment to dying. Given his high overall risk, averting an inpatient admission will be challenging. Yet within CAMS, we will attempt to do just that. We next endeavor to develop a treatment plan that can be used to safely guide suicide-specific outpatient care that is expressly designed to help save Bill's life.

CHAPTER 5

CAMS Treatment Planning

Coauthoring a Suicide-Specific Treatment Plan

As we all know, there are hundreds of different types of psychotherapies and clinical treatments represented in the mental health treatment literature. When I first taught courses in our graduate program, it was common to think in terms of the three major schools of theory: psychoanalytic, behavioral, and humanistic. Today, these major schools have further evolved and blended. For example, psychoanalytic theory has evolved into a variety of "psychodynamic" schools of thought, including ego psychology, drive theory, object relations, and self psychology, to name but a few. There are still enthusiastic practitioners of humanistic, patient-centered, and existential psychotherapies, and there is pervasive use of constructs and ideas from these traditions. Behavioral treatments (particularly behavioral activation; see Dimidjian et al., 2006; Martell, Dimidjian, & Herman-Dunn, 2013), combined with cognitive approaches, have clearly been in ascension over several decades and tend to have the best data overall. Within the cognitive-behavioral tradition, a new generation of "third-wave" psychotherapies emphasizing mindfulness are now fully taking center stage. Examples of such therapies include mindfulness-based cognitive therapy (Segal, Williams, & Teasdale, 2012), acceptance and commitment therapy (Ducasse et al., 2014; Hayes, Strosahl, & Wilson, 2011), and other similarly oriented integrative therapeutic approaches (Kahl, Winter, & Schweiger, 2012; Roemer & Orsillo, 2009).

Beyond considerations of different schools and kinds of psychotherapies, there are countless other forms and modalities of treatment in the tool kit of mental health providers. Innovations using prolonged exposure (PE; Foa, Hembree, & Rothbaum, 2007; Powers, Halpern, Ferenschak, Gillihan, & Foa, 2010), cognitive processing therapy (CPT; Matulis, Resick, Rosner, & Steil, 2014; Resick & Schnicke, 1992), and eye movement desensitization and reprocessing (EMDR; Shapiro, 1996) are available for treating various kinds of trauma. Bateman and Fonagy's (2006, 2009) mentalization is another novel approach used to treat patients with complex personality disorders (see also Allen, Fonagy, & Bateman, 2008). Biofeedback (Nestoriuc, Martin, Rief & Andrasik, 2008; Siepmann, Aykac, Unterdörfer, Petrowski, & Mueck-Weymann, 2008) and clinical hypnosis (Patterson & Jensen, 2003) have been available for some years to treat a spectrum of problems and psychosomatic concerns. From the medical field, there are numerous psychotropic medications (Mark, 2010), electroconvulsive therapy (Kayser et al., 2011), transcranial magnetic stimulation (Slotema, Blom, Hoek, & Sommer, 2010), and the intriguing use of intravenous ketamine infusion (Price, Nock, Charney, & Mathew, 2009). In terms of mental health treatment modalities, there is of course individual psychotherapy, group therapy, couple therapy, family therapy, and behavioral *in vivo* exposure treatments that may be done in public or in the privacy of a patient's home. Finally, there is an extensive assortment of clinical treatment settings, ranging from clinics, to counseling centers, to crisis units, to inpatient settings, community mental health settings, partial/day-treatment environments, and the like.

As a pragmatic clinician, I endorse whatever theory, treatments, and modalities (or any combination thereof) that effectively treat mental disorders, reduce symptoms, and ultimately alleviate the pain and suffering of my patients. As an academic clinician-researcher, I tend to strongly favor those interventions and modalities that are supported by data, even though I know from 25 years of clinical experience that there are many effective treatments that do not yet have the support of research evidence. All things being equal, I have an obvious bias for treatments that clinically work and have empirical support as well.

Given the full array of treatment options and the various "truths" in mental health about what works, I could never imagine myself being deeply encamped in one particular school of thought or restricting my practice to staying within any one particular lane of theory or treatment. I was originally trained to conceptualize cases psychodynamically and applied this perspective to understanding suicidal risk (refer to Jobes, 1995b; Jobes & Karmel, 1996). Over the years I have remained particularly appreciative of psychodynamically oriented defense analysis (see McWilliams, 2011). But my actual clinical practice is now interspersed with insight-oriented and cognitive-behavioral techniques as well a generous sampling of humanistic, interpersonal, and existential approaches. Obviously, like many in the field, I am integrative in my clinical approach to care. Moreover, I know the tremendous value of group psychotherapy, the valuable effects of well-prescribed and monitored psychoactive medications, the value of couple work, and the power of clinical hypnosis.

Upon reflection, one of the most memorable experiences in my professional youth was observing the transformative power of electroconvulsive therapy (ECT) with a severely depressed and suicidal inpatient. Unable to care for himself, this once proud and distinguished senior federal government worker became incontinent each night (of stool and urine), and his personal hygiene deteriorated significantly. Much to our collective shock, this same man quite literally came bounding out of his room early in the day after his third ECT treatment greeting the staff at the front desk with a broad smile and the salutation "Good morning, everyone! Isn't it a wonderful day?" When one has seen the therapeutic power of the full spectrum of treatments for some of the most severe of mental health conditions, it is hard to not pragmatically appreciate the virtues of therapeutic flexibility and the full use of the array of available treatment options. For my part as a mental health provider, I want to use every therapeutic arrow I can find in my mental health quiver in the singular pursuit of helping my patients who suffer.

Yet I do know that many clinicians do not embrace an integrative approach to care. Indeed, the fact that many mental health professionals deeply identify with a particular clinical approach or theoretical orientation poses an exacting test for the wide professional embrace and routine use of an approach to suicide like CAMS. As noted in Chapter 1, a primary goal in developing CAMS over the years has been to purposely build an intervention that can be broadly used to treat suicide risk, regardless of the clinician's theoretical orientation, preferred treatment approach, mental health discipline, or clinical setting. While CAMS does have some front-end requirements for clinical engagement and assessment, the suicide-specific treatment planning that is a signature feature of CAMS may encompass any theory or treatment that is deemed appropriate to successfully treat patient-defined suicidal drivers. In this regard, I have consistently contended (e.g., Jobes & Drozd, 2004) that CAMS neither usurps clinical judgment nor dictates the theory or type of treatment that must be used. This chapter will thus describe broad conceptual aspects of CAMS-informed treatment planning before transitioning to a more step-by-step description of CAMS treatment planning procedures.

AN OVERVIEW TO CAMS TREATMENT PLANNING

As a general matter in relation to suicide-specific treatment planning, you must ask yourself, "If suicide is the best option for this patient to cope with his or her pain and suffering, *why then is this person talking to me—a mental health professional—about this topic?*" The answer invariably is that the patient is talking to you because he or she has not yet decided that suicide *is* the best way of coping with their pain and suffering; the patient is *ambivalent,* which creates a portal through which the dyad can pass to discover a life-saving clinical intervention together.

While a suicidal patient is usually ambivalent, the potential seduction of suicide can feel formidable and urgent. In this regard, the clinician must skillfully manage the temporal aspects of negotiating the treatment plan with any suicidal

patient. Time considerations are crucial because it is unreasonable for a highly suicidal person to "give up" suicide as an option for coping *indefinitely*. Alternatively,
I would argue that it is reasonable for the clinician to negotiate a discrete time
period in which clinical treatment is given a fair chance. We thus propose pushing
the option of suicide onto the patient's psychological back-burner. My foot-in-the-
door argument to the patient is this:

> "Before you take your life to end your suffering, let's try to give an evidence-
> based suicide-specific treatment a reasonable chance to help you find other
> ways of coping. Obviously, there are countless other options—such as suicide—
> that you can reflect on later without my support."

The last portion of this statement may sound unnecessarily provocative. But in
a clinical context with the proper tone and emphasis, such a statement is not only
reasonable, it is both empathic and usually deescalates a potential power struggle
over suicide. Perhaps most notably, this statement and position does not eliminate
from the already vulnerable patient his or her sense of power and autonomy that
the option of suicide psychologically assures. In my mind, one of the most powerful clinical interventions one can make when working with a suicidal person is to
overtly negotiate with the patient the notion of putting off suicide to a later point
in time. The inherent issues are summarized as follows: What is reasonable for
the clinician to expect of a suicidal patient? Conversely, from the suicidal patient's
perspective, what is reasonable regarding further enduring seemingly unbearable
suicidal suffering for the prospect of a potentially effective treatment that may
ultimately prove to be life-saving?

I assert to my suicidal patients that it is clinically reasonable and necessary
to negotiate finite suicide-specific outpatient treatment plans. In CAMS, patients
are asked to commit to a mutually negotiated suicide-specific treatment plan for
an exact period of time. Moreover, within CAMS we discourage clinical or moral
coercion or an open-ended approach to treatment planning. As noted earlier, when
I negotiate a suicide-specific treatment plan with a patient, I forthrightly acknowledge that the patient can obviously take his or her life *later* (when not otherwise
engaged in treatment focused on saving that life). But I emphatically insist that
while the patient is engaged in our suicide-specific and time-specific treatment,
he or she must be fully committed—as I will be—to that life-saving treatment.
Invariably this treatment thoughtfully explores whether there are, in fact, viable
alternatives to the finality of suicide.

Beyond these considerations, I am explicit with my patients that if they become
a clear and imminent danger to self or others (as described in the HIPAA-compliant
consent form that they read and signed at the start of care), I will not hesitate exercise my professional duty to hospitalize them as per legal statutes that require
clinicians to intervene in this manner (Jobes & O'Connor, 2009). But anything short

of this most extreme medico-legal threshold leaves plenty of room for the clinician and patient to thoughtfully maneuver as they collaboratively endeavor to negotiate a potentially life-saving treatment plan. I usually point out that the patient has everything to gain, and really nothing to lose, by giving treatment a chance.

To succeed in these treatment-planning negotiations, it is imperative that patients believe and feel that they are maintaining some sense of control by understanding that they can take their life later, *after* they have given treatment a fair and reasonable chance. Whenever I say things along these lines, I remain absolutely clear that I do not endorse suicide as a viable option and that I will never "sign off" on suicide as the optimal way to respond. I will not do that. Consequently, my suicidal patients are presented with a profound choice: Do they want to live a bit longer to see if treatment can help make their life livable without pain? Or do they choose not to be in this treatment and to continue to be subjected to unbearable suffering, with the obvious implications therein? It is a weighty choice, but I think it must be plainly posed to the patient. The clinician must therefore skillfully pose to the suicidal patient a time-specific treatment choice that typically inspires an intentional decision to *choose to live*—at least for now—to find out what might be possible (which invariably inspires a flicker of *hope*).

Similar to the spirit of the "pitch" I described in Chapter 1, I often use the following therapeutic metaphor as approach describing CAMS-specific treatment planning:

> "I want you to consider taking a therapeutic road trip with me. On this trip you will be the driver and I will be the navigator. I have taken this trip many times before, I know the roads well, and I have excellent maps and a GPS. But the journey is never the same route for any two drivers. It is unique to the driver and the way we decide to travel together—which roads to take, when to stop, and how fast or slow we decide to go. For this road trip to be successful, you must, like me, commit to the trip we plan. I know that our desired therapeutic destination can be hard to find, and frankly we may take some wrong turns along the way. But I nevertheless remain confident that we can get to where we want to go if we work together as a traveling team.
>
> "Because I know you suffer deeply, I am only asking that you travel with me for a specific period of time, a minimum of 3 months. After that, we can decide together whether we should continue our travels together or perhaps part ways so that you can drive on your own or perhaps travel with a different navigator. Despite your suffering, I still believe this is a reasonable request to ask of you, given both the promise of our desired destination and the seriousness of the alternative you are considering.
>
> "If you agree to take this trip with me, for a period of time to which we both commit, then it requires that we both seriously promise to fully take this journey. That means you must get completely in the car, with the door closed

and locked, seatbelt on, both hands on the wheel. This journey will fail if you insist on leaving your door ajar so that you may jump out of the car if the road gets bumpy. If that is something you need to do, we need to find you another navigator or perhaps we should acknowledge that you are not yet ready to take this kind of trip with a person like me.

"As your navigator, I will stay right beside you with my expertise, maps, GPS, and my experience to facilitate this trip for the period of time we are both committing to so that we may find the therapeutic destination that we both seek for you. I can assure you that the destination is a much better place than where you now reside, it will be a place where your pain and suffering are meaningfully decreased and your ability to cope with life is meaningfully improved."

I want to emphasize that to properly take this metaphorical journey, both parties must be fully seated in the car—no doors are left ajar, no metaphorical feet are allowed to hang out. We are asking the patient to commit, and in turn, the patient can anticipate that we will commit as well, with both doors closed, locked, and seatbelts securely fastened. We both pledge to taking this therapeutic trip together in search of a prized destination that the patient has clearly not been able to find up to this point traveling solo. For patients who are not up for taking this type of therapeutic trip under these travel conditions I indicate that there are basically three options: (1) an inpatient hospitalization if they are in imminent danger, (2) referral to another clinician who travels in a different manner with different traveling conditions, or (3) for the patient—*if not in imminent danger*—to continue driving on his or her own without my help or guidance (i.e., the obvious but often overlooked option of not being in mental health treatment—Jobes, 2011).

As I have discussed elsewhere (Wise, Jobes, Simpson, & Berman, 2005), what I call "time-specific contingent treatment planning" with suicidal patients may not be suitable for every potential patient the clinician encounters (particularly those with developmental disabilities, acute psychosis, or severe personality disorders). But clinicians have an obligation to transparently provide to any prospective patient (particularly if suicide is in the picture) a clear message about what in their professional opinion is a reasonable plan for clinically proceeding, with a focus on pursuing care that is in the patient's best interest. Whether the patient-consumer agrees and chooses to "buy" this treatment should be up to the patient-consumer, with no latent threats or clinical arm-twisting. As an aside, let me note that even though I am not an enthusiast of coercive approaches to clinically preventing suicide, I still believe that there are occasions when suicidal patients should be hospitalized, sometimes even against their will. As previously noted, I follow and comply with any and all legal duties that statutes require when a patient who poses a *clear and imminent* danger to self and/or others. But short of this most dire presentation, I am ardent about conducting reasonable negotiations with the patient that are designed to buy crucial time and trust, thereby creating a stronger alliance that may in turn help increase the patient's motivation to fight for his or her life.

Let me conclude this particular discourse by underscoring something central to the CAMS approach. The book you are reading is about the collaborative assessment and *management* of suicidality. I specifically decided years ago that this approach should emphasize the word *management* versus *treatment* in relation to dealing with suicidal risk. CAMS is not CATS. Obviously, there are treatment implications throughout this chapter and the entire book. But the emphasis in CAMS is on clinically managing the potential for suicide, until the patient has been fully "won over" to the side of wanting to live. CAMS-guided care succeeds when patients uncouple themselves from their suicide attachment. The truth is that suicidal people only really give up on suicide when the purpose and value of suicide in their lives is made obsolete, not because we have told them they cannot have it. Rendering suicide obsolete in patients' lives is a central goal in CAMS as they shift their thinking and fully attach to life.

Clinical Treatment Planning in the Face of "Suicidal Blackmail"

A common struggle clinicians have with suicidal patients is the fear that if they do not accommodate or bend over backward for the patient, the patient may attempt suicide or actually die by suicide, and then they will be blamed and possibly sued for malpractice. In the first edition of this book I bluntly referred to this phenomenon as "suicidal blackmail." Based on that initial foray into this thorny topic, I wrote an entire chapter about the tricky ethical and risk management issues related to suicidal blackmail (Jobes, 2011). The cases to which I refer may start out unremarkably only to later escalate into a situation in which the clinician becomes the proverbial "deer in headlights" facing the prospect of a patient's suicide. In other cases, the struggle may be immediately obvious. Invariably in such cases, the clinician ends up fielding phone calls at all hours, changing his or her usual and customary practices, modifying boundaries, and spending inordinate amounts of time on a single, terrifying, even harrowing case. Believe me, I know about this kind of experience firsthand (see Jobes, 2011, for a full case description).

Even an otherwise conscientious clinician can lose perspective in the face of an escalating suicidal risk. As just noted when dealing with the risk, clinicians may feel compelled to do things that feel uncomfortable, to bend their rules and modify their customary practice. Then, before they know it, the treatment is off the rails and may career out of control. Treatments of this type can become reactive and chaotic—think of the story of the little Dutch boy racing around trying to plug the leaks in the dike. More critically, however, is the fact that such treatments are rarely in the patient's best interest. Such frantic treatments often burn out competent and conscientious clinicians, leaving them feeling miserable and incompetent. All of these considerations have at least in part led to the fairly structured, transparent, and forthright approach that is manifest within CAMS.

a contention that *not* being
the suicidal patient, which
ınd clinician alike. While I
teadfast on this point and
ıtive therapeutic outcomes.
ıirical research is that for
ed and willing to proceed
e properly motivated in a
ıg a clear and transparent
the patient can make his
eatment (see also Street,

ːidal person (in particu-
ılanning on doing with
ion about what is in the
ıt clearly to the patient.
ɪues should be plainly
bout engaging in that
icide is in the picture
ɪat it must be directly
e must have a direct
ʲoing to deal with the
ınɪɛxɪʋɪe—certain conditions must be
ɪɪɪ ʋ pɪuceed with a suicidal patient in good faith. The patient, in
turn, can then decide how to proceed (or not) in response to my professional judgment and my experience-based optimal conditions for care.

As an example, let us consider an especially contentious issue that may arise
between a clinician and a suicidal patient. Imagine a scenario in which a highly
suicidal patient is seeking treatment and acknowledges ready access to a firearm in
the home. In the course of discussing this access, the patient makes it known that
he or she will not remove this weapon from the home environment at the request
of the clinician, even for a relatively short-term period (e.g., a month). This standoff
is difficult. On the one hand, the patient may legitimately own a firearm. On the
other hand, surveillance data from the Centers for Disease Control and Prevention and other researchers have shown the clear lethal threat of a firearm in the
home (CDC, 2010; Lahti, Keränen, Hakko, Riala, & Räsänen, 2014; Stroebe, 2013).
As the clinician, I can gamble and acquiesce to the patient's refusal. Alternatively,
I can make this issue a "deal breaker" and tell the patient I do not feel comfortable
proceeding with care in the face of the risk posed by the weapon and the patient's
refusal to remove it for the period of time in which we will pursue treatment. I
choose to interpret the patient's refusal as therapeutic bad faith. In my view, such
a position on the patient's part is a direct threat to our treatment plan, fundamentally undermining our treatment efforts to preserve his or her life. Furthermore,

I may be compelled to terminate the case and refer the patient on to another provider. Let me be clear: This is not a political or constitutional issue; this is clinical judgment about what is in the patient's best interest. I am not saying a patient of mine may not own a firearm. Rather, I am saying for the period of time that we have agreed to work on the issue of suicide, I reserve the right to assert a basic ground rule in order for therapy to proceed. I do not want to clinically compete with the temptation of a gun.

At this juncture, it is important to address legitimate concerns about the ethical issue of clinical "abandonment" (Jobes, 2011). The central ethical concern about abandonment centers on any unilateral action by the clinician of suddenly discontinuing clinical care, leaving the patient in the lurch. In cases of clinical abandonment, the patient has been suddenly dropped from clinical care, leaving the patient vulnerable with no effort extended by the clinician to ensure any ongoing therapeutic care or support. It is, however, a different situation when a clinician takes a thoughtful and principled position in the patient's best interest that may ultimately compel the clinician to end the treatment. In cases in which a patient's abject refusal to abide by certain necessary conditions of appropriate treatment compel the clinician to potentially bring the care to an end, it is important to (1) transparently work in the best interest of the patient, (2) be absolutely clear about the necessary elements of treatment (and why they are necessary), (3) make every reasonable effort to make referrals that would bridge the patient to other appropriate care, (4) seek professional consultation, and (5) carefully document one's decision making about the patient's best interest (documenting the input of one's professional consultant is also wise).

Consider the following case example. Some years ago, a senior colleague of mine sought consultation on a particularly difficult case. I was quite familiar with this complex case from previous consultations. My colleague had been seeing this woman for almost 3 years; she was diagnosed with dysthymic disorder and borderline personality disorder. The treatment had been notably stormy and contentious, with ongoing threats of suicide, two overdose attempts, and one psychiatric hospitalization. The situation that compelled him to seek me out yet again involved a new wrinkle in their embattled treatment relationship. The patient announced after missing a week of sessions (she was seen twice a week) that she had fired her psychiatrist and was now seeing a new psychiatrist who was completely changing her extensive medication regimen. My colleague, a clinical psychologist by training, was shocked by the sudden development and insisted that she sign a release for him to make contact with the new psychiatrist. The patient refused, insisting that she did not want him talking to her new psychiatrist, and she insisted that the new doctor was fine with this arrangement. My colleague explained that standard professional practice and ethics required a coordinated clinical effort and that his inability to consult with the other member of her treatment team was not in her best interest and this new arrangement was ultimately unacceptable to him. She would not budge; in fact, he noted that she appeared to "enjoy" defying him in this manner. After discussing the history of the case, the ethics, his countertransference, and various other issues, we concluded that he had to take a strong position that his work with her would need to end if she was unwilling to let him coordinate her care with the physician. He reasonably gave her 3 weeks to change her mind. But at the end of 3 weeks, she remained steadfast and their tumultuous work together came to a necessary end. In their final session, he reviewed the basis for this course of action and offered to refer her to other providers. He was even willing to take her back if she changed her mind. However, she did not change her mind, and she left in an angry snit, announcing that she would be seeing her psychiatrist for both her medicine and her psychotherapy. While this case is not satisfying from an outcome standpoint, I believe my colleague had little choice and he proceeded in a completely ethical and appropriate manner in bringing this case to a necessary close.

The point in all this is that it is crucial to know and assert one's clinical judgment about how certain aspects of the treatment *must* proceed. When working with a patient who refuses to meet certain necessary conditions of treatment, I have said, for example:

> "Your position that you reserve the right to kill yourself during your treatment is untenable to me; it simply won't work for us to proceed in that fashion. To that end, you may need to find another therapist—which I will of course help you do—or maybe you should reconsider your overall readiness to engage in psychotherapy at all."

Clinicians in my workshops are often shocked when I take this kind of position with the patient. In response, I clarify that I am not trying to use a paradoxical intervention or be provocative with the patient. I am simply being clear about my limits and the constraints of the treatment that I am able and willing to offer and why this is so. I recommend to suicidal patients that they should seriously consider engaging in a clinical treatment that endeavors to pursue their best interest *before* the more drastic option of suicide. But if they are to be in treatment with me, I want them to be fully in treatment—not ready to jump out of the "treatment car" while it is moving. It is, therefore, important to be transparent about the process of the clinical engagement, to develop treatment plans and contracts carefully, and to work within specific time frames. We cannot let the patient's problems, suicidal threats, or personality pathology be the "tail that wags the dog" of proper treatment that is in the patient's best interest. Critically, at the end of each treatment contract time period a mutual discussion ensues as to whether we should clinically proceed for another discrete period of time.

I am often asked, "What happens if you take this rigid approach and tell the patient that she is not ready for therapy because she refuses one of your conditions and then she proceeds to go home and kill herself that very evening. Aren't you liable?" Such a scenario would undoubtedly be a tragedy, and I would feel horrible if it happened, of course. But frankly, such a prospect comes with the territory and can happen with any suicidal person, regardless of whether one uses the approach I am advocating. It is a risk we all face. However, irrespective of whether I suggested that the patient was a poor candidate for treatment (e.g., by virtue of refusing to comply with a key treatment condition), the determination of liability will rest on one critical hindsight question: Was the patient at the moment he or she left my office in clear and imminent danger? If the answer is yes, that person should have been sent to the hospital—voluntarily or involuntarily if necessary—to ensure that the person does not engage in a self-harm behavior. A failure to effect a hospitalization under these circumstances may well make the clinician liable. But if the answer is no, we have a tragic situation to be sure, but nevertheless a situation in which a prospective patient was neither able nor willing to accept a reasonable time-limited treatment proposal that was designed to save the patient's life. There are no guarantees that one will not be sued in such a scenario, and I am impressed by the willingness of plaintiff attorneys to explore malpractice even in extremely weak cases. But clinicians must be clear about their usual and customary practices—why they made the decisions they made and how they must loop back to what was in their patient's best interest. If this position can be further bolstered by theory or especially data, it is even more defendable in a hindsight situation. As I note repeatedly in Chapter 8, the role of detailed and thorough documentation is key in relation to the "Monday-morning quarterbacking" that invariably occurs in malpractice cases where the wisdom of hindsight is plain.

Experience has demonstrated to me that the alternative to my way of thinking is simply indefensible—that a clinician would knowingly begin (or continue) a therapeutic relationship with a patient giving up on critical and necessary conditions of treatment. It is metaphorically akin to knowingly embarking (or continuing) on a potentially dangerous boat trip with the suicidal patient in spite of a large hole in the hull of the vessel; it is a lose–lose scenario for the clinician and the patient. If, however, a clinician acquiesces on basic conditions of appropriate care, it is akin to telling the patient that it is acceptable to be unreasonable (i.e., it is okay to not meet the clinician halfway in good faith to pursue a reasonable time-specific treatment that is designed to save the patient's life). Like many of you reading this book, I have been there and done that. Such an approach does not work for the patient and it certainly does not work for the clinician. Such acquiescence on the part of clinician in the face of suicidal blackmail is not in the best interest of the patient and I cannot abide it. (For more information on this topic, see Stefan, 2016.)

FILLING OUT SECTION C OF THE SSF

Now that we have considered the broader conceptual aspects of the general CAMS approach to suicide-specific treatment planning, let us now examine some of the more concrete procedural aspects of CAMS treatment planning. In Chapter 4, we left off with the collaborative completion of Section B of the SSF suicide risk assessment (within the first CAMS session). As discussed, the clinical dyad should spend roughly 30 minutes working through the SSF assessment, Sections A (in the patient's hand) and B (in the provider's hand). Completion of this collaborative risk assessment process now sets the stage for CAMS suicide-specific treatment planning proper, which involves completing Section C of the SSF (which also includes completing the CAMS Stabilization Plan as part of the treatment plan).

Overview to Negotiating the Treatment Plan

Following are key elements that should guide any CAMS-based clinical negotiation of a suicidal patient's current and future stability and safety:

1. The CAMS clinician should be forthright with the patient about any relevant legal statutes pertaining to confidentiality and the potential threat of imminent danger to self. This important information is usually handled within the informed consent process. Relevant forms related to this process should be handled *prior* to direct clinical contact and therapeutic engagement. It is incumbent on the licensed provider to fully address and answer any questions related to this information.
2. The CAMS clinician embraces the importance of mutual give and take—there are reasonable expectations that each party should have of each other.
3. The CAMS clinician should communicate *empathy* for the patient's suicidal wish—appreciating the patient's feeling that suicide may be a tempting means for dealing with *seemingly* unbearable pain. However, the clinician can subsequently and sensitively ask: Is suicide the *best* way to cope and get your needs met?
4. The CAMS clinician should negotiate current and future care in relation to time-based considerations and persist in exploring all possibilities for *delaying* the need to rely on suicidal behavior.
5. The CAMS provider fundamentally seeks a reasonable, good-faith, time-specific, agreement with the patient to give treatment a fair chance of making a difference. I typically request 3 months (12 sessions), knowing from the research the most patients respond to CAMS in six to eight sessions (Jobes, 2012).

As noted earlier, within standard CAMS-guided care there is an overt emphasis on developing a viable *outpatient* treatment plan during the first session, which by its nature will justify pursuing outpatient work together, thereby averting the need to hospitalize. The exception, however, is when CAMS is used with suicidal inpatients, wherein the treatment planning emphasis centers on appropriate discharge and disposition (Ellis et al., 2015).

In standard outpatient CAMS, I typically introduce SSF Section C, Treatment Planning, by saying something like the following:

"Now we need to develop your treatment plan. To do this successfully we need to fully consider all the information we have learned about your pain and suffering and potential risk for suicidal behavior. To create an effective plan, we can refer to Sections A and B of the assessment we just did to help us shape problems, goals, and objectives for our work together. Since we must take the issue of suicide seriously, we must first consider how we are going to deal with your self-harm potential and then how we will treat the problems that led you to consider suicide. Let me be plain: We will try to develop a treatment plan that will keep you *out of the hospital*. But to achieve that goal, we must develop a suicide-specific outpatient treatment plan that we are both committed to pursuing together for a certain period of time."

In specific reference to the first-session SSF Section C (see Figure 5.1), we see that the treatment-planning portion of the form is organized into the following four major heading sections: (1) Problem # and Problem Description, (2) Goals and Objectives, (3) Interventions, and (4) Duration.

The Section C treatment plan section should be completed by the clinician in consultation with the patient, remaining in the side-by-side seating arrangement. In this spirit, we say that the CAMS patient functions as a *coauthor* of his or her own treatment plan. It is important to underscore that within Section C, Problem #1—"Self-Harm Potential"—is actually *not* negotiable if we are intent on avoiding an inpatient psychiatric admission. In the important first session of CAMS,

Problem #	Problem Description	Goals and Objectives	Interventions	Duration
1	*Self-Harm Potential*	*Safety and Stability*	*Stabilization Plan Completed* ☐	
2				
3				

Section C (*Clinician*):   TREATMENT PLAN

YES ____ NO ____   Patient understands and concurs with treatment plan?

YES ____ NO ____   Patient at imminent danger of suicide (hospitalization indicated)?

Patient Signature   Date   Clinican Signature   Date

FIGURE 5.1. First-session SSF Section C Treatment Plan.

the initial treatment planning process begins with a singular focus on self-harm potential and the subsequent development of a crisis-specific and suicide-specific stabilization plan.

CAMS Stabilization Planning

A major initial focus of CAMS-based treatment planning is the thoughtful and thorough development of a stabilization plan that is used to facilitate patient safety and stability. Within standard use of CAMS, I recommend the use of the "CAMS Stabilization Plan" (which appears as the next page within the SSF-4). Alternatively, a similar stabilizing intervention can be achieved by using Stanley and Brown's (2012) Safety Plan Intervention, or Rudd and colleagues' (2001) Crisis Response Plan. Each of these three interventions achieves similar goals—they are fundamentally designed to increase the patient's ability to cope with current and future crises and in so doing, averting or at least delaying suicidal behaviors. In other words, each of these plans provide pre-established steps to help guide a suffering person through his or her suicidal dark moments that may avert the need to resort to self-harm behaviors. Importantly, these suicide-specific and coping-oriented stabilizing plans are emphatically *not* variations of "no-suicide" or "no-harm" contracts. For decades in both outpatient and inpatient mental health care settings, getting a suicidal patient to "commit to safety" (sometimes with direct coercion) has been the clinical standard of care. Unfortunately, no-suicide contracts and commitments to safety are still used despite being roundly criticized and eschewed by experts in clinical suicidology (e.g., Jobes et al., 2008; Stanley & Brown, 2012), who point to the absence of empirical support and potentially increasing liability (see further discussion by Lewis, 2007; Rudd, Mandrusiak, & Joiner, 2006). But there is a compelling difference between focusing on what the patient *will do* if he or she gets into a suicidal crisis (stabilization steps) versus focusing on what the patient *will not to do* (promising to not attempt suicide) in some ephemeral manner.

All the above noted stabilization planning interventions are close cousins; while differently formatted, they typically include a focus on means restriction, self-soothing, coping strategies, distraction techniques, methods for seeking relational support, and how to seek professional help if needed in a life-or-death situation. Within CAMS-guided care, stabilization planning is the first step in developing a larger suicide-specific treatment plan. Over the course of CAMS-guided care, stabilization planning is routinely revisited along with the systematic treatment of patient-defined suicidal drivers within each session until the patient meets CAMS criteria for clinical resolution (i.e., three consecutive sessions where the overall suicide risk is meaningfully reduced and any remaining suicidal thoughts or feelings are effectively and reliably managed).

Stabilization planning can be done in a variety of ways, and the CAMS clinician is free to be creative with coping interventions that make sense. On the front end of CAMS stabilization planning, there is an initial and primary focus on the importance of reducing access to lethal means. It is the essential first step for effective stabilization planning. In many cases, this focus centers on literally securing and/or removing lethal means from the patient's direct access or environment. For example, a gun must be transferred to a trusted friend or dismantled; a stash of pills must similarly be removed from the patient's reach. Bryan, Stone, and Rudd (2011) have thoughtful ideas about using a "receipt" to verify the removal of means signed by a third party; alternatively, a third party can leave a message on the clinician's voicemail verifying the means have been removed. For means that cannot be literally removed from the patient's environment (e.g., jumping or carbon monoxide), efforts can focus on reducing access to those locations by avoiding a particular bridge or ensuring car keys are kept secure by a spouse when the car is not in use. While removing or blocking access to lethal means is sometimes not possible, creating a psychological buffer can reduce the risk of impulsive attempts and it demonstrates a good-faith effort by the patient to take some responsibility for reducing lethal temptations.

Within CAMS-guided care, the collaborative discussion of means restriction is often a moment of truth between the patient and clinician; it tests the resolve of both parties to join forces for a discrete period of time to earnestly embrace a goal of saving the patient's life from suicide. It can be a tense and contentious discussion. Patients often refer to the stash of pills as the "security blanket" and actually feel frightened by the prospect of not having their lethal stash to fall back on if needed. The CAMS clinician must empathically appreciate the attachment to this kind of comfort, but gently challenge patients to consider an alternative comfort that does not cost them their life. I often say that the access to lethal means is *competition* to a life-saving treatment like CAMS. To me, the good-faith willingness to remove or decrease access to lethal means is a critical milestone in the therapeutic relationship. Alternatively, intransigence on removing or decreasing access to lethal means might call into question the viability of proceeding in outpatient clinical care. Sometimes a standoff on this issue may necessarily take us down an unpleasant path to pursue a voluntary or even involuntary inpatient hospitalization; something I am loath to do for all but for the most lethal situations.

Beyond securing lethal means, it is also important to ensure that the patient has a specific plan in place in case suicidal ideation or urges arise. One way to accomplish this is through the use of a coping hierarchy. On the CAMS Stabilization Plan, we work to generate five responses to the prompt "Things I can do to cope differently when I am in a suicide crisis." These types of things usually include different distracting or redirecting behaviors, ways of seeking support, or specific activities that engage the patient if they feel unstable. Such coping strategies can be listed on the form or perhaps transferred to the back of the clinician's business card, which is small enough to fit in a wallet or purse pocket so that the patient can have ready access to the crisis card at all times. Others in the field have written eloquently about coping strategies (e.g., Linehan, 2014; Najavits, 2002).

Generally speaking, this coping-oriented strategy fits nicely into the CAMS philosophy of collaborative empowerment of the patient. Specifically, in the course of treatment planning, it is important that the patient know that there is a reliable preplanned stepped approach to coping with a difficult situation should an emergency situation arise between sessions. On the appropriate section of the CAMS Stabilization Plan I propose that we come up with five things the patient can do should a crisis occur. Ideally, these ideas come from the patient and must be protherapeutic, typically involving behavioral activation and different distraction techniques. For example, going out and getting drunk is not an acceptable item for the stabilization plan. Alternatively, activities such as exercising, therapeutic writing, or talking to a supportive friend are all excellent examples of helpful coping strategies. If the patient is stuck with no good ideas, I chime in with some suggestions. Indeed, patients can sometimes get upset about being stumped by reflections on healthy coping. Often a patient coping repertoire amounts to drinking or getting stoned, which of course is problematic. Consequently for patients who are discouraged, I simply acknowledge the obvious: saving your life will require developing a tool kit for coping differently and better. I then jump in and begin to propose various tried and true coping strategies, encouraging the patient to give them a try so that we can see what works and what does not work. What follows is short list of protherapeutic coping strategies that I have routinely seen work with suicidal patients:

1. Going for a walk
2. Writing in a journal
3. Taking a hot bath
4. Doing my nails
5. Watching some sports on TV
6. Walking my dog
7. Listening to music
8. E-mailing a supportive friend
9. Taking a nap
10. Doing some artwork
11. Reading one of my therapeutic books
12. Brushing out my hair 100 times
13. Going to church to pray
14. Meditating
15. Playing a video game
16. Reading a magazine
17. Watching the Animal Planet channel on TV
18. Writing a letter to an old friend

19. Playing Sudoku
20. Watching YouTube videos

This list represents the kinds of activities that one looks for on a sensible stabilization plan—protherapeutic activities that engage, redirect, and behaviorally activate the patient to self-soothe or engage others. Critically, after the process of identifying five coping strategies, I rather ceremoniously add a sixth item: an emergency phone number where the patient can receive direct clinical care. In my own case, this is my business phone number or personal cell number (my own "usual and customary" practice, but not for everyone I know). For those working in an agency with coverage or hospital centers, this number may be an emergency coverage number. In the United States we can offer the National Lifeline number (800–273–TALK) with well-trained crisis center paraprofessionals in a crisis care system that is supported by an evolving evidence base (Gould, Kalafat, Harris-Munfakh, & Kleinman, 2007; Gould, Munfakh, Kleinman, & Lake, 2012). Clinicians may feel conflicted about giving access to their personal phone, which I most certainly understand. Yet I find when this number is offered as part of a life-saving treatment and properly contextualized as *privilege,* it is not abused as much as one might think. Across the evidence base of effective clinical treatments, providing means for reaching out for support when coping fails is axiomatic (e.g., Linehan, 1993a, 1993b; Wenzel et al., 2009).

Whatever the case, it is my strong contention that there should be a way for a suicidal patient to access a clinician or paraprofessional in the event of a true emergency. In relation to this topic, I routinely say to the patient something along the lines of:

"Okay, this is your suicide coping list—a critical component of your stabilization plan. Your commitment to me and to your overall treatment is that you will do each item on this coping list should you find yourself in a crisis state— feeling impulsive, really upset, or suicidal. The goal here is for you to learn to cope in different ways than you are used to and to develop ways of getting out of trouble on your own. If you do each of these items on your coping list and you are still in a crisis state, then you contact me on my cell phone. If I do not respond or answer, you can leave a voicemail and I will typically get back to you as soon as possible. But if you still need to talk to someone immediately, call the Lifeline and they will help you until I can get back to you. The point is that I am interested in being available to you if you are in a true life-or-death emergency state. You will know that the situation is a true emergency by virtue of having gone through all five ways of coping on your list and you feel that you are still in serious, life-threatening trouble. To be clear, you are only to call me after you have done the five preceding coping ideas; if none of those seems to work, then you know to contact me."

The beauty of this suicide coping list approach is that it clearly communicates a crucial therapeutic message to the patient: You *can* learn to cope with your crises; if that does not work, I will endeavor to be directly available to you for true emergency support. Rudd and colleagues (2001) conceptualize this as self-regulation training—the five crisis coping items are designed to improve the patient's *internal* resources to manage a crisis before turning to *external resources*—direct engagement of professionals or paraprofessionals. These are cardinal features of Stanley and Brown's (2012) safety plan intervention as well. The treatment idea here emphasizes the importance of the patient developing a "thicker psychological skin," to better withstand the ups and downs of life—the disappointments, hurts, and injuries that happen to us all. Earnestly using a predeveloped suicide coping list is an excellent way for the patient to directly learn about developing a thicker psychological skin.

When I discuss the use of the suicide coping list at my professional workshops, I am often asked whether patients actually use this strategy—what is to stop them from skipping items 1–5 and going right to calling me directly? In response, I note that the vast majority of patients use the intervention appropriately if it properly presented and framed. Although all patients may not use it perfectly, most catch on to the intent of the strategy, which in part is to help clarify for the patient what is and what is not a mental health emergency. In more than 25 years of clinical practice I have only been forced to change my unlisted number twice, not an inordinate number given how many suicidal patients I have worked with over these years.

As an elaboration of the suicide coping list idea, I sometimes transfer the list to the flip side of my business card, creating a Crisis Card that is more easily transportable. Carrying such a card has been highly effective for many of my patients over the years, many times in different and unexpected ways. For example, many years ago I worked with a patient who simply took out the card and looked at the items, which made her feel better. She did not do any of the coping items; just looking at the card was all she needed. Another example involves a teenage patient whose eyes filled with tears when we completed the card. She could not believe that I cared so much that I was willing to give my personal phone number. Another successful use of the Crisis Card approach was by a patient who was completely skeptical about using the intervention. The weekend following our developing her Crisis Card was marked by a series of conflicts and disappointments. She warily took out her card and began marching through each item, certain that this effort was a complete waste of time and that she would soon be calling me as the only option to deal with her evolving crisis. This patient first took a walk and then had a long talk with her roommate—neither helped. In good faith she pursued item 3, which was to take a nap. She stretched out on her bed at 7:00 P.M. and much to her shock, woke up the following morning at 7:00 A.M.—a 12-hour nap! She could barely wait to tell me in our next session that the Crisis Card had worked exceptionally well—she had gotten through a tough night on her own when she was virtually certain that she was going to need to call me. I would further note that carrying a card may not be necessary if the patient takes a picture of the stabilization plan and coping list on a smartphone to access as needed.

The CAMS Stabilization Plan also seeks to strengthen relational supports within the patient's life. The dyad can note names of supportive friends, family, clergy, and so on who might play a supportive role. Contact information can be recorded and a release can be obtained to contact these people in case it is necessary to locate the patient or deal with an acute suicidal crisis.

Finally, as with any effective intervention, it is essential that the patient attend sessions regularly and not drop out prematurely. Even with the best of intentions, practical issues may interfere with reliably attending treatment. It is therefore important in the initial session to identify as many barriers to treatment as possible and brainstorm strategies to address them. For instance, with low-income patients, access to bus passes or other transportation may be needed. Alternatively, sessions may need to be scheduled when a substance abuse patient is least likely to be intoxicated or when a patient with insomnia is most likely to be alert. Talking in advance about strategies for dealing with potential barriers to care is thus important.

Problems #2 and #3 and the Treatment of Suicidal Drivers

Beyond the obvious importance of establishing a thoughtful stabilization plan, CAMS "driver-oriented" treatment properly begins in the first session, when the clinician asks the patient to identify Problem #2 and Problem #3 in Section C of the SSF. The patient should identify these problems as the two foremost concerns that fundamentally compel him or her to consider suicide. Identifying these two suicide-causing problems in the first session thus launches an ongoing clinical discussion across CAMS-guided care of what exactly contributes the patient's risk for suicide. Within CAMS-guided care it is important to "connect the dots" in the suicidal patient's thought process. In other words, there are legitimate reasons at the root of any suicidal state. In CAMS, our goal is to effectively identify and thoroughly flesh out and understand these reasons for suicide. Then we clinically endeavor to treat these reasons such that the patient no longer needs to take his or her life because these particular causes for suicide have been therapeutically eliminated.

The two patient-identified "suicidogenic" problems are thus noted in the SSF treatment-planning section with corresponding treatment-related goals/objectives and various proposed interventions that can be used to treat these problems, respectively. For example, a traumatized combat veteran may say, "My combat-related PTSD and my marriage falling apart make me want to kill myself." In such a case, the CAMS clinician might work with the patient to develop corresponding goals and objectives related to decreasing PTSD-related distress with appropriate interventions (e.g., with prolonged exposure or cognitive processing therapy). The failing marriage would have related goals and objectives for improving communication and saving the marriage, which could prompt treatment interventions of communications skills and the initiation of couple therapy. As a final treatment-planning consideration, the potential "dose" of care is noted under duration (e.g., four sessions, or 3 months of one session per week—whatever seems reasonable to address the problem).

Within ongoing CAMS care these major problems typically continue to evolve as we further develop the idea of "suicidal drivers." This will be discussed in more depth further on, but generally speaking, suicidal drivers within CAMS-guided care are of two types. There are "direct drivers" of suicide, which are psychological forces idiosyncratic to the patient (e.g., various thoughts, feelings, and behaviors) that may propel the patient into acute suicidal states. In other words, direct drivers are patient-specific idiosyncratic suicide warning signs (Tucker et al., 2015). Suicidal patients are not acutely suicidal 24 hours a day/7 days a week. Instead, there are moments when a suicidal person's direct drivers are triggered or engaged, placing him or her on the path to suicidal coping. In contrast, "indirect drivers" of suicide are those issues or stressors that regularly influence the patient but are not immediately connected to acute suicidal states. Examples of potential indirect drivers might be homelessness, unemployment, or even mental illness—stressors that are in the patients' lives, yet do not necessarily propel them to suicide. Nevertheless, indirect drivers can make the patient feel vulnerable to either the insidious or sudden activation of direct drivers that may catapult the patient into an acute suicidal crisis. In any case, driver-oriented treatment is a signature treatment approach that is unique to CAMS-guided care and is discussed further in Chapter 6.

Commitment to Treatment

A final step on the heels of successful CAMS treatment planning in the first session is the notation (Yes or No) for two final treatment plan items: (1) "Patient understands and concurs with treatment plan?" and (2) "Patient is at imminent danger of suicide (hospitalization indicated)?" If these are answered "Yes" and "No," respectively, the patient is asked to sign at the bottom of Section C, as will the clinician. In turn, the patient will be given a photocopy/printout of the first and second page of the SSF along with his or her CAMS Stabilization Plan and then is free to go. We routinely encourage the patient to create a file folder of the copied SSF documents. In our Army randomized controlled trial, we customarily had the clinicians ask the soldiers to fold up the forms from each session and place them in their utility pocket on their sleeve. My favorite patient in the study would subsequently post his SSFs on the refrigerator at home and review with his wife his most recent SSF assessments and driver-oriented treatment plans after each session. His wife was reassured that her husband's suicidal risk was being routinely tracked and treated, and she proved to be a great ally over the course of his care. Again, hard copies of the SSF may not be needed if patients keep pictures of these documents on their smartphones, a consideration that may be especially relevant to younger patients.

If collaborative efforts to negotiate stabilization plans go poorly, and the patient seems highly ambivalent about pursuing an outpatient course of suicide-specific treatment, then the clinician may be compelled to initiate an inpatient psychiatric hospitalization. But again, within CAMS-guided care, hospitalization is the last resort (vs. the first response), and this course of action can be noted at the bottom of the treatment plan section and on the HIPAA page as well.

A WORD ABOUT SELF-HARM

This chapter on the treatment of suicide would be remiss if it did not attend to the ubiquity of self-harm behaviors that often interface with suicidal risk in complex ways. As many clinicians encounter, there is a wide range of self-harming behaviors in which many patients engage. These behaviors may be indirectly self-harming—for example, my VA patient who smoked three packs of cigarettes and drank a fifth of vodka per day, routinely driving in excess of 100 miles per hour on the Washington beltway. Other behaviors may be much more directly self-harming, such as an inpatient I worked with whose arms were shredded by severe cutting, leaving large welting scars and permanent damage to her ligaments and tendons. Her chest and legs were also covered with scars of severe self-administered cigarette burns. Historically, these notorious behaviors were referred to as "parasuicidal" behaviors; more recently, the term "nonsuicidal self-injury" (NSSI) has been proposed and appears in the exploratory section of DSM-5 (American Psychiatric Association, 2013). While self-harm behaviors can prove to be nightmarish to practitioners, these behaviors are not typically intended to end the patient's life. For example, many patients with borderline personality disorder experience highly dissociative states that they can rapidly and dramatically remit using cutting behaviors. In such cases, a person can feel terribly lost and disconnected from reality, and the cutting functionally serves to reconnect the person with reality. Obviously, the "functional" cost of the disfiguring behavior is extremely problematic. Nevertheless, these behaviors can be exceptionally seductive to certain suffering patients. But similar to an addictive drug, there is a distinct "high" connected with these behaviors, as well as psychological habituation and withdrawal. Patients often find they must cut more and deeper to get the same effect, and it is hard to quit cutting or burning once one is hooked on the behavior (American Psychiatric Association, 2013; Nock & Prinstein, 2004).

While self-harm behaviors are not suicidal per se, they are obviously problematic and not altogether disconnected from actual suicidal behaviors. Unfortunately, there tends to be a tricky and significant degree of overlap between self-harm and frank suicidal thinking and behaviors. Sometimes, patients engage in NSSI and may get carried away or miscalculate behaviorally. Moreover, while individuals with borderline personality disorder are infamous for frequently engaging in sublethal self-harm, they also may suffer terribly, become acutely suicidal, make attempts, and die by suicide. This complex overlap can be quite confusing and exceptionally challenging from a clinical perspective.

The CAMS approach was not specifically developed to work effectively with self-harm per se; rather, CAMS is better suited to working with issues of suicidal ideation and behaviors. In cases in which the patient's suicidal risk is confounded with various self-harm behaviors, it is important to try to assess and treat both the suicidality and the sublethal self-harm behaviors. In this sense it is my recommendation that a separate self-injury treatment strategy be layered into the CAMS treatment plan. In this regard, I would recommend the outstanding treatment approaches developed by Linehan (1993a, 1993b, 2014) and Walsh (2014); each provide excellent and practical ideas pertaining to clinical care and treatment of self-harm behaviors.

FILLING OUT SECTION D OF THE SSF:
THE HIPAA PAGE

Section D of the SSF used in the first session is generally referred to as the "HIPAA page"—it is the page of the SSF that includes the main elements of what is required according to the Health Insurance Portability and Accountability Act (U.S. Department of Health and Human Services, 1996). HIPAA is a federal law that describes key aspects of clinical record keeping, particularly in relation to the maintenance and completion of the "medical record." Consequently, the full documentation of the CAMS-guided assessment and treatment planning requires the completion of this documentation after the session has occurred.

While there are different uses of the SSF across clinical settings, my clear recommendation is to use the SSF documentation as *the* medical record for high-risk suicidal patients. To this end, the use of the SSF HIPAA form clearly completes a full and comprehensive medical record for suicidal patients over the course of a suicide-specific treatment. Once the patient meets CAMS criteria for "resolution" (or other outcomes and dispositions), the intervention can be discontinued; the clinician can revert to the routinely used medical record documentation. In my view, use of the SSF is the best approach for creating a thorough suicide-specific level of documentation, which invariably helps to significantly decrease the potential for malpractice liability (see Chapter 8). The following brief discussions of the main features of the SSF HIPAA page should further clarify the importance of this particular aspect of CAMS-related medical record documentation.

Mental Status Exam

Under HIPAA guidelines there is an expectation that mental health clinicians will routinely assess and document information related to the patient's mental status. Within Section D of the first-session SSF, the evaluation of mental status is made relatively simple, such that the clinician needs only to circle certain items and add a few words of explanation. Please note for those not familiar with psychiatry shorthand, "WNL" stands for "within normal limits."

DSM/ICD Diagnostic Impressions

Even though I have critiqued the overemphasis on diagnosis in relation to suicide risk (Jobes, 2000), I am not anti-diagnosis by any means. Diagnoses are crucial for giving clinicians a common language and understanding the treatment possibilities and prognosis. It was therefore important to be able to record diagnostic impressions within the nosology's of the DSM-5 (American Psychiatric Association, 2013) or the International Classification of Diseases, Tenth Revision (ICD-10; World Health Organization, 1992) diagnostic systems.

Overall Suicide Risk Level

It is also important from a clinical conceptualization perspective to make a professional judgment about the patient's overall suicidal risk (Maltsberger, 1994). At the end of the assessment day, the clinician must make an informed judgment about the relative risk of suicide and document that clinical formulation in a clear and definitive fashion. As noted in Chapter 2, there are data that can greatly inform this judgment. Based on the empirical work conducted on Wish to Live versus Wish to Die and Reasons for Living versus Reasons for Dying (Brown et al., 2005; Corona et al., 2013; Jennings, 2015), there is a data-informed way to judge the patient's overall risk in terms of those lower-risk suicidal patients who remain attached to living (i.e., high wish to live and more reasons for living than dying). In contrast, there are the moderately at-risk patients (i.e., their relative ratings of wish to live vs. die and reasons for living and dying are essentially equal). Finally, there is the high-risk group that is more attached to dying than living (i.e., more wish to die and more reasons for dying than for living). These are not the only reference points for thinking about the three reliable tiers of overall risk, but these data should be duly considered when formulating and documenting the overall risk of prospective suicide.

Case Notes

Finally, the clinician should routinely write a case note related to overall issues of diagnosis, functional status, treatment plan, symptoms, prognosis, and progress to date. This entry should be akin to a general progress note that would routinely be entered into a standard medical record.

CASE EXAMPLE:
FIRST-SESSION TREATMENT PLANNING WITH BILL

After successfully working through the CAMS SSF assessment sections (A and B), treatment planning with Bill proved to be a bit contentious at the outset. On the one hand, Bill made it clear that he prefers to not be hospitalized. On the other hand, when we embarked on developing his CAMS Stabilization Plan, he strongly balked at my insistence of securing his guns as a necessary first step to keeping him *out* of the hospital. The conversation went as follows:

CLINICIAN: Okay, great, we have learned so much important information about your suicidal pain and suffering . . . now as we shift our attention to your treatment plan, I would like for us to find a way to safely keep you out of the hospital if at all possible.

BILL: Damn right, I have zero interest in going to the loony bin!

CLINICIAN: Fair enough, it sounds like we share this goal . . . but to keep you out of the hospital we have to carefully develop a stabilization plan, and as you can see, this plan begins with reducing access to your lethal means, which in this case would require securing your all your firearms . . .

BILL: (*visibly angry*) Now hold on, you are not taking away my guns, I know my Second Amendment rights! These are my guns and no shrink—no offense, doc—or government agent is taking away my constitutional right to bear arms!

CLINICIAN: (*long pause, calm but firm*) Now Bill, let me be clear, this is not a constitutional issue, this is not about your legal rights . . . this is about saving your life! And I am not going to debate your constitutional right to own firearms. But I have a solemn duty as a licensed provider under the laws of my jurisdiction to protect a patient of mine from clear and imminent danger to self and others. And in my judgment based on our assessment here, you may well pose just such a danger to yourself right now!

BILL: (*less angry*) Yeah, things are really a mess and I have been feeling really desperate . . .

CLINICIAN: I hear that and I see that, and yet something brought you here in spite of everything! Shouldn't we try to honor the part of you that brought you in and try to do what we can to save your life? You see right now, that handgun in your desk drawer is competing with our potentially life-saving treatment, and we need to remove that temptation if we intend to save your life . . . I can say without a doubt that this treatment doesn't work if you shoot yourself!

BILL: (*chuckling softly*) Yeah, I guess that makes sense, you got a point there . . .

CLINICIAN: Okay, so to keep you out of the hospital, we need to make your situation and your environment is less lethal, which means securing your firearms for, say, the next 3 months while we try to save your life with our treatment. In addition, I want you to seriously cut back on—or stop altogether—your drinking, because it clearly puts you at more risk. You have told me that your most suicidal moments are when you are intoxicated, right? I am just asking for 3 months of earnest mutual work to save your life. You really have everything to gain and nothing to lose.

BILL: (*calmer and conciliatory*) Yeah, I see what you are saying . . . okay I'm on board for now, but this is really hard for me. How do you propose we deal with my guns?

While this interaction is a bit testy, it is nevertheless an example of a clinician asserting a life-saving treatment agenda that is unequivocally in the patient's best interest. Moreover, it also illustrates what I call "therapist backbone"—the firm resolve, even insistence, on working in the patient's best interest in accordance with the law, professional ethics, empirical research, and the best clinical practices. As noted earlier, clinicians too often back down in the face of suicidal blackmail, which is neither in the best interest of the patient nor the clinician (Jobes, 2011). Fortunately, Bill rather quickly saw the light in the face of my resolve around this agenda. But if we had not satisfactorily negotiated this crucial issue, I may have moved to hospitalize Bill either voluntarily or even involuntarily, given his obvious high risk and potential lethality. Importantly, Bill called his brother on his cell phone during our session to stop by his house to pick up all his guns later that evening, and he agreed to leave me a voicemail by 9:00 P.M. to verify that the guns had been removed. While his brother seemed curious about this request, he did not hesitate to agree, and I felt comfortable within my budding alliance that this would indeed be done and trusted his leaving a voicemail to verify. But I nevertheless said that if I did not get this verification call, I would interpret that behavior as a clear and imminent emergency and call the police to intervene accordingly. Bill understood these conditions, and the voicemail verification indeed came around 6:00 P.M., with Bill noting that he actually felt relieved!

With this important and contentious issue behind us, Bill's affect actually brightened slightly as we worked through the stabilization plan together. As shown in Figure 5.2, one can see that Bill's proposed coping strategies involved a lot of behavioral activation and distracting techniques. As part of my customary practice, I gave Bill both my personal cell phone number (with my discussion

CAMS STABILIZATION PLAN

Ways to reduce access to lethal means:

1. *give guns to my brother — will leave voicemail by 9:00 P.M.*

2. *decrease my drinking/consider AA?*

3. _____

Things I can do to cope differently when I am in a suicide crisis (consider crisis card):

1. *take dog for a walk*

2. *watch ESPN*

3. *go out and shoot some hoops*

4. *do some journaling*

5. *try to talk to my wife or kids*

6. **Life or death emergency contact number:** *555-123-4567   DJ cell*
   Lifeline 800-273-TALK

People I can call for help or to decrease my isolation:

1. *my brother*

2. *my neighbor Fred*

3. _____

Attending treatment as scheduled:

Potential barrier: Solutions I will try:

1. *I'll come*   *(not applicable)*

2. _____

FIGURE 5.2. Bill's stabilization plan.

of privilege and its use in a true emergency) and the National Lifeline number (800–273–TALK) as well.

Buoyed by the completion of a sensible stabilization plan, we moved to consider Bill's two primary treatment problems (see Figure 5.3). Without hesitation, Bill stated that the two problems that put his life at risk were (1) his failing marriage (Problem #2) and (2) his hopelessness (Problem #3). As you can see, my proposed treatment interventions for these two suicidal problems/drivers included possible couple therapy, some insight-oriented and supportive psychotherapy, behavioral activation, and some specific hope-related interventions that would be pursued over 3 months of CAMS-guided treatment.

In addition, Bill's completed HIPAA page from our first session of CAMS can be seen in Figure 5.4.

SUMMARY AND CONCLUSIONS

This chapter has traversed the philosophy and the concrete clinical procedures of suicide-specific (driver-oriented) treatment planning that is a hallmark feature of CAMS-guided care. I hope it is plain that CAMS emphasizes a fundamentally different approach to the entire clinical endeavor of working with suicidal risk. As noted throughout this chapter, CAMS can be used across theoretical orientations and clinical techniques; the approach is designed to accommodate the full spectrum of treatments that clinicians may use to treat the patient's self-defined

Section C (Clinician):   **TREATMENT PLAN**

Problem #	Problem Description	Goals and Objectives	Interventions	Duration
1	Self-Harm Potential	Safety and Stability	Stabilization Plan Completed ☑	3 mo.
2	failing marriage	save marriage improve communication	couples therapy, insight, CBT, BA therapy	3 mo.
3	hopeless	↑ hope	Hope Kit, read "Choosing to Live"	3 mo.

YES ✔ NO ____   Patient understands and concurs with treatment plan?

YES ____ NO ✔   Patient at imminent danger of suicide (hospitalization indicated)?

FIGURE 5.3. Bill's SSF Section C treatment plan.

Section D (*Clinician Postsession Evaluation*):

MENTAL STATUS EXAM (Circle appropriate items):

ALERTNESS: (ALERT) DROWSY LETHARGIC STUPOROUS

OTHER: _____

ORIENTED TO: (PERSON) (PLACE) (TIME) (REASON FOR EVALUATION)

MOOD: (EUTHYMIC) ELEVATED DYSPHORIC AGITATED ANGRY

AFFECT: FLAT BLUNTED CONSTRICTED (APPROPRIATE) LABILE

THOUGHT CONTINUITY: (CLEAR & COHERENT) GOAL-DIRECTED TANGENTIAL CIRCUMSTANTIAL

OTHER: _____

THOUGHT CONTENT: (WNL) OBSESSIONS DELUSIONS IDEAS OF REFERENCE BIZARRENESS MORBIDITY

OTHER: _____

ABSTRACTION: (WNL) NOTABLY CONCRETE

OTHER: _____

SPEECH: (WNL) RAPID SLOW SLURRED IMPOVERISHED INCOHERENT

OTHER: _____

MEMORY: (GROSSLY INTACT)

OTHER: _____

REALITY TESTING: (WNL)

OTHER: _____

NOTABLE BEHAVIORAL OBSERVATIONS: *generally cooperative, testy around gun issue*

DIAGNOSTIC IMPRESSIONS/DIAGNOSIS (DSM/ICD DIAGNOSES):

deferred
R/O major depression, generalized anxiety
monitor alcohol use and insomnia

PATIENT'S OVERALL SUICIDE RISK LEVEL (Check one and explain):

☐ **LOW (WTL/RFL)** **Explanation:**
☑ **MODERATE (AMB)** *Fairly high risk, but is on board with CAMS treatment,*
☐ **HIGH (WTD/RFD)** *giving gun to his brother decreases his risk*

CASE NOTES:
Bill is a 50-year-old white male who complains of marital distress and hopelessness.
Poor mental health compliance. He is depressed and is drinking. He is willing to give up
his gun and give CAMS a go. Explore the use of couples therapy, possible Rx, CBT,
Behavioral Activation.

Next Appointment Scheduled: _____ Treatment Modality: _____

Clinican Signature Date

FIGURE 5.4. Bill's Section D HIPAA page.

suicidal drivers. Within CAMS, the first-session engagement and process is critical to success over the course of care. CAMS treatment-planning success rests on successful engagement and the initial collaborative assessment of suicidal risk that is guided by the SSF. Administered side-by-side with the patient, the assessment process in CAMS is meant to underscore the importance of a team approach to care wherein the clinician sees things through the patient's eyes. Subsequently, this unique assessment sets the stage for the development of a suicide-specific treatment plan that includes establishing a stabilization plan and identifying problems that cause the patient's suicidality. As noted, the SSF documentation is crucial to clinical success within CAMS care, and this thorough documentation is formally concluded by completion of the HIPAA page of the SSF after each CAMS session. The collaborative spirit of CAMS is sparked in the index session, launching a non-adversarial treatment trajectory and the formation of a strong clinical alliance. When well formed, this clinical alliance has the power to inspire both hope and crucial motivation within patients to discover new and better ways to meet their legitimate needs as the drivers of their suicidal risk are therapeutically targeted and treated in the course of CAMS-guided clinical care.

CHAPTER 6

CAMS Interim Sessions

Tracking Suicide Risk Assessments and Treatment Plan Updates

Within CAMS-guided care, there is a great deal of focus on the first session. As noted earlier, future dismantling studies of CAMS will likely underscore the importance of the first session with its emphasis on empathic and collaborative assessment and treatment planning. Still, CAMS is much more than just the first session. Upon reflection, as the development of the intervention matures, what happens within the "interim sessions" of CAMS is now becoming better understood and is increasingly more central to successful CAMS care. To be clear, the interim sessions are those that follow the first session and precede the final "outcome-disposition" session. There is no prescribed number of CAMS interim sessions. There are as many interim sessions as necessary to realize CAMS resolution criteria or other clinical outcomes and dispositions (as I discuss in depth in Chapter 7). From the perspective of our clinical research, we know that the vast majority of CAMS cases will resolve within 12 sessions (Jobes, 2012), with the modal response occurring in six to eight sessions (e.g., Comtois et al., 2011; Jobes, Kahn-Greene, et al., 2009). Subsequent to the first edition of this book, perhaps no part of CAMS has evolved more than what is done during the interim sessions as we continue to research, develop, and clinically craft what constitutes CAMS "driver-oriented" treatment and intervention (Jobes et al., 2011, 2016).

We will first consider a broad overview of how to adherently conduct CAMS interim sessions before shifting attention to how we more specifically target and treat patient-defined suicidal drivers across the course of CAMS interim care. Within this discussion, we will also examine the optional use of the CAMS Therapeutic Worksheet (CTW), which can be used to further flesh out and focus CAMS driver-oriented treatment (see Appendix E). Finally, the chapter ends with a review of the CAMS interim sessions for our case study of Bill.

OVERVIEW TO CAMS INTERIM SESSIONS

While there is still an overall structure to adherently conducting all CAMS interim sessions, this intervention embraces a flexible, adaptive, and nondenominational approach to clinical treatment of suicidal risk that makes CAMS care unique in comparison to other evidence-based approaches to suicide prevention. Instead of following a highly structured step-by-step manual-defined approach (e.g., Wenzel et al., 2009), CAMS-guided clinical care is characterized by adherence to broad components of ongoing suicide-specific care. CAMS interim sessions begin with tracking the ongoing suicide risk and end with a treatment plan update that involves both the further refinement of the CAMS Stabilization Plan and the "sharpening" of patient-defined suicidal problem/drivers and evolving corresponding interventions.

Interim Tracking of CAMS Suicide Risk Assessment

Following the first CAMS session, described at length in the preceding chapters, every CAMS interim session begins with a relatively quick SSF-guided check-in pertaining to current suicidal risk. The clinician thus starts sessions by handing a copy of the SSF Interim Session form (page 4 of the SSF-4) to the patient. The dyad specifically focuses on Section A of the document, entitled CAMS Suicide Status Form–4 (SSF-4)—Tracking/Update (Interim Session). The patient completes the SSF Core Assessment at the start of each interim session. This usually takes about 30 seconds and can be done side-by-side or from a normal seating position. Whether you change seating positions to update the Core Assessment each session is up to you, but interim sessions should end with the side-by-side seating arrangement for updating the CAMS treatment plan. Upon completion of the SSF Core Assessment, there is a need to thoroughly review and discuss the patient's ratings of pain, stress, agitation, hopelessness, self-hate, and overall risk of suicide. Many clinicians (and patients) value reviewing the SSF Core Assessment items from session to session to track relative progress or setbacks over the course of care. The routine ratings of the SSF Core Assessment are akin to taking the patient's suicidal "vital signs" at the beginning of each session, and patients quickly become familiar with and often come to prize this assessment routine. In our Seattle study, there was a schizophrenic patient with an extensive abuse history who appreciated both the focus and concreteness of completing and reviewing the SSF Core Assessment in each session and then comparing his ratings across the course of his care. I would hasten to point out that many recent studies emphasize the clinical importance of treatment-progress monitoring as a valuable component of evidence-based assessment and clinical care across the spectrum of psychotherapy (Dozois et al.,

2014; Hunsely, 2015). These studies underscore the utility of progress monitoring for clinicians. For example, this kind of monitoring offsets clinicians' tendency to overestimate positive treatment outcomes and helps inform case conceptualization and treatment planning. There is also clear therapeutic value in progress monitoring for patients (Lambert & Shimokawa, 2011; Unsworth, Cowie, & Green, 2011).

Naturally, we hope to see the ratings of the SSF Core Assessment drop over the course of CAMS care. For some patients, there can be rapid reductions on certain ratings; for others, some constructs may change while others remain relatively static. Within CAMS-guided care, there is a particular set of SSF-based ratings to which we pay particular attention because they directly relate to criteria for "resolving" CAMS as a desired and optimal clinical outcome. Specifically, discontinuation of CAMS is based on the *three consecutive sessions* wherein the following three SSF-based criteria are obtained:

1. The patient rates either "0" or "1" on the final SSF Core Assessment ("Rate Overall Risk of Suicide") over three consecutive sessions.
2. The patient reports "Yes" on the SSF-based query " Managed Thoughts/ Feelings" (in the past week) over three consecutive sessions.
3. The patient reports "No" on the SSF-based query "Suicidal Behavior" (in the past week) over three consecutive sessions.

In contrast to the resolution criteria described in the first edition of this book, the CAMS resolution criteria that we now use have been modified based on our clinical trial research. We came to appreciate that the previous criteria developed as part of the initial use of the SSF (Jobes et al., 1997) were just too extreme: *three consecutive sessions of no suicidal thoughts, feelings, and behaviors.* While the spirit of these original criteria has been retained, we observed that CAMS patients can meaningfully "resolve" and move on from CAMS without using such absolute and extreme criteria (i.e., the complete "exorcism" of suicidality). In contrast, these newer criteria for resolving CAMS emphasize *managing* suicidal thoughts and feelings—distinctly turning away from a reliance on suicidal coping—or, in the words of one suicidal soldier who was successfully treated in our CAMS randomized controlled trial at Ft. Stewart, "When I first came suicide filled my windshield, but I have come to see that suicide is not the best way to deal. So now it's like suicide is behind me, in my rearview mirror—I can still see it, but it is fading away as I drive forward by getting better!"

Hence a CAMS clinician can "tolerate" occasional suicidal thoughts even in the course of resolving CAMS. We must be mindful that for many patients suicidal thoughts have been around for many years, much like an unwelcome but still present "old friend" from childhood. It is therefore unrealistic to aspire to the complete elimination of such thoughts in the course of a dozen sessions. Notably, this modification is consistent with the mindfulness-based therapy mindset, in which the ability to gain awareness, acceptance, and remain "unhooked" by unwanted thoughts is the goal rather than to completely eliminate such thoughts. Accordingly, the key to CAMS resolution is the effective and sustained management of suicidal thoughts (and related behaviors) and moving toward a full embrace of adaptive coping and living, thereby leaving behind suicidal coping and an overall attachment to suicide. While the particulars of CAMS resolution criteria have shifted based on clinical trial research, the value of using three consecutive sessions to demarcate resolution has not changed. Across decades of clinical studies of CAMS, three consecutive sessions has held up well in terms of defining resolution, with a small number of SSF-defined resolved cases relapsing. From our various clinical trials of CAMS I would estimate fewer than 10% of resolved cases relapse (Jobes, 2012).

Given this discussion, the CAMS clinician closely tracks the patient's ongoing and shifting experience of his or her attachment to suicide and overall management of suicidal thoughts, feelings, and behaviors. For many cases, there is a steady and linear reduction on the SSF Core Assessment ratings as criteria for resolution are relatively quickly achieved. For some other cases, a suicidal patient may be tracked for many sessions until criteria for resolution are obtained. I once tracked a chronically suicidal patient in my private practice for 63 sessions until criteria for resolution were realized—a momentous accomplishment for this particular patient! Generally speaking, the SSF Core Assessment ratings often wax and wane but tend to move in a therapeutic direction in the course of adherent and effective CAMS-guided care. Sometimes there will be two consecutive sessions wherein resolution seems on the horizon, only to have a setback that dashes that prospect, which means restarting the resolution "clock" to work toward the three-session criteria again. In some other cases, criteria for CAMS resolution are clearly met, but at the clinician's discretion, the patient may continue for another session or two beyond the third session of CAMS resolution to fully safeguard that the apparent resolution outcome holds firm. In any event, every interim session of CAMS-guided care is defined by the initial check-in on the SSF Core Assessment with a continuous and watchful eye to the CAMS resolution criteria that define clinical outcomes and dispositions within CAMS-guided clinical care.

Interim Treatment Plan Updating

After completing the initial assessment, all interim sessions mostly focus on treating problems/drivers. All CAMS interim sessions end with a side-by-side reconsideration of the suicide-specific CAMS Treatment Plan Update (Section B on the SSF interim form). Interim session treatment plan updating is designed to recapture the spirit of collaboration that was established in the initial session of CAMS. To this end, the dyad should reconsider the CAMS Stabilization Plan—was it used and did it work? Does anything need to be modified going forward? After consideration of the stabilization plan, there is another check-in pertaining to Problems #2 and #3 on the treatment plan—the patient-defined suicidal drivers. For many cases, the patient's problems/drivers may remain the same across the course of CAMS-guided care. Alternatively, drivers can evolve or be displaced by new suicide-causing problems.

For example, a suicidogenic problem/driver of "my failed relationships" in CAMS Session 1 may evolve into a more specific driver in Session 6 with the emergence of "sexual trauma history" that fundamentally damages the patient's ability to trust and be intimate in her relationships and takes center stage of treatment. In another case, the problem/driver of "chronic unemployment" addressed in Sessions 1–3 may displaced with a new driver in Session 4, when the patient's home is repossessed and homelessness seems imminent. Whatever the case, we should never assume that patient-defined suicidal drivers will remain static, which is exactly why we double-check at the end of every interim CAMS session when we update the treatment plan. Beyond verifying with the patient the problems/drivers at the end of each interim session, we also complete the related "Goals and Objectives," "Intervention," and "Duration" portions of Section B that further elaborate CAMS driver-oriented treatment. After both parties sign at the bottom of the interim session SSF, the patient should receive a hard copy of the SSF interim form at the conclusion of each tracking/update session (or perhaps take a picture of it on his or her phone).

Interim HIPAA-Page Documentation

Similar to the HIPAA documentation that is done after the first session of CAMS, each interim session should have SSF HIPAA-page documentation (Section C). The format of the SSF HIPAA page is the same across the entire course of CAMS-guided care and can be quickly completed after all interim sessions. As noted, this page of additional clinical documentation provides valuable comprehensive progress information that reflects a thorough and complete HIPAA-compliant medical record.

TARGETING AND TREATING SUICIDAL DRIVERS

Now that we have broadly reviewed the routine components of CAMS interim sessions, it is important to spend a bit more time focusing on the treatment of the patient's suicidal drivers. The emphasis on "driver-oriented treatment" is a unique aspect of CAMS-guided care and sets it apart from both "traditional" and other evidence-based treatment approaches for suicidal risk. As discussed in Chapter 3, traditional approaches typically reflect a directive, clinician-as-expert attitude that emphasizes the treatment of mental disorders presumed to be etiologically relevant to suicidal risk. Within CAMS-guided care we never presume that a mental disorder lies at the heart of a patient's suicidal risk (unless the patient explicitly states as much in the CAMS discussion of suicidal drivers). Alternatively, if one is using a well-researched therapy approach for treating suicidal risk (e.g., Wenzel et al., 2009), there are several theoretically based a priori assumptions that are made about the patient's suicidal risk (e.g., the central CBT construct of the "suicidal mode"). Using the CBT example, we see an approach to suicide that uses a highly structured phasic methodology that emphasizes learning about the suicidal mode, systematically developing coping strategies, and ultimately using a relapse prevention strategy to effectively deal with prospective suicidal risk.

But considering the range of available clinical interventions for suicidal risk, only CAMS thus far offers the idea of using a flexible therapeutic framework that fundamentally relies on what the *patient* says puts his or her life in peril. It is a simple idea. Rather than relying on a mental disorder diagnostic bias or using an a priori theoretically driven treatment model, why not directly ask the person who most intimately knows about the suicidal struggle? "What problems, issues, or concerns most make you want to take your life?" Having watched literally hundreds of videos of CAMS clinicians within our clinical trial research, I am fascinated by how responsive most suicidal patients are to this simple and direct query. I would note that many patients act surprised that the clinician actually cares about what they think! Subsequently, when patients comes to realize that their view of things is actually *central* to CAMS treatment planning, they often become engaged—even animated—because of the truly pivotal role they play in the development of their own treatment plan. As a "coauthor" of their treatment plan, it is interesting to see how quickly many suicidal CAMS patients latch on to the idea of targeting and treating their suicidal drivers. Many such patients start explicitly referring to their suicidal drivers (and various other SSF constructs) within sessions as they begin to internalize the language of CAMS into their own descriptive lexicon. Because suicidal drivers have become so fundamental to CAMS-guided care, it is important to more fully flesh out the construct and further appreciate the differences between what we call "direct" and "indirect" drivers of suicide.

Direct Drivers

As noted in Chapter 5, CAMS driver-oriented treatment truly begins when the clinician asks the patient to identify the two problems (#2 and #3 on the CAMS treatment plan) that most compel the patient to consider suicide. Within "standard of care" mental health practice, it is routine that treatment "problems" are duly identified and noted within the treatment plan. However, in typical mental health practice, the identification of treatment problems is usually based on the *clinician's* judgment and observations. But in CAMS treatment planning, the patient is directly drawn into the treatment-planning discussion by identifying suicide-causing problems, which opens the treatment door to the whole notion of suicidal drivers. The feeling of being "driven" to suicide is ubiquitous among many suicidal people. A patient of mine once described the feeling as follows: "I feel like I am a reluctant passenger on an inevitable death ride with no say so or control over the inescapable final destination—suicide."

While the notion of drivers is unique, conceptually compelling, and clinically useful, there is sometimes confusion about what exactly we mean when we talk about suicidal drivers within CAMS. For example, how are suicidal drivers different from treatment plan problems? And what differentiates a direct from an indirect driver? Let me endeavor to explain through a case example. I once saw a suicidal patient—"Larry"—in CAMS who, when asked what made him suicidal (Problems #2 and #3 of the CAMS treatment plan) said, "My life and I suck and I have no girl-friend." Larry's first suicide-causing problem ("my life") is too broad, inexact, and not readily treatable. So a treatment-oriented discussion ensued to become a bit more precise: What exactly about your life is most pressing and causes you to want to end it? In turns out that what troubled Larry most was a lack of meaningful and successful employment—he had been vocationally lost since graduating from col-lege 8 years prior. In relation to "I suck and I have no girlfriend," we further clari-fied that Larry had major self-esteem issues and felt "unlovable." Thus Problem # 2 on the CAMS Treatment Plan was "Vocational Uncertainty" and Problem #3 was "Poor Self-Esteem." With these suicide-causing problems now established in Lar-ry's first CAMS session, the interim sessions focused on how these problems were actually functioning as "direct drivers" within a series of acute suicidal crises that had plagued Larry in recent years. In other words, Larry became suicidal when he ruminated over his lack of vocational direction and focused on his self-loathing (that invariably focused on his regrets and his sense of being a failure and unlov-able in terms of romantic relationships).

Indirect Drivers

Within CAMS-guided care, "indirect drivers" are issues, or problems, or concerns that make the patient vulnerable to his or her direct drivers but do not in them-selves cause suicidal states. By definition, these issues are not actually linked to suicidal states but can nevertheless "set the stage" for the patient's direct drivers to become activated, thereby creating a potentially acute suicidal crisis. Indirect driv-ers may be things such as drinking behavior, isolation, homelessness, insomnia, depression, or a trauma history—issues that the patient lives with every day but do not necessarily cause suicidal thoughts. In Larry's case, his indirect drivers tended to center on various self-defeating and demoralizing behaviors, including overeat-ing when he felt depressed and "Facebook stalking" his apparently successful high school friends. Over the course of successful CAMS care, he came to appreciate how his indirect driver behaviors could trigger and activate his direct drivers, thereby increasing his suicidal risk. His CAMS-guided interim treatment psychotherapy focused on vocationally oriented work, joining Weight Watchers, and getting back into martial arts (which he had enjoyed in high school). He ultimately got in much better physical shape, changed his career focus, and got into graduate school where he met and dated one of his classmates (whom he ultimately married).

Interventions for Suicidal Problems/Drivers

CAMS-guided care emphatically does not prescribe any specific interventions for treating a patient's suicidal drivers. Instead, the CAMS clinician is encouraged to use familiar clinical strategies within interim sessions, particularly any evidence-based approaches that may be used to address a particular suicidal driver. CAMS-guided treatment is thus problem focused and flexible rather than strategy focused and rigid. Importantly, CAMS clinicians do not have to learn an entirely new theoretical approach to care, to develop a whole new repertoire of interventions, or to stop using techniques in which they already have expertise. As long as they are thoughtfully using interventions that target and treat patient-defined suicidal drivers in the interim sessions, they remain adherent to the CAMS framework while still using skills, techniques, and interventions that are familiar to them within their professional discipline and training. Accordingly, relationally oriented problems/drivers can be treated with CBT, insight-oriented psychodynamic therapy, behavioral activation, or couple therapy—whatever seems appropriate to the clinician (and patient). Similarly, trauma-related drivers can be treated with exposure therapy, insight-oriented work, clinical hypnosis, EMDR therapy, cognitive processing therapy, and the like. Again, a signature feature of CAMS is never telling clinicians *how* to do treatment. Instead, within CAMS interim sessions there is plenty of room for a broad spectrum of treatments and related interventions as long as they focus on the systematic elimination of those concerns that fundamentally lead to the patient's suicidal thoughts, feelings, and behaviors.

Clinical Case Consultation

An additional treatment consideration that I find remarkably undervalued in general clinical practice is the importance of clinical consultation. From our process improvement projects and our clinical trials we have come to appreciate the indispensable value of having access to clinical case consultation. Yet many providers—and systems of clinical care—do not have regular case consultations. As described in depth of the first edition of this book, I strongly recommend a standing meeting for staff to routinely discuss all ongoing CAMS cases within their system of care. Not only are "two heads better than one" in terms of creative ideas and suggestions about treatment and interventions, case consultation is also ethically encouraged and highly protective from a liability perspective (Archuleta et al., 2014) and important to providing evidence-based treatments, particularly in terms of supporting clinical behavior change in using an empirically supported treatment (Beidas, Edmunds, Marcus, & Kendall, 2012; Karlin et al., 2010). For two evidence-based treatments for suicidal risk, clinical consultation for clinical team members is an expectation of adherent care (e.g., Brown, Have, et al., 2005; Linehan, 1993a; Wenzel et al., 2009).

The CAMS Therapeutic Worksheet

One last CAMS interim treatment consideration is the optional use of the CAMS Therapeutic Worksheet (CTW) that can be introduced in Session 2 but can be used later or revisited as needed over the course of CAMS interim care (see Appendix E). Developed by my research collaborator Stephen O'Connor in the course of one of our CAMS randomized controlled trials (Comtois et al., 2011), the CTW is still a work in progress and will be further modified based on our clinical research. Critically, the CTW can be used as a potential tool for further elucidating and deconstructing the patient's suicidal drivers. As can be seen in Appendix E, the CTW begins with a query for the patient to describe his or her "Personal Story of Suicidality," which creates a narrative opportunity to describe how, when, and where the concept of suicide first came into the patient's mind. Initial awareness of suicide may be inspired by a movie, a relative who died by suicide, or a book reference; invariably, some historical experience usually marks the genesis of suicidality within the patient. We want the patient to become curious about how suicide has become a part of his or her life and a coping solution. It does not come out of the blue. There is usually a useful story to uncover and explore. Next on the CTW, there is an examination of the patient's suicidal drivers/problems through a systematic deconstruction driver-related thoughts, feelings, behaviors, and potential driver-oriented themes that may emerge. Then there is a further consideration of potential indirect drivers on the CTW that may additionally contribute to an increasing over-all awareness of suicidal risk that is unique to the patient's experience.

The CTW ends with a suicidal conceptualization using a flow diagram that serves as a visual aid of how indirect drivers may create instability and vulnerability to potential suicidal suffering, which may then lead to the activation of direct drivers that may push the patient toward suicide as the ultimate coping option. Use of the diagram can help the patient and clinician discover that contextual, behavioral, and motivational factors that can and do play a major role in exacerbating or reducing suicidality. To this end, we document potential "bridges" that psychologically propel the patient toward suicide. In turn, we also note potential "barriers" that may help avert the patient from traveling further along the fatal path that ends with suicide. Ultimately, we are endeavoring to help the suicidal patients develop a deeper psychological understanding of how various factors may contribute to his or her escalating into a highly suicidal state. Furthermore, patients can also see that *they* often play a pivotal contributory role in either maintaining their attachment to suicidal coping or changing their relationship to suicide and attaching to life instead. It all helps make the patient an expert on his or her own struggle (i.e., we help the patient become a suicidologist, an expert on their own suicidal struggle).

As noted elsewhere (Jobes et al., 2016), the optional CTW tool serves three primary functions within CAMS-guided care. First, it replicates the collaborative intimacy established in the initial CAMS session. Second, it is designed to build on—and then extend—the assessment and treatment planning aspects of CAMS pertaining to our singular preoccupation on suicidogenic problems and the patient's idiosyncratically defined suicidal drivers. Third, the CTW helps reduce drift from the CAMS agenda by underscoring the driver-oriented treatment.

Finally, beyond these primary functions, there is the added virtue of supplemental clinical documentation related to suicide-specific assessment and treatment.

CASE EXAMPLE: BILL'S INTERIM CAMS-GUIDED CARE

Bill was notably steadied early on by our carefully developed CAMS Stabilization Plan. With his guns secure, Bill began attending AA meetings and looked up his old sponsor, who helped him considerably. Beyond his increased stabilization, Bill's interim CAMS-guided care primarily focused on his two stated suicide-causing problems—namely, his failing marriage and his overwhelming sense of hopelessness. Bill's wife was quite receptive to my suggestion and referral for couple therapy, until their third couple session, which created a whole new suicidal crisis. It turns out that Bill had had an affair with a coworker over 20 years ago and fathered a daughter who was now 19 years old. While the affair had ended many years prior, he nevertheless provided substantial financial support to his former coworker for their daughter. The mother and daughter had moved to Canada, and Bill's only contact with the mother was through an arrangement to wire her money each month—he had never met the daughter, and he had kept the secret from his wife because he feared that disclosing his infidelity (and his fathering of the child) would end his marriage.

The disclosure of this significant deception and dramatic revelation sparked a new suicidal crisis early in Bill's CAMS care, which almost led to a hospitalization when Bill's wife found him doing Internet research on lethal dosages of over-the-counter medications. Bill was desperate to save his marriage but was convinced that he could not win back the trust of his understandably furious wife. Fortunately, a skilled couple therapist bought some time by developing a strict behavioral contract for Bill to follow that was designed to systematically earn back his wife's trust. The contract focused on better communication, sobriety from alcohol, and his wife being more directly involved in their finances (she was particularly upset about financial deceptions that Bill had used to hide the money he sent to support the daughter). Bill also agreed to pursue spiritual direction with their priest to more fully understand and address his moral failings in relation to his historic infidelity and financial deceptions. In hindsight, the 6-month behavioral contract developed by the couple therapist likely saved Bill's marriage and perhaps his life. I should note that Bill's Problem #2 of "Failing Marriage" was "sharpened" in his fourth session of CAMS to "Betrayal and Trust Issues with Wife," which shows a more focused issue that may drive him to suicide.

In terms of Bill's #3 problem of hopelessness, the impact of this particular suicidal driver was closely linked to the various ups and downs of his extremely fragile marriage and the crisis created by revelation and deception related to the affair and fathering a daughter outside his marriage. We nevertheless developed a Virtual Hope Kit during one interim session on his smartphone that featured pictures of his kids and he routinely used various distraction activities (Bush et al., 2015). We also held a separate family meeting that included his grown children, and he studiously read *Choosing to Live: How to Defeat Suicide through Cognitive Therapy* (Ellis & Newman, 1996) that fueled much discussion in our interim sessions. In addition, we did a fair amount of historical insight-oriented work that centered primarily on his relationship with his father, who was himself depressed, secretive, had a serious drinking problem, and likely had numerous affairs over the course of his marriage.

Bill's CAMS Stabilization Plan proved to be quite useful; he faithfully used his coping strategies and the document was routinely revised and updated based on his various efforts to successfully cope. By Session 6, we actually drew up a completely new stabilization plan, taking a fresh look at what was working in our efforts to build Bill's coping repertoire. Bill faithfully carried the stabilization plan in his breast pocket and actually would pat it with his hand in sessions when he talked about his efforts to cope.

In summary, Bill's interim care was dominated by the dramatic revelation of his 20-year infidelity secret that plunged his marriage into serious crisis. Bill's increased drinking, depression, and personal decline fueled an escalating risk of suicide that was deeply rooted in his hopelessness and his assumption that his marriage was over. What also emerged over his interim care was that he had taken out a large life insurance policy that would generously compensate his wife, whom Bill believed would be unburdened by his suicide death. He was simply waiting for the double indemnity clause for suicide to expire at the 2-year mark. It turns out that I first saw Bill in CAMS within a week of that date. For the complete SSF documentation for the full course of CAMS with Bill, refer to Appendix H.

SUMMARY AND CONCLUSIONS

CAMS interim care is defined by ongoing tracking of suicidal risk assessment and driver-oriented treatment. After the first session of CAMS, each interim session is defined by checking the suicidal "vital signs" of the SSF Core Assessment at the start of each session. The treatment focus of all CAMS interim sessions is a singular preoccupation with treating, managing, and addressing the patient's suicidal problems/drivers. Each interim session ends by revisiting the CAMS treatment plan, which requires double-checking the effectiveness of the stabilization plan and checking on whether there is any need to modify the drivers or related interventions as CAMS treatment evolves. When three consecutive sessions of meaningfully managing suicidal thoughts, feelings, and behaviors are realized, interim CAMS care is poised to move into the final outcome/disposition phase.

CHAPTER 7

CAMS Clinical Outcomes and Disposition

Lessons in Living and a Postsuicidal Life

Bill's clinical care progressed significantly over the course of eight sessions. We veered near to a potential hospitalization relatively early on, when his historic infidelity was revealed. But we were nevertheless able to stabilize him quite quickly because his wife, Kathy, did not immediately move to end their marriage. Kathy's willingness to give Bill a second chance was pivotal; the couple therapist artfully bought time and psychologically averted an imminent suicidal crisis for Bill. The behavioral contract that was hammered out in the couple therapy, established a valuable framework that helped to fashion a way forward in a focused effort to rebuild their relational trust given Bill's betrayal. By Session 6 of CAMS, we saw marked reductions on Bill's SSF Core Assessment ratings—his overall risk score was a 2 and he was readily able to manage some lingering suicidal thoughts and feelings with no evidence of suicidal behaviors and he was guardedly hopeful about getting a second chance with his wife. In Session 7, Bill talked about the behavioral contract required him to "check in" with his wife every morning before the start of their day. He laughed that on a couple of occasions their check-in turned into some deep discussions that caused them to both be late for work! After only a handful of sessions with the couple therapist, Bill was delighted that his tentative proposal for dinner and a movie (a "date night" homework assignment that he had been avoiding) for an upcoming weekend led to an unexpectedly enthusiastic response by Kathy. There were still some tense moments in their marital life, yet the combination of Bill's solid program of sobriety (his AA sponsor was key player in his recovery) and his earnest efforts to abide by the behavioral contract and make amends with Kathy was appreciated by her, even as she remained understandably wary. The couple therapy in particular seemed to buoy them significantly, and their emotional and physical intimacy improved in increments. Toward the end of Session 7, I noted the prospect of potentially "resolving" Bill's care because he was consistently meeting criteria for CAMS resolution. If the overall risk remained low and if he effectively managed any lingering suicidal thoughts, feelings, and behaviors in his forthcoming session, we could formally end our CAMS-related work. Bill was both surprised and intrigued by my observation that perhaps he had meaningfully turned a corner in his relationship to suicide; poised to resolve CAMS in his next session, Bill actually cracked an appreciative smile at the apparent prospect of rejecting suicide and fully attaching to his life.

OVERVIEW TO CAMS OUTCOMES AND DISPOSITION

As noted early on, the CAMS approach to suicidal risk has a beginning (the index first session of initial assessment and treating planning), a middle (the interim sessions of CAMS that begin with SSF Core Assessments, focusing on treating suicidal drivers, and treatment plan updates), and an end (the final session of CAMS and the completion of the Outcome/Disposition SSF). In this chapter, we consider in more depth the outcome and disposition phase of CAMS-guided care. As in the preceding chapters, we will initially consider the conceptual aspects of CAMS clinical outcomes and dispositions before shifting our attention to the specific procedural aspects of endeavoring to bring CAMS to an optimal clinical close.

Within our clinical research we have consistently seen uniform improvements among patients using the SSF and CAMS (Comtois et al., 2011; Ellis, Green, et al., 2012; Ellis et al., 2015; Jobes et al., 1997, 2005). Replicated data clearly show that CAMS is associated with improvements in overall symptom distress, rapid reductions in suicidal ideation, and changes in suicidal cognitions over the course of clinical care (Jobes, 2012). The majority of patients in our studies resolve their suicidal risk within 6 to 12 sessions. Moreover, we know there are various index-session SSF quantitative and qualitative data that can be used to predict different aspects of treatment outcomes (e.g., Brancu et al., 2015; Corona & Jobes, 2013; Fratto et al., 2004; Jobes & Flemming, 2004). There are also promising data that show the CAMS may be related to decreases in primary care and emergency department visits (Jobes et al., 2005) and may have an impact on suicide-attempt and self-harm behaviors as well (Andreasson et al., 2016). We are also beginning to understand what successfully treated CAMS patients found to be helpful within their care. In a study of 50 successfully treated CAMS patients, Schembari, Jobes, and Horgan (2016) reliably coded written patient responses to the prompt: "Were there any aspects of your treatment that were particularly helpful to you?" The patients in this study reported that the following aspects within their CAMS-guided care were helpful: "therapeutic process," "action-oriented techniques," "mind-focused techniques," "the clinician," "supportive resources," "validation," and "CBT/DBT techniques." Further replication of these outcome data is needed and an increasing focus on the mechanisms of change within CAMS-guided care will be pursued in the years ahead.

Optimal Clinical Outcomes

When I refer to "optimal" clinical outcomes in relation to CAMS-guided care, I am referring to ideal suicide-specific treatment-based outcomes that include (1) no completed suicide, (2) no suicide attempts, (3) the elimination of suicidal ideation, (4) the meaningful reduction of general symptom distress, (5) the clear development and internalization of alternative ways of coping, and (6) the development of reasons for living, improved ability to think about the future, and the development of existential purpose and meaning. But beyond desirable suicide prevention outcomes, we must also consider the full range of clinical outcomes that may occur during care.

Post-CAMS Continued Care

One potentially important disposition after CAMS-guided care is the mutual continuation of psychotherapy beyond the CAMS resolution of suicidal risk. Over the years, I have known many patients—and clinicians—who eagerly seek to build on their initial CAMS-based therapeutic success. In the course of potentially conquering their life-and-death struggle, many such patients often remain highly motivated to continue in psychotherapy. In such cases, the patient and clinician may move seamlessly into an ongoing line of psychotherapy as CAMS comes to a close. Often such dyads continue to address direct and indirect drivers that were initially identified within their CAMS-guided care. While the original work may have been launched by CAMS, other issues naturally come to the forefront as the spotlight on suicidality fades.

Referral to Alternative Care

Alternatively, making an appropriate professional referral after a successful course of CAMS can often be a desirable clinical outcome. Once suicide risk has effectively receded, there is often an opportunity for a patient to seek further care with another provider or perhaps a more specialized form of care. For example, in our Seattle randomized controlled trial (Comtois et al., 2011), we had a subset of suicidal patients who met criteria for borderline personality disorder that were quickly and effectively stabilized using CAMS, which prompted a subsequent referral to dialectical behavior therapy. These were among some of our best outcome cases. There are optimal ways to effect appropriate referrals such that a patient does not feel "dumped" but rather appreciates that he or she has been carefully evaluated, prepared, and then transitioned to the best possible indicated care. As a general matter, making effective clinical referrals is often an underappreciated professional skill. Doing it well requires skilled informed consent about the potential benefits of an excellent and properly facilitated clinical referral.

Mutual Termination of Care

Another positive outcome is the mutual termination of psychotherapy as CAMS care comes to a close. In our various research studies across samples I would estimate that approximately 20–50% of CAMS patients chose to not pursue additional psychotherapy beyond resolution of suicidality (this is particularly true for our military samples). It has been my experience that for certain patients, a short-term course of care that has a positive outcome and ends on the patient's timetable may be the best way to promote further treatment at a later point in time, if needed. This kind of outcome is theorized (and has some empirical support) to prevent dropouts from treatment (Ogrodniczuk, Joyce, & Piper, 2005). In my experience, many clinicians may fall into a presumption that more psychotherapy is desirable. I can think of many patients I have seen who describe themselves as not being a "therapy-type" person. When such a person has a short-term success, particularly in a life-and-death struggle with suicidality, I mention the possibility of termination to ensure that they do not feel trapped in an endless course of therapy. In a related sense, I usually offer clinical "tune-ups" or "booster" sessions as an option to consider if they are inclined to terminate. I take this approach because experience has taught me that control and autonomy are often cardinal concerns of the suicidal mind. I am therefore particularly sensitive to respecting and honoring those sentiments, a view that is shared by proponents of self-determination theory and motivational interviewing for suicidal treatment (Britton, Patrick, Wenzel, & Williams, 2011; Britton, Williams, & Conner, 2008). Usually I tend to err on the side of not pushing things further than what we set out to do—in the case of CAMS-guided care, this often means having established a stabilization plan and alternative ways to cope with pain and suffering. Upon reflection, something quite profound has been achieved when we succeed in systematically rendering suicide functionally obsolete in the patient's life. And sometimes, that is enough.

Other Clinical Outcomes

Dropouts

Perhaps among the most worrisome and least desirable of clinical outcomes are unilateral terminations, which are better known as dropouts. Within in our study samples, dropouts may range from 7% (Comtois et al., 2011) to almost 20% (Jobes et al., 1997). Upon reflection, clinical dropouts are a subsample of suicidal patients who actually sought care, acknowledged some degree of suicidal thinking, and subsequently exited that care—invariably not responding to phone calls, letters, or e-mails encouraging them to return. These outcomes often leave the clinician feeling like a failure because a connection clearly was not made with the patient; there was an obvious failure to "hook" the patient to the treatment process. Again, this concern goes to the heart of CAMS philosophy and structure with its clear emphasis on the collaborative involvement of the patient in clinical assessment and treatment planning process—from start to finish. Fortunately, there is clear empirical evidence that CAMS achieves better treatment retention to care with fewer dropouts than usual care (Comtois et al, 2011).

Given the high risk level of CAMS patients, it is good to have a "usual and customary practice" related to dropout cases. At a minimum, there should be thorough documentation about the suicidal risk when last seen and your efforts to reconnect with the patient to encourage at least one more session or the completion of care. Within my practice, I usually send a follow-up e-mail, make a phone call, and document these efforts respectively. In some cases, I have sent a registered letter again attempting to reconnect and include other possible referrals and resources along with a specific deadline date for "closing the case" in the event that I do not hear back from them. I once consulted on a case where a colleague had a high-risk suicidal dropout and made no fewer than six different efforts to reengage that were thoroughly documented. When a suicide of this patient tragically occurred, the family's plaintiff attorney began to pursue malpractice litigation but ultimately dropped the case probably because the clinician used CAMS and made so many documented efforts to reconnect with the patient (more will be said about this in Chapter 8). Ideally, all your clinical practice and procedures (such as what you do in cases of unilateral termination) is disclosed in your routine informed consent at the start of treatment.

Hospitalization

As CAMS has primarily been designed as an approach to keep suicidal patients *out* of the hospital, it follows that an inpatient psychiatric hospitalization is usually not a desired outcome. Of course, the obvious exception to this outpatient emphasis is when CAMS is used within an inpatient setting (Ellis et al., 2010, 2015; Ellis, Daza, & Allen, 2012; Ellis, Green, et al., 2012; Jobes, 2012). It should be noted that inpatient use of CAMS is singularly focused on getting a suicidal patient stabilized and prepared for *discharge* to further engage in suicide-specific outpatient care. For the record, I do not have a preexisting bias against psychiatric hospitalization; in fact, much of my early career and ongoing work involves inpatient care for suicidal patients. But I am aware of contemporary limitations in standard inpatient treatment, with remarkably little of that treatment being suicide specific (refer to the discussion on this topic in Chapter 1). Given this state of affairs, I do not believe that typical contemporary inpatient care offers much salvation for perhaps the majority of suicidal patients and I am further sobered by the fact that hundreds of patients still die by suicide every year on locked inpatient psychiatric units (The Joint Commission, 2013, 2016).

It is my sense—based on clinical experience and our research—that most suicidal cases are *best* handled on an outpatient basis. Nevertheless, my impression is that most mental health providers still consider inpatient psychiatric care the optimal clinical response. Problematically, research has repeatedly shown increases in potential suicide risk following discharge from inpatient psychiatric care (Bostwick & Pankratz, 2000; Meehan et al., 2006; Qin & Nordentoft, 2005), particularly in the weeks immediately following discharge. Some have argued persuasively that the use of contemporary inpatient psychiatric hospitalization for preventing suicides has no empirical support and may actually be *harmful* in many cases (e.g., Linehan, 2015).

When I reflect on my days working on an inpatient unit, it sure *felt* like we did some life-saving work. And I still harbor a belief that if a hospitalization is the *only* thing that can be done to save a patient's life (particularly if he or she is in a state of psychosis), then I can support trying any clinical interventions we have to offer to prevent a premature death by suicide. I would feel somewhat differently if genuine and reliable suicide-specific care actually occurred during a typical inpatient stay, wherein a patient would be at less risk by virtue of receiving an effective suicide-specific intervention prior to discharge. Along these lines, I enthusiastically support the work of Marjan Holloway (Ghahramanlou-Holloway, Cox, & Greene, 2012), who has developed and is studying an inpatient version of CT-SP for inpatients called postadmission cognitive therapy (PACT). Naturally, I also support the innovative inpatient use of CAMS by Tom Ellis and colleagues (Ellis, Daza, et al., 2012; Ellis, Green, et al., 2012, Ellis et al., 2015) at the Menninger Clinic (otherwise known as CAMS-M).

Safely maintaining a suicidal person in the outpatient world (which keeps the patient with family, friends, gainful employment, or school) is intuitively preferable and compelling. All too often within our culture, inpatient care may prompt the unfortunate scourge of stigma as the person might now be seen as "crazy." To this end, we are now increasingly hearing powerful first-hand testimonials and accounts from members of the "attempt survivor/lived experience" community about how negative, shaming, iatrogenic, and even punitive some inpatient psychiatric experiences can be (Yanez, 2015). There will likely be a continued need for inpatient psychiatric care, but changes in that care over the past 30 years is dramatic. Now in a heath care reform era, I would predict that the operative buzzwords for suicide-related mental health care going forward will increasingly be *least restrictive, evidence based,* and *cost effective* (Jobes, 2013a; Jobes & Bowers, 2015). Hence, there are now many clear and convincing incentives for endeavoring to keep suicidal patients out of inpatient care if possible.

Chronic Suicidal States

In the first edition of this book, I readily acknowledged that CAMS may be less suited for more chronic suicidal states, particularly in association with border-line personality disorder (BPD). I further noted that Marsha Linehan's dialectical behavior therapy (DBT) is the obvious and empirically proven treatment of choice for self-destructive borderline patients with an extensive literature of empirical validation (Linehan, 1993a, 1993b, 2005, 2014; Linehan et al., 2006, 2015; Linehan, Armstrong, Suarez, Allmon, & Heard, 1991; Neacsiu, Rizvi, & Linehan, 2010; Stoffers et al., 2012). Having argued for DBT as the optimal treatment choice for sui-cidal patients with BPD, I still made the anecdotal case for the use of CAMS with certain chronically suicidal and BPD patients (such as we saw in our Seattle RCT noted earlier). Indeed, a number of providers over recent years have told me that their chronically suicidal patients who were treated within CAMS-guided care demonstrated less of a need to act out or further "amplify" their emotional distress through suicidal threats and behaviors because their self-destructive impulses were so closely and faithfully monitored within CAMS at every interim session.

Beyond clinical anecdotes, there is now a growing body of evidence that CAMS may be effective for some chronic suicidal states and patients with BPD traits (Andreasson et al., 2014, 2015, 2016). In this regard, we are currently studying suicidal college students using a "SMART" (i.e., sequential, multiple assignment, randomized trial; refer to Collins, Murphy, & Stecher, 2007) RCT investigating the effectiveness of sequential or alternative uses of CAMS and/or DBT (Pistorello & Jobes, 2014). In recent years, I have heard many diehard and adherent DBT provid-ers note the value of integrating CAMS with DBT, as these patients often lapse into seriously suicidal states. Thus at this juncture, the evidence remains clear that DBT is the best approach possible for chronic, personality-based suicidal states; how-ever, for providers who may not have access to DBT care, the use of CAMS shows promise as well. In coming years we will investigate the differential use of these evidence-based treatments, ideally matching different treatments to different sui-cidal states within our RCT investigations.

Suicide Attempt

We all know there are no guarantees in this business. It is unlikely there will ever be a clinical approach or treatment that will work for every clinician and suicidal patient. Having said that, however, I would still contend that a clinical assess-ment and treatment that specifically targets suicide is going to be more effective than a treatment targeting mental disorders wherein suicidality is understood as a mere symptom. It seems self-evident that a treatment that does not focus on the risk of suicide completions or attempts has a much higher likelihood of missing these potentially lethal behaviors altogether. While suicidal behaviors remain a low base-rate event in the grand scheme, there are going to be cases where even the most conscientious clinician and approach may not avert attempt behaviors that remain largely outside our direct influence and control. While discouraging, a suicide attempt does not necessarily mean that treatment is futile. Rather, it means the treatment has yet to be fully effective, meaning it is time to redouble our efforts and get it right.

In the progression of our research trials there have, of course, been CAMS patients who have made suicide attempts. One particularly poignant case within our Seattle RCT was of a patient who was a few weeks into his CAMS care. Haunted by chronic alcoholism, this patient "fell off the wagon"—ironically, on his way to an AA meeting. His intent was to just have "one drink" after a particularly tough day. Needless to say, one drink turned into many, and the patient ultimately cut himself on his arms and was hospitalized on an inpatient unit for 10 days. When the patient sheepishly returned to CAMS care, the clinician faithfully abided by the therapeutic adage that Marsha Linehan has noted to those she trains: "The patient never fails the treatment; only the treatment fails the patient." With this sentiment in mind, the CAMS clinician skillfully navigated the tricky waters of shame and embarrassment as the patient could barely make eye contact with the therapist for having "failed" to follow his stabilization plan. His averted eyes welled with grateful tears when his clinician gently pointed out, "We are in this together. You need to get that, and we have to improve our stabilization plan so that you never have to go back into that dark place again." With this level of support and acceptance, the patient rallied and turned out to be among our best outcome cases in the study. Even in the hands of a skilled practitioner, suicide attempts do happen, and they can be scary. But within every suicide attempt, by definition, there is still a living person, and lessons can be learned and lives may ultimately be saved in turn (refer to O'Connor et al., 2015, about his notion of a "teachable moment" intervention).

Completed Suicide

Finally and tragically, there are completed suicide deaths. We know that among the average 110 or more people who typically die each day by suicide in the United States (Drapeau & McIntosh, 2014) roughly 35% will have previously sought mental health care (Cavanagh, Carson, Sharpe, & Lawrie, 2003). Plainly stated, no mental health professional is immune—no matter how expert, no matter how earnest we are in our efforts to save a life, we cannot guarantee any patient or their family that a suicide will not ultimately occur. I have written at length about my own personal, professional, and ethical struggles working with a particularly high-risk suicidal patient (Jobes, 2011). It follows that mental health professionals must reconcile and ultimately process the fact that they may one day lose a patient to suicide, no matter how hard they try. Within my own struggles to deal with the gravity of working with serious suicidal risk, I have been compelled to find a sensible way to proceed so that I am not clinically paralyzed as the proverbial "deer in headlights" in the face of a patient's suicidal struggle. In case you are wondering about my solution, you are currently reading all about it.

No suicide treatment or intervention is perfect. At least when using CAMS, one has the reassurance of knowing that this approach works with the vast majority of suicidal patients with whom it is used (Jobes, 2012). And while I never foolishly promise a patient or family that I can guarantee CAMS will work and save a patient's life, I do proffer the prospect of providing *the best possible care* for suicidal risk that I know to provide, using an approach steeped in hard-earned clinical wisdom and extensive clinical research. It is the best I know to offer, and it helps me endure something that I know that I can never control: the ultimate life or death of another human being. There will be more on this topic in Chapter 8.

CAMS SUICIDE TRACKING OUTCOMES: PROCEDURAL CONSIDERATIONS

In terms of specific CAMS procedures related to outcome and disposition, there are two primary domains of clinical outcomes to consider: (1) CAMS resolution and (2) various unresolved clinical outcomes and dispositions. Each of these domains of clinical outcomes will now be considered, with a particular emphasis on relevant CAMS-related procedures.

Clinical Resolution of CAMS

As I noted in Chapter 6, resolving the use of CAMS requires three straight sessions of meaningfully reducing the patient's suicidal risk. In the first edition of this book, the criteria for CAMS resolution was three consecutive sessions with absolutely *no* suicidal thoughts, feelings, and behaviors. But as we delved into our large RCT with suicidal Soldiers, we came to realize that these criteria were just too stringent. In many of our cases, the total eradication of any vestige of suicidality was just too extreme. We began to appreciate that a meaningful CAMS clinical resolution corner had been turned when a patient with relatively modest suicidal thoughts or feelings described the ability to reliably and effectively *manage* any such thoughts or feelings (in conjunction with no suicidal behaviors). Hence our revised operational definition for CAMS suicide resolution became three sessions wherein the SSF Core Assessment overall risk variable was 1 or 2, and the patient was able manage any suicidal thoughts and feelings while exhibiting no suicidal behaviors over the past week. These modified criteria have worked well in our recent RCTs and reflect a more realistic resolution for CAMS (vs. eradication of suicidality).

Procedurally, patients on the cusp of resolution in the penultimate CAMS session (i.e., the second consecutive session where resolution criteria are met) should be made aware that if the resolution criteria are met in their next session, the

Outcome/Disposition version of the SSF will be used to bring CAMS-guided care to a close. It follows that in that next session, if the patient's overall risk indeed is a 1 or 2, and they have managed any suicidal thoughts and feelings with no suicidal behaviors, then resolution can formally occur, if the clinician concurs. There were occasional cases in our clinical trials where, on a consultation call, we would advise the clinician to give the patient another week or two of CAMS just to make sure that the apparent resolution in fact holds. A patient who is responsive to CAMS usually sees that he or she is on the road to recovery and often is eager to achieve this goal. Alternatively, there are patients who may have two consecutive resolution sessions but then experience a setback the next week that spikes their overall risk rating or challenges their ability to effectively manage their suicidal thoughts and feelings. When this occurs, it must be taken in stride; the dyad merely regroups on their CAMS driver-oriented treatment and the resolution "clock" starts over. For a subset of patients, shaking their attachment to suicide can be both scary and difficult. Accordingly, we must be clinically patient, understanding, and supportive about how the CAMS clinical resolution process plays out. To the best of our ability, we must earnestly endeavor to not rush or pressure the patient into resolution prematurely because of *our* needs.

Suicide Resolution: Section A

Given the preceding considerations for setting up for a possible CAMS resolution session, the clinician should begin by checking in with the patient to verify whether resolving CAMS makes sense. If all seems in order, then the clinician gives the patient the CAMS SSF-4—Outcome/Disposition (Final Session) document to complete. By this time, the SSF Core Assessment ratings in Section A should be familiar to the patient. Generally speaking, I recommend the use of side-by-side seating for all interim sessions, but I do think this seating arrangement is optimal in the final resolution session, as there is a fair amount of collaborative work being done in relation to outcome and disposition.

As with all interim sessions, reviewing the SSF Core Assessment items is indicated to ensure that third-session resolution criteria have indeed been met (and marked as such in Section B of the Outcome/Disposition SSF). During the CAMS resolution session, the patient and clinician may benefit from a review of previous interim SSFs, and the first-session SSF in particular, to fully appreciate the changes in assessment scores over the course of care. After the patient completes the final set of SSF Core Assessment ratings, there are two open-ended prompts at the end of Section A. The first question asks about what aspects of treatment were helpful to the patient. The second question asks about what has been internalized should suicidal risk return in the future. These two queries were adapted from those used in the famous National Institute of Mental Health (NIMH)–funded Collaborative Study of Depression (Elkin et al., 1989) and can obviously be used to further generate a reflective discussion between the clinician and patient about what has been accomplished and internalized and how any future relapse into suicidality may be averted (for more on the research of these patient responses to these "relapse-prevention" oriented questions, refer to Schembari, Jobes, & Horgan, 2016).

Suicide Tracking Outcome/Disposition Form: Section B

Patients are responsible for completing Section A of the Outcome/Disposition SSF (just as they have since the first session). In turn, the clinician is responsible for completing Section B, which begins by confirming that indeed a third session of resolution has been achieved. The clinician should then lead a general discussion about the outcome and disposition of the case with the patient. Usually, potential next steps for care and disposition should be discussed in advance of this resolution session, but Section B provides an opportunity to further discuss and formally document CAMS-related outcomes and disposition on the SSF. For any resolving cases there are four obvious clinical dispositions: (1) continued psychotherapy, (2) mutual termination, (3) the patient's unilateral termination from care, or (4) a professional referral. With each of these potential clinical dispositions, I proceed as I would with any case: following my best professional judgment and standard clinical practices. As previously noted, I am usually fairly supportive of a patient's desire to end care. However, if in my judgment termination is not in the patient's best interest, I clearly share that opinion but inevitably honor the patient's desire to end care unilaterally if he or she wishes to do so. In cases of unwise unilateral termination by the patient it might be worth considering providing some form of "non-demand" caring contact in the form of letters, e-mails, or follow-up phone calls given the empirical support for this kind of intervention (see review by Luxton, June, & Comtois, 2013; Motto, 1976; Motto & Bostrom, 2001).

Whatever the specific clinical disposition might be, I *always* commend the patient who successfully resolves CAMS-guided care. A CAMS resolution session is a prime opportunity to celebrate a potentially life-saving course of care, and fully acknowledging this accomplishment can be an important thing to do. Even after 25 years of researching resolution of suicidal states using the SSF and CAMS I am still stirred by the significance of this achievement.

Suicide Tracking Outcome/Disposition Form: Section C

Similar to previous phases of CAMS-guided care, the resolution session is followed by the completion of the final "HIPAA page" (Section C). Completion of this final SSF document is particularly relevant after the resolution session because it now formally completes and records an extremely thorough medical record of the CAMS-guided care. As previously noted, the extensive documentation that is built into CAMS is a signature feature of the intervention that should help significantly reduce the risk of malpractice vulnerability should a patient die by suicide and the surviving family pursues litigation for wrongful death.

Suicidal Relapse

Of course, it is possible that a once-resolved suicidal patient may become suicidal again. This has happened within my own clinical caseload and in our clinical trial research too. Based on the clinician's judgment, if a once-resolved suicidal patient later becomes actively suicidal, one can delve back into interim session tracking and make a deliberate shift in focus back to driver-oriented treatment. But in certain cases, starting from scratch with the SSF first-session assessment and treatment planning may have virtues as well. While clinicians and patients may not relish the prospect of redoing the whole CAMS procedure, I would argue that seeing suicidal states as episodic is better than simply labeling a patient as "chronically" suicidal. I think it is important to impress upon the suicidal patient that one can get better (even episodically), which contrasts the perception that things will never be better (the hallmark of a chronic suicidal state that may spawn a kind of *identity* that can make successful treatment even harder).

Unresolved Clinical Outcomes

There are many alternative clinical outcomes to resolution of CAMS that must be accounted for within a complete and HIPAA-compliant medical record. Therefore, the SSF Outcome/Disposition can be used for outcomes that are generally linked to a discontinuation of the relationship with the CAMS clinician. These outcomes include (1) hospitalization, (2) mutual termination between clinician and patient (even without the resolution of CAMS), (3) unilateral termination on the patient's part (dropping out of care or terminating against the wishes of the clinician), (4) a clinician's referral to other care or a different provider, and (5) tragically, even a completed suicide can be documented under the heading "Other." Such outcomes have been discussed throughout this chapter. As an important aside, clinicians are encouraged to seek consultation as indicated to make their best professional recommendations for care. Such consultations should be thoroughly documented under Section B (under "Referral to" or "Other") or perhaps under "Case Notes" on the final SSF HIPAA page.

A POSTSUICIDAL LIFE: LESSONS IN LIVING

In the course of conducting various RCTs of CAMS, and literally watching hundreds of hours of clinicians endeavoring to adherently use CAMS with seriously suicidal people, something has struck me. On many occasions, I have observed potentially lethal suicidal patients who respond remarkably well to CAMS, some-times in astonishingly short order (e.g., four to six sessions). We also see patients even with lengthy histories of suicidal behaviors and long-term suicidal ideation come around to the notion that perhaps suicide may not be the best way to deal with their circumstances. Within this realization there is the real prospect of detaching from suicide, attaching to life, and embracing the prospect of hope. Interestingly, many of these patients' lives remain extraordinarily chaotic—a Soldier with four young children in and out of wedlock with multiple mothers, significant finan-cial debt, and intrusive combat-related trauma. A young college student who acts out sexually, cuts herself regularly, drinks and uses drugs, and has made multiple overdoses since middle school. A middle-aged homemaker who raised five kids and now hates her "empty nest" life; she is overweight and anxious—her hus-band interrupted a near-fatal attempt when he wrestled away a gun pointed at her head. Stabilized by CAMS and effectively persuaded to give up on suicide, such patients may have little sense of how to proceed beyond their suicidal reality. Such patients sometimes describe a sense of "comfort" in their suicidal contemplations. Suicide may be seen as a "warm blanket" of control and security; a patient once described to me her "relationship" with suicide as a kind of love affair with death. Cases like these have more recently given me pause to consider what might be pos-sible beyond suicide for many such people—those who have seriously danced with death as their potential solution, their personal deliverance and salvation. How exactly does such a person actually go about pursuing a *postsuicidal life*?

As I reflect on the 10 years since the first edition of this book I am aware that the front end of CAMS was well researched and fleshed out in 2006—the back end of CAMS, not so much. A decade later, I am appreciating the maturation and evolution of the intervention and how much we have learned in the treatment of patient-defined suicidal drivers over the course of the interim CAMS sessions. In fact, Tucker and colleagues (2015) have argued that the construct of suicidal "driv-ers" is a major innovation in conceptual and clinical thinking about suicide risk. In their important paper, these authors make a compelling case for the evolution in suicidology over the past decades wherein hundreds of psychosocial "risk fac-tors" for suicide dominated the field early on (Maris et al., 2000). This was followed by a later argument for the merits of more proximate temporal markers of risk within the construct of suicidal "warning signs" (Rudd, 2008; Rudd, Berman, et al., 2006). Tucker et al. now make the make the case for suicidal drivers as a form of "personal warning signs"—patient-defined problems that propel a person into an acute suicidal state. We now understand a great deal more about treating the suicidal patient within the CAMS interim sessions, particularly in relation to our focus on targeting and treating patient-defined suicidal drivers. But it is clear that the back end of CAMS-guided care has been the least evolved part of the inter-vention. To this end, I will conclude this chapter with some current reflections and considerations about CAMS-guided outcomes and dispositions with distinct implications for a postsuicidal life.

Relapse Prevention

What is plain within the evidence-based treatment literature, both broadly defined and specific to suicide, is an understandable emphasis on the importance of "relapse prevention" (Apil, Hoencamp, Judith Haffmans, & Spinhoven, 2012; Brown & Chapman, 2007; Dimidjian, et al., 2014; Gleeson et al., 2011; Huijbers et al., 2012; Piet & Hougaard, 2011). In fact, within the highly effective cognitive therapy for suicide prevention (CT-SP) approach, the final sessions use a guided-imagery relapse prevention protocol as a signature feature of the treatment intervention (Wenzel et al., 2009). Within this phasic approach to treatment, there is an initial emphasis on identifying and recognizing the suicidal mode. Valuable coping skills are then imparted within CT-SP that help prepare patients to respond differently when their suicidal mode is activated at any point in the future. But what really carries the day are the final sessions in which the suicidal mode is activated in session through guided imaginary exposure exercises that includes the patient rehearsing suicidal coping behaviors he or she has learned. It is a beautiful thing, and the data clearly show that suicide attempt behaviors are significantly decreased in turn (Brown, Have, et al., 2005; Rudd et al., 2015).

Consequently, I have come to appreciate the singular importance of relapse prevention, particularly in relation to suicide. As previously noted within CAMS, the two final open-ended questions in Section A of the outcome/disposition SSF directly embraces the spirit of relapse prevention: "Were there any aspects of your treatment that were particularly helpful to you?" and "What have you learned from your clinical care that could help you if you became suicidal in the future?" and we are beginning to harvest valuable information from these questions (Schembari et al., 2016). While it is obviously crucial to not *fall back* to one's previous suicidal ways, in more recent years I have become increasingly preoccupied with the importance of *going forward*. How exactly does a resolving CAMS patient find a way to leave suicide behind and move forward to endeavor to pursue a life worth living, a postsuicidal life? How do we as mental health providers help such patients to earnestly pursue a life with purpose and meaning?

Lessons in Living

One concept that I have been mulling over is the process of sending a formerly suicidal patient on his or her way with a simple therapeutic orientation to "lessons in living." What I mean by "lessons in living" are basic transtheoretical ideas that can impart some basic guidance about how best to proceed. It is important to offer some kind of a therapeutic springboard to help a once-suicidal person begin to develop the essential building blocks of a life worth living. Along these lines, what I find most compelling are intuitively appealing models that tend to emphasize the importance of psychological balance. For example, Bonanno and Castonguay (1994) wrote a fascinating article that that talked about the importance of balancing the constructs of psychological "agency" and "communion." Agency is a primary focus on one's internal life, performance, achievement, and a sense of purpose (i.e., "doing"). Communion is a focus on one's relational life, concentrating on communicating, connecting, interacting with others, and an appreciation for "being." These authors persuasively argued that relative mental health might be best pursued by developing a healthy balance between agency and communion—having both a meaningful internal life focused on the self and a meaningful relational life focused on attachments to others.

Carl Rogers (1957) posited another favorite simple construct many years ago within his notion of "congruence." More recent scholars similarly talk of "self-discrepancy" theory (Higgins, 1999; Higgins, Roney, Crowe, & Hymes, 1994). The essential idea is a kind of psychological consistency between the person one aims to be and the person one actually is. When there is relative congruence between these, a person is probably functioning well in life. When there are significant gaps in who we aim to be and who we are, there is invariably distress and suffering, as we are not living up to our aspirations.

Finally in this vein, I have appreciated Zimbardo's (Zimbardo & Boyd, 1999) notion of psychological orientation in terms of time. We have all known people who are rooted psychologically in the *past* (perhaps preoccupied with historic trauma or an overattachment to certain periods of life, such as high school or college). There are others who psychologically live for *now,* following a personal credo to focus on the existential present moment at hand, not wasting time ruminating over the past or speculating about an unknowable future. In turn, there are still other people who are psychologically rooted in the *future,* working hard to get the right education, job, spouse, friends, home, and life circumstances to one day live that life. Zimbardo argues that relative psychological health exists when one is relatively psychologically aware of the past, present, and future aspects of one's life. Drawing wisdom from the past, appreciating the current moment, and planning for the future intuitively seems like a sensible way to think about how we should pursue a life with purpose and meaning.

Admittedly, I am perhaps a bit out of my league on such matters, and I do not pretend to have special insights on the meaning of life. But when one studies suicidal people for 30-plus years, it does provide for some interesting perspectives and gives one pause to think about purpose, meaning, and other lofty things. But the idea of developing or elaborating rather simple ideas that create a foundation for moving beyond suicide is compelling, and there is remarkably little on this topic within the suicidology literature. One might readily argue that this line of thinking ventures into the field of "positive psychology" or is nothing more than what the humanistic movement tendered in the 1960s by Maslow, Rogers, Frankl, and May. Yet the application of such ideas specifically to people who have been suicidal has not been a particular focus heretofore and is certainly worth further clinical consideration and empirical research. For a potential next edition of this book there may be an optional document, perhaps called the "Living Status Form," that could mirror the first-session first page of the SSF. Such a form could be used for certain patients who have successfully resolved their CAMS care, but need some guidance—a springboard—to their next steps exploring simple lessons in living. Such a form could help orient the patient to postsuicidal life in the larger pursuit of existential purpose and meaning. This line of thinking is akin to some of the values-oriented work that is involved in behavioral activation (Martell et al., 2013), acceptance commitment therapy (Hayes et al., 2011), and motivational interviewing (Britton, Conner, & Maisto, 2012; Britton et al., 2011).

SUMMARY AND CONCLUSIONS

In this chapter we have examined the final phase of CAMS-guided care—the point at which outcomes occur and clinical dispositions are realized. Optimally, we hope to see a suicidal patient successfully reach criteria for "resolving" suicidal risk, which then brings CAMS care to a close. There are, of course, alternative clinical outcomes to this optimal scenario that we have reviewed in this chapter as well. At its best, the resolution of CAMS marks a significant therapeutic achievement—the systematic deconstruction of a patient's suicidality such that a patient's attachment to suicide can be thoroughly understood and appreciated. When suicidality is understood in this manner, meaningful stabilization and CAMS-guided treatment of patient-defined suicidal drivers can ensue to systematically eliminate suicide from the patient's life. Even when our most desired outcomes are not realized, there can be comfort in knowing that CAMS and the SSF can still guide a therapeutic process and accommodate the full range of possible clinical outcomes, providing important documentation that reflects excellent suicide-specific clinical practice that rises far above the standard of care for most mental health care providers. Finally, we briefly explored some new ideas about how CAMS ends both in terms of relapse prevention and the pursuit of a postsuicidal life through the possible exploration of simple orienting ideas—lessons in living—that may help formerly suicidal patients leave suicide in the rear-view mirror, as they forge ahead to intentionally pursue a life they mean to live.

CHAPTER 8

CAMS as a Means of Decreasing Malpractice Liability

No clinical assessment and treatment can guarantee that an otherwise determined patient will not take his or her life. All we can do is all we can do. But the material issue is this: Did the patient receive the best possible evidence-based assessment and suicide-specific treatment? This must be our creed, something that we can earnestly aspire to and actually offer: the *best possible care* that is evidence based and suicide specific. Our patients—and their families—should be able to count on it.

Unfortunately, there are strongly held fantasies among our patients (and their families) that we clinicians can do more than we can do. In turn, if we fail to live up to those fantasies, particularly for a patient who ends his or her life, things can get ugly and legal in the form of malpractice litigation. Thus the prospect of being sued for malpractice "wrongful death" in the aftermath of a patient's suicide has become a major preoccupation for many clinicians (at least in the United States, but increasingly elsewhere as well). Some survey data confirm that such concerns are warranted. According to Peterson, Luoma, and Dunne (2002), the *majority* of family survivors of a loved one in clinical treatment at the time of a suicide death considered contacting an attorney, and 25% actually did!

To flesh out the issues we discuss in this chapter, consider two clinical case examples:

> A 20-year-old female junior business major who is attending a large Midwestern university is found by her roommate, hanging from a belt attached to a hook in her bedroom closet. The student's mother—a divorced wealthy real estate agent from Chicago—was stricken and infuriated by her daughter's

death. Shortly following her daughter's funeral, knowing her daughter had been previously seen in the university's counseling center, she made an appointment with the center's director and the clinical social worker who had seen the daughter in 23 sessions of CAMS-guided care. The daughter had suicidal ideation on and off since her freshman year and into her sophomore year, but was never hospitalized through the steady and successful use of CAMS. However, following summer break after sophomore year, the student never reengaged her clinician upon returning to campus (as had been mutually planned). The clinician made no fewer than *four* documented efforts—two by phone and two by e-mail—to reconnect the student back into care. The mother came to the meeting with the director and clinician accompanied by her attorney prepared to "burn down this institution with litigation!" In the meeting, the director calmly gave the attorney the patient's file, which was filled with SSF documentation and clear notations about the efforts to reengage the patient back into care. To the mother's fury, he declined the case by simply stating, "There is no negligence here." The distraught mother ended up contacting three more plaintiffs' attorneys, who all similarly agreed—there was no basis for a claim of any malpractice in this tragic case.

A 25-year-old economist working in a research think tank on the East Coast was being seen in a private practice setting by a clinical psychologist. The young man had an extensive history of clinical depression and anxiety and had a previous 10-day hospitalization that he described as a negative experience. He had gotten into a dispute with his boss over a particular research project and had been placed on probation. In addition, a recent breakup with a longtime girlfriend had put him into a depressive tailspin. The patient was seen for a total of six CAMS sessions. There had been extensive discussion about his plan to obtain a gun for his suicide, and he agreed to forgo this plan as part of his CAMS Stabilization Plan. Tragically, he shot himself 2 days after his last CAMS session and died. Some 10 months after the death, the clinician got an e-mail and subsequent phone call from the patient's brother in California. He had been going through his brother's belongings and had come across a file folder marked "Mental Health." He was both surprised and intrigued to see a collection of SSF documents that the patient had apparently collected. The clinician and brother ended up having a 90-minute phone call about the patient and the use of CAMS. During the call the brother disclosed that in the file there was a receipt for the gun the patient used to take his life, bought 2 weeks prior to his first CAMS appointment. The clinician was shocked by this revelation and pointed out the extensive documentation about the issue of buying a gun. The brother noted that the patient never would have tolerated another hospitalization, which must be why he lied. Their conversation ended with the brother actually *thanking* the clinician, saying, "At least I have the comfort of knowing that the person who last worked with my brother did not have his head in the sand about suicide—I'm sorry for us both that he was obviously so determined to die!"

These are difficult case examples, but they reveal both the heartbreak and the central challenge at hand. They also illustrate some ways surviving family members and others may respond to the death of their loved ones and seek explanations from clinicians who treated them before they took their lives.

This chapter considers various aspects of malpractice tort actions secondary to a patient's suicidal death. Consequently, we will consider how using CAMS with a suicidal patient may assuage various concerns related to clinical negligence that decreases the prospect of malpractice liability. I am quite aware that this topic can quickly veer toward an overemphasis on protective or defensive practice versus the singular importance of clinically saving lives. Nevertheless, we must endeavor to fully explore and consider the inherent issues of this chapter because they are so imperative to well-informed and competent clinical practice, which actually *does* help save lives (Roberts, Monferrari, & Yeager, 2008; Smith et al., 2008).

OVERVIEW TO MALPRACTICE

Malpractice laws vary from state to state. In truth, the determination of wrongful death malpractice liability may often be determined not by what a clinician actually did in the course of treating a patient, but by the relative credibility of the engaged experts and litigation skills of the participating lawyers who influence the sentiments and sympathies of nonexpert jurors and the judge. So, while the relevant laws may vary and the relative impact of experts and lawyers cannot be predicted, what is clear in this arena is that the responsible, systematic, and well-documented care of a patient is helpful in dissuading plaintiffs' attorneys from suing for malpractice in the first place (Bender, 2014).

As discussed by Berman, Jobes, and Silverman (2006), malpractice wrongful death litigation following a suicidal death is a tort action whereby the plaintiff (usually the surviving family members) seeks to pursue malpractice litigation against the clinician-defendant. A plaintiff's complaint is typically filed in civil court, usually listing an abundance of clinical failures attributed to the care provided by the clinician-defendant. Within this unpleasant scenario the alleged clinical failures on the part of the clinician—acts of omission or commission—are purported to be either a direct or proximate cause of death or significant injury. The burden of proof lies with the plaintiff.

Whether a clinician is judged to be guilty of malpractice is determined through the lens of the "standard of care." This standard is defined by what one should expect of a reasonable and prudent clinical practitioner, in similar circumstances, with a similar patient (Melonas, 2011; Michaelsen & Shankar, 2014). Notably, the standard of care is *not* what the expert practitioner would be expected to do; rather, it is what the reasonably prudent and generally competent clinical practitioner would do. The process of litigation proceeds with court orders (subpoenas) to produce all relevant written materials related to the case, a process referred to as discovery. The progression of litigation then continues with both sides of the case engaging foren-sic experts who will evaluate the written record and often interviews of various parties (depositions) to determine with the wisdom of hindsight whether the clini-cian did not or did meet the professional standard of care (Hashmi & Kapoor, 2010).

From my own experience and from discussions with other suicidology foren-sic expert-colleagues, the vast majority of these cases do not go to trial. This is pri-marily due to the nature of this type of litigation. Plaintiff attorneys spend a great deal of time developing and pursuing cases of malpractice for wrongful death, cases that are typically undertaken on contingent arrangement. While plaintiffs pay for costs related to pursuing the case, the lawyer's full compensation for their considerable billable hours is contingent on the outcome of the case (i.e., a favorable settlement or a monetary award that arises from a guilty verdict). In other words, the prospect of not recouping billable hours that typically range from $40,000–$50,000 for an average case makes plaintiff attorneys cautious about pursuing just any case (Wise et al., 2005). Thus many cases initially pursued by grieving families do not progress much further because plaintiff attorneys are understandably wary of expending significant amounts of time for which ultimately they may not be compensated—it is just bad business. While clinician fears and anxieties about malpractice liability are understandable and do have a basis in reality, only a rela-tively small number of wrongful death malpractice cases ever see the inside of a courtroom (Berman et al., 2006; Ellis & Patel, 2012).

Frankly, the experience of going to court to fight for one's professional life is dreadful. But even if the case does not go to court, the tortured experience of being accused of malpractice invariably takes its toll on the clinician's professional reputation and personal life. As noted by Hendin, Haas, Maltsberger, Szanto, and Rabinowicz (2004), a patient's death by suicide is in itself experienced as a cata-strophic event in the clinician's life, sometimes causing severe emotional distress in the clinician-survivor. Add to that understandable grief the possibility of mal-practice litigation for wrongful death, and you have an abjectly miserable experi-ence, making the loss of the patient just that much more difficult for the clinician-survivor.

Having clearly established the aversive nature of the malpractice litigation, it is incumbent on us to be aware of the process to fully appreciate what is expected of clinicians who work with suicidal patients in the eyes of the legal system. As noted by Berman and colleagues (2006; see also Sher, 2015), in order for a plaintiff to prove malpractice wrongful death after a suicide has occurred, four elements must be demonstrated throughout the process of litigation:

1. Evidence must be presented that the mental health clinician had a duty to care (which is typically self-evident through the nature of the professional relationship).
2. Evidence must be presented that there was a dereliction in the clinician's performance of that duty.

3. It must be shown that damages occurred (e.g., various secondary losses such as future income, pain and suffering, and the loss of companionship).
4. Critically, while the specifics vary from state to state, it must be established that these damages were *caused* by the alleged dereliction of the clinician's duty (e.g., through negligence).

Over two decades ago we (Jobes & Berman, 1993) published a paper that specifically focused on decreasing malpractice liability through competent practice (see also Melonas, 2011; Roberts et al., 2008). In our article we argued that competence in relation to the clinical care of a suicidal patient is defined by three overarching principles of professional practice with suicidal patients that emphasize the importance of (1) foreseeability (assessment), (2) treatment planning (ideally that is suicide specific), and (3) clinical follow-through (including the importance of consultation and appropriate documentation—see Simpson & Stacy, 2004). This organizing focus for decreasing malpractice liability has directly shaped the development of key features of CAMS. Let us therefore generally consider each of these principles in a bit more depth, particularly as they each relate to cardinal features of CAMS.

THE IMPORTANCE OF FORSEEABILITY

The concept of foreseeability pertains to the idea that the clinician anticipated the risk of suicide and consequently performed a competent and thorough suicide risk assessment. But the relative thoroughness of the assessment is often a critical issue within malpractice cases. For example, is it *reasonable* for a clinician to ask a 14-year-old with a history of conduct disorder and previous suicidal ideation and behaviors, "Are you suicidal?" to which the teenager simply responds, "No"? On the one hand, a defendant can legitimately argue, "A suicide ideation question was asked and answered." The plaintiff attorney might effectively argue, "Yes, but can you truly take at face value the yes/no answer of this boy, given his history?" Depending on the circumstances of each case, I have made arguments on both sides of this kind of debate; it depends on the particulars of the case as reflected in the medical record. In reference to the case just mentioned, yes, it is good that the clinician at least asked the 14-year-old about suicide and documented that fact in the medical record. Candidly, most clinicians do not even do this (Coombs et al., 1992). But is it sufficient to convince a judge or jury that the clinician provided an *adequate* level of assessment for suicide risk that meets the standard of care? This question is impossible to answer in any cut and dried way; each case has its own unique elements and circumstances. But in any event, do you really want to take the risk? Thus the best strategy for averting the contest of dueling forensic experts opining on your professional fate is simply ensuring that you have conducted a thorough assessment of suicidal risk that is well documented within the medical record (Bender, 2014; Smith et al., 2008). To this end, the CAMS-based SSF initial and interim assessments of suicidal risk are thorough, consistent, and extremely well documented.

Beyond an initial assessment of risk, there is undeniable further value of consistently assessing suicidal risk over the course of care and making an overall formulation of risk explicit within your documentation. Within CAMS-guided care, the overall formulation of suicide risk is specifically noted on every "HIPAA page" under the section "Patient's Overall Suicide Risk Level" (with three levels of risk and a written explanation for your determination therein). Moreover, suicidal risk should be explicitly indexed to the medico-legal issue of "clear and imminent danger," with specific reference to the need for hospitalization (or not). Notably, the SSF-4 does this exact thing at the end of first-session treatment-planning section. Furthermore, the ongoing prospect of hospitalization is a clinical option under the "Patient Status" (Section B) of the SSF for all CAMS interim sessions. Finally, the option of hospitalization is similarly noted on the final Outcome/Disposition SSF documentation as well. It is generally important to document why hospitalization is or is *not* indicated based on clinical judgment, which should be rooted in the best interest and overall welfare of the patient.

Years ago, I had a challenging case of a high-risk suicidal young man who as a teenager had been repeatedly hospitalized over three successive summers. According to the patient, his parents would go on vacations while he was in the hospital. In the course of each of these hospitalizations, the patient was brutally and ritualistically sexually abused by two members of the psychiatric nursing staff. Given this particularly traumatic history, I did not believe an additional hospitalization when he was suicidal as an adult was remotely in his best interest. Fortunately, the patient was successfully treated through some seriously suicidal episodes by using an early version of CAMS. Given these unique historic circumstances, my documentation for not hospitalizing this patient was extremely thorough and comprehensive, with extensive discussion of my professional reasoning as to what was truly in this patient's best interest.

Thus documentation is crucial when it comes to issues of malpractice liability. As any plaintiff attorney will tell you, "If it was not written down, it did not happen." Among the clinicians I know and train, the importance of documentation is often seen as an onerous and unduly burdensome demand. Yet in malpractice wrongful death scenarios, insufficient documentation can be cruelly turned against the clinician-defendant by a skilled plaintiff attorney. With the wisdom of hindsight, the plaintiff attorney will pointedly argue that explanations about what the clinician did and did not do have no credibility. It is the clinician's faulty memory and self-serving word against the fact of a dead patient—an "obvious victim" of failed clinical care. The adversarial tactics, for which plaintiff attorneys are infamous, never put the clinician-defendant in a flattering light. A skillful attorney can easily foment sympathy among the jury for the grieving family in the face of the "rich and heartless" provider (often an untrue and unfair characterization), who was obviously derelict in caring for the patient by virtue of the fact that the patient died. It has been argued that 80–90% of what determines, in the mind of the attorney, whether a malpractice case should be pursued depends principally on the *quality of the written medical record* (Simpson & Stacy, 2004; Wise et al., 2005). There is nothing more protective in terms of malpractice liability than competent, well-documented clinical care.

As noted since Chapter 1, the idea of identifying any current suicidal risk at the earliest possible point in a clinical encounter and thoroughly assessing that risk is a signature feature of CAMS-guided clinical care. This is particularly true if the clinician routinely uses some kind of standardized symptom-based assessment tool to screen and identify potential risk through a simple self-report assessment at the outset. If current suicidal risk is quickly picked up and identified, triggering the subsequent use of CAMS, then there is no hindsight dispute that the clinician failed to recognize the potential suicidal risk and promptly respond to it—which is the fundamental contention that lawyers argue when there was a *lack* of fore-seeability. It would then be hard to later criticize the routine and ongoing clinical assessment of suicidal risk that is central to CAMS-guided care. Let us be plain: No matter what a plaintiff attorney may argue from the vantage point of 20:20 hindsight, mental health clinicians cannot infallibly foresee the future or necessar-ily predict human behavior. However, the failure of a clinician to sense or detect and thoroughly assess the prospect of suicidal risk is the issue upon which many malpractice cases turn. Reliably using CAMS and the SSF with a suicidal patient should essentially eliminate this particular malpractice concern.

THE IMPORTANCE OF TREATMENT PLANNING

A second major malpractice consideration is the key role of treatment planning in averting any sense of negligence on the part of the clinician that the plaintiff attor-ney argued was a proximate cause of the patient's demise. In the first edition of this book, I wrote about this notion rather broadly. Some 10 years later I can write about this topic much more specifically. What the research literature now shows quite clearly is that successful treatment of suicide risk should involve treatments that are *suicide specific*. Indeed, the clarity of this is now manifest from replicated RCT treat-ment research for DBT (Linehan et al., 2006; Neacsiu et al., 2010; Stoffers et al., 2012), cognitive-behavioral therapy for suicide prevention (Brown, Have, et al., 2005; Rudd et al., 2015; Wenzel et al., 2009), and CAMS (Andreasson et al., 2016; Comtois et al., 2011). As noted in Chapter 2, there is little to no evidence that treating mental health disorders reduces suicidal ideation or behaviors; consigning suicide to the role of symptom simply misses the mark from a suicide treatment standpoint. Yet, based on my experiences in the field, this is exactly what most practitioners still do—treat mental disorders, thinking that is the best way to reduce suicidality. While such non-suicide-specific treatments may technically meet the contemporary "standard of care," this kind of treatment approach may become increasingly less defensible in the face of the mounting empirical evidence. Obviously, CAMS-based clinical care far exceeds the general standard of clinical care given its extensive evidence base as an effective treatment for suicidal risk (Jobes, 2012).

As noted throughout this book, no aspect of CAMS has evolved more in the past 10 years than our "driver-oriented" approach to suicide, which is described in depth in Chapter 6. Not only is CAMS treatment planning unabashedly suicide specific, we have further elaborated a whole new model for thinking about the etiology of suicidal risk with distinct and direct implications for suicide-specific clinical care (Jobes et al., 2011, 2016; Tucker et al., 2015). Hence, the suicide-specific nature of CAMS treatment planning is highly protective in any 20:20 hindsight consideration of malpractice negligence. Beyond this general consideration, there are specific components of the CAMS SSF treatment planning that are important to consider in a bit more depth.

Treatment Plan Problems

From Session 1 though all subsequent interim sessions of CAMS-guided care to final outcome and disposition, there is no ambiguity about what is the principal problem that fundamentally defines the CAMS treatment planning: Problem #1, Self-Harm Potential. This chief focus makes plain that there is nothing more important within CAMS-guided care than managing this concern. In turn, this primary consideration is also pivotal in relation to our focus of endeavoring to *not* hospitalize suicidal patients whenever possible. Beyond this fundamental treatment focus, the balance of CAMS treatment planning centers on the aforementioned suicidal drivers under Problems #2 and #3, which are described in depth in Chapter 6.

Treatment Goals and Objectives

Any good treatment plan should clearly articulate both the treatment goals and objectives. Moreover, the plan should ideally also identify both short- and long-term treatment goals. In the cases of suicidal risk, there must be an immediate short-term focus and strategy for effectively managing outpatient stability (i.e., getting patients through acute suicidal "dark moments"). Within CAMS, the goals and objectives are readily achieved through the satisfactory completion of the CAMS Stabilization Plan. Beyond this immediate need for short-term stability, a thorough treatment plan should also address longer-term, overarching goals that are central to successful care. In CAMS-guided care, this consideration is achieved through the identification and elaboration of patient-defined suicidal drivers under

Problems #2 and #3. Most CAMS-based suicidal drivers tend to be bigger picture and broader concerns that usually take more time to effectively target and treat during interim sessions, ultimately rendering suicidal coping obsolete.

Treatment Interventions

As noted in Chapter 6, a hallmark feature of CAMS-guided care is a general receptivity to the full spectrum of treatment interventions that might be available to effectively target and treat a patient's suicidal drivers. CAMS is not limited to any one theoretical approach or set of interventions; quite literally, anything that clinically works can be imported into fully adherent CAMS-guided care. This may include different treatment modalities, diverse types of psychotherapeutic techniques, case management, medication, vocational counseling, and so forth. I once trained a group of Native American mental health care providers who relished the thought of integrating traditional native medicine and spirituality into their use of CAMS for suicidal youth.

One common complaint that is often seen in malpractice litigation is the alleged failure of the clinician to recommend any and all appropriate and necessary treatments. Again, the "Monday-morning quarterbacking" of the plaintiff's expert tends to argue that the "kitchen sink" of care should have been offered, given the eventual fatal outcome. For example, not referring a patient with significant symptoms of a mental illness for a psychiatric medication consultation could be viewed as a major act of clinical omission in hindsight. Even if a clinician is skeptical about the value of psychotropic medications for certain cases, that same clinician may nevertheless be found liable for having failed to recommend a medication consultation. The current position of most forensic experts would be that referrals for medication consultation reflect the professional standard of care. Thus the failure to make such a referral could have significant malpractice implications—whether the patient takes the referral is another matter altogether and may be immaterial to perceived liability.

Beyond the issue of treatment omissions, the clinician's consideration and use of referrals to the full spectrum of treatments generally demonstrates a broader and more comprehensive approach to clinical care. In hindsight, such an approach appears more protective in contrast to a narrower approach that relies on only one treatment (particularly when there is evidence that an additional referral or an alternative treatment *could* have made a difference). For example, with suicidal adolescents the failure to have substance abuse separately evaluated by a specialist might be argued in hindsight by the plaintiff's expert as a significant failure. This would be particularly true if substance abuse was an obvious significant contributor to the suicidal risk. Failure to follow post-discharge plans following an inpatient admission can be expose a clinician to increased liability as well (Bender, 2014; Hashmi & Kapoor, 2010).

It is important to routinely revise and update a patient's treatment plan across the course of care. Sometimes when a case is going poorly, there is a need to overhaul the entire treatment plan (see Jobes, 2011). This discussion points to the importance of staying on top of the treatment and not settling into an open-ended and static version of care. This open-ended approach is vulnerable to the retrospective review of the plaintiff's forensic expert, who will render an opinion that the treatment plan was outdated, inadequate, and not appropriately modified to address the evolving needs of the patient who ultimately died under the care of an inattentive clinician. Clinicians who can demonstrate that their treatment was creative and evolving in the face of shifting clinical needs are much less vulnerable to malpractice liability.

Treatment Duration

Suicidal patients should be engaged in time-limited, not open-ended, treatment. Time is a huge point of leverage within treatment in general, but particularly in cases of suicidal risk. It is important for increasing motivation and for creating expectations that meaningful relief can be delivered in a reasonable time frame. To this end, there may be specific treatment protocols for certain drivers that last for 10 sessions—good to know. When I do not have a duration that specific, I propose in the first session of CAMS a 3-month course of care as a reasonable time frame to execute an effective course of CAMS treatment. We know from research that most patients respond within 12 sessions (not forever), which may be seen as a compelling alternative to the time frame for suicidal coping which is, in fact, forever.

A Word about Consultation

Beyond the constant refrain about the importance of documentation, there is a need to routinely seek professional consultation (which of course must be carefully documented). The importance of professional consultation cannot be overstated. Professional consultation is critical because it demonstrates good clinical judgment and the appropriate use of one's resources. It also makes clear that the clinician was not operating as a "lone ranger" on the case. On the SSF-4, such consultation can be noted in the Case Note section of the HIPAA page. A final general intervention consideration is the potential importance of seeking a release from the patient to obtain collateral information and support from family members and possibly other significant people in the patient's life. For example, within our military research we often observe the significant positive impact of engaging the patient's first sergeant or commanding officer in an effort to problem solve job-related problems or interpersonal issues within the patient's unit. Alternatively, engaging parents and siblings of a suicidal teen can be crucial in creating a supportive safety network around the patient. Spouses can be similarly engaged to great effect, particularly if they are involved within a "Crisis Support Plan" intervention (refer to Bryan et al., 2011). Although there are exceptions, one should routinely consider the virtue of pursuing collateral information and support as a standard part of good clinical care.

THE IMPORTANCE OF CLINICAL FOLLOW-THROUGH

A final concept of competent practice, with distinct implications for decreasing malpractice liability, pertains to the importance of clinical follow-through. Competent clinical treatment (which should be reflected in the written record) requires the clinician to execute the treatment as planned and to professionally follow through, working in the best interest of the patient. An obvious and important forensic question within malpractice litigation is the retrospective determination of whether the treatment was actually implemented as planned. As a forensic consultant/expert witness, I have been involved in several cases in which the treatment plan that appeared in the medical record reflected an appropriate and adequate approach to the case, but the clinical care that actually ensued was not consistent with the plan. Such a failure in treatment plan follow-through may be seen as a direct cause of the patient's demise and may reflect negligence and liability on the clinician's part when examined in hindsight.

Another major complaint that is routinely seen in malpractice cases is a failure to sufficiently coordinate with other providers involved in the patient's overall clinical care (Bender, 2014). Relatedly, failure to adequately review a patient's chart or obtain records from prior providers regarding self-harm history can be seen as malpractice pitfall (Melonas, 2011). Thus one should at least attempt to make contact with the patient's previous care providers to obtain information or appropriate care-related records. Naturally, such efforts should be thoroughly documented. A common breakdown that occurs is between psychotherapists and practitioners who are prescribing and monitoring the patient's psychotropic medications. All appropriate releases, signed by the patient, authorizing this coordination of care should appear in the medical record as well. In addition, provisions for emergency coverage should also be noted in the medical record. Documentation about clinical coverage and mindfulness about potential emergencies reflects a larger professional awareness, conscientiousness, and clinical competence as expected within the standard of care.

When effecting a referral to another mental health professional, one should be careful to develop the rationale and timetable leading up to that referral. Obviously, the ethical issue of clinical abandonment must be carefully considered and managed (particularly if suicidal risk is involved). This concern is especially true in cases in which the patient is reluctant to accept a referral from the clinician. If the clinician's judgment is that this referral is in the best interest of the patient, then the rationale for the referral must be developed and documented in the record. Any follow-up documentation that notes the outcome of the referral (e.g., whether the patient accepted the referral) is important information to include in the medical record too.

In some jurisdictions, there may be provisions within state law that make it possible to maintain notes that are separate from the medical record progress notes, which are required and may be discoverable. It is therefore important to be aware of jurisdictional statutes as to whether under HIPAA provisions and state law the clinician is allowed to maintain a separate set of nondiscoverable "psychotherapy notes." If the clinician is allowed to maintain such notes, he or she should consider doing so because these notes typically provide a much more detailed level of practice information that can later be produced to verify the depth and thoroughness of care, which may not be typically reflected in a standard medical record progress note. However, the clinician must be sure to follow the relevant rules or state statutes that pertain to maintaining psychotherapy notes. For example, such notes should be stored in a completely separate file (i.e., these notes must be physically stored in a different location away from the patient's medical record). These kinds of notes tend to be more narrative and can accommodate a much more detailed level of subjective information than the typical medical record progress notes, which tend to highlight just the objective facts of the case and the care rendered.

Obviously within CAMS-guided care, the notion of clinical follow-through is paramount. Indeed, within CAMS the issue of suicide should never "fall through the cracks" of clinical care as suicide risk is specifically identified early, tracked and treated during interim sessions, and completely accounted for within CAMS outcome/disposition. In other words, the SSF basically functions as a follow-through treatment plan guide. If the clinician and patient faithfully complete each section of the SSF at the beginning, through the interim sessions, and then at the end of CAMS, they have been compelled to routinely and thoroughly assess suicidal risk, develop a suicide-specific treatment plan, and consider the appropriate use of referrals and seeking of professional consultation. The routine use of the SSF means that the clinician's medical record is fully HIPAA compliant, and by using CAMS the clinician has produced a remarkably complete and thorough suicide-specific medical record, *par excellence*. More important, however—which is the whole point of this undertaking—the clinician will have provided outstanding evidence-based clinical care to the suicidal patient that our clinical trial research shows actually works.

SUMMARY AND CONCLUSIONS

As noted throughout this chapter, competent clinical practice, working in the patient's best interest and being mindful of potential malpractice liability are not mutually exclusive concepts. If a clinician works to thoroughly assess suicide risk, thoughtfully develop a treatment plan specific to that risk, and follows through on clinical care, the clinician will have provided a level of quality care that far eclipses the "standard of care"—the lens that is used to examine what happened in the course of malpractice litigation. If the clinician uses CAMS, competent suicide-specific clinical practice will be abundantly documented within the SSF-based medical record. By its nature, CAMS lays out a reliable, evidence-based course of action for the clinical dyad to pursue together. It is my sense that this kind of suicide-specific care can and will make a difference in the life of the struggling patient by fundamentally helping to stabilize and preserve that life while treatment of suicidal drivers ensues. While such a treatment cannot guarantee a non-fatal outcome, it does nevertheless provide the basis for ensuring the best possible care that is evidence based and suicide specific. This is all we as mental health professionals can and should aspire to do. And it is among your best options to make your practice relatively "bulletproof" from the distinct unpleasantness of malpractice tort litigation. More important, it is one of a handful of available approaches for the singular and noble pursuit of endeavoring to bring the best we have to offer to help save a patient's life.

CHAPTER 9

CAMS Adaptations and Future Developments

In this final chapter we will review various adaptations and uses of CAMS across a range of clinical settings and modalities. In addition, I will close out the chapter with a look at future developments pertaining to CAMS-based clinical care. As noted early on, the development of the SSF and its ultimate use within CAMS arose out of various real-world clinical needs. The initial need was to improve suicide risk assessment and management for outpatient providers working in university counseling centers with suicidal college students (Jobes, 1995b; Jobes et al., 1997). Later, the use of the SSF was extended to U.S. Air Force mental health providers working with suicidal active-duty personnel in outpatient clinics (Jobes, Wong, et al., 2005). This rather modest beginning use of the SSF ultimately led to an extensive line of clinical research and the ongoing development of CAMS described in this book. Today, CAMS is a living, breathing, and continuously evolving clinical intervention that is used in an expanding range of clinical settings around the world and with a broad spectrum of suicidal patients. It is used across professional disciplines, theoretical orientations, and clinical techniques. I fully expect CAMS to continue to evolve as a result of ongoing clinical research and particularly in relation to a remarkably fluid period of change within mental health care delivery in the United States and abroad.

ADAPTATIONS OF THE CAMS FRAMEWORK

Since its inception, I have intended for CAMS and the SSF to be flexible and highly adaptable to a range of clinical settings and suicidal populations (Jobes, 2000). As noted throughout this text, the use of CAMS has been primarily concentrated on outpatient clinical settings for use by licensed mental health providers of varying disciplines. But since the first edition of this book, many interesting adaptations of CAMS have emerged. This may be due to our determined efforts to situate CAMS as both a *philosophy* of care and a flexible suicide-specific therapeutic *framework*, instead of a new psychotherapy for treating suicidal risk (Jobes et al., 2011, 2016). These adaptations across settings and modalities are worth reviewing.

Using CAMS across Different Treatment Settings

What follows is a sampling of the use of CAMS across a range of settings that sets the stage for our discussion of CAMS use via different treatment modalities and other adaptations.

General Outpatient Settings

Because the SSF was originally developed for outpatient care, its use and the later development of CAMS has been naturally well suited to general outpatient clinical settings. In this regard, CAMS has proven to be particularly valuable in situations where there might be concerns about suicidal patients "falling through the cracks." For example, in settings where less experienced clinicians may be seeing patients under supervised practicum training, the use of CAMS can provide valuable structure and support for both patients and novice providers. Moreover, the routine use of interim tracking of ongoing suicidal risk requires a clinician perforce to stay on top of these cases, with continuous attention to suicide risk. In many settings where CAMS is reliably used, agency directors can take comfort that potentially worrisome suicidal cases are being appropriately identified, assessed, managed, and treated in a suicide-specific way. As noted in Chapter 8, even when suicides occur, SSF documentation generated through the adherent use of CAMS typically significantly decreases the risk for litigation.

University Counseling Centers

There are now many university and college counseling centers using CAMS across the United States and abroad. We know from epidemiological research that being a college student is suicide protective when compared to non-university-based cohorts (Schwartz, 2011). Thus many unique features of the typical campus environmental can facilitate the effective use of CAMS. For example, resident advisors (and under the proper circumstances even dorm roommates) can be thoughtfully engaged to help provide support and companionship for a suicidal college student in a residence hall setting. Coordination between counseling center mental health work and health care services (e.g., in terms of medications or the medical monitoring of eating disorders) is usually possible with relative ease. Invariably, there are many other campus-based resources such as reading and study skills services, a campus ministry, countless clubs, organizations, and student-run causes that can be used to therapeutically involve a suicidal student and help the patient become behaviorally activated. Over the years we have published a number of articles about the campus-based use of CAMS and the SSF, providing a rich set of resources for mental health providers working within higher education (Jobes et al., 1997, 2004; Jobes & Jennings, 2011; Jobes & Mann, 1999).

Community Mental Health Centers

I have provided training and consultation to a number of community mental health centers (CMHCs) for decades. Through my interactions with these professionals I have gained a sense of the unique needs and challenges of these treatment settings and have seen the singular value of using CAMS within community mental health care. However, one problem raised by some community mental health professionals is that the CAMS may be too sophisticated for work with the severely mentally ill or developmentally delayed patients. Although this is an understandable concern, I would contend that clinicians can still use the SSF as a valuable clinical guide even with severely disabled mentally ill patients. However, for CAMS to be used successfully with more severely mentally ill patients, it will likely require more time and an active and somewhat directive level of involvement by the clinician. Within my own practice, I have successfully used CAMS with delusional and psychotic patients—but it has required more patience, time, and perseverance on my part. For cognitively disabled patients, or for those who do not read, clinicians can use the approach, but again must simply be much more active in terms of walking patients through each element of the SSF and they may need to do the writing for them. I understand that many clinicians may not have the luxury of time that might be required to administer the SSF and CAMS to such patients. This may be particularly true for clinicians in CMHC settings who may have inordinately large caseloads of patients who might be quite sick. But we have nevertheless seen CAMS flourish within CMHC settings both in the United States and abroad once it becomes ingrained within the clinical culture of these treatment environments (e.g., Comtois et al., 2011; Corona et al., 2013). As discussed later in this chapter, the potential use of CAMS groups (CAMS-G) is promising way to provide care that maximizes limited resources while treating more suicidal patients.

Private Practice Settings

It is my belief that CAMS—and this book—may be particularly well suited to clinicians working in private practice settings. I know from my workshop training experiences that private practitioners report feeling especially vulnerable when working with suicidal patients. Depending on the nature and scope of the practice, many private practice clinicians may feel uniquely isolated; as such providers often do not have various services, a staff of colleagues, or administrators to help provide resources, structure, and professional support. Private practitioners may feel at a loss or overwhelmed with a new suicidal patient or when an existing patient becomes suicidal as they scramble to figure out what to do. Even with the best of intentions and a genuine desire to help, some practitioners may find themselves overrun by a suicidal case and thereby vulnerable to "suicidal blackmail" (see Chapter 3).

In such situations, CAMS may offer a meaningful remedy because it provides a clear procedural roadmap, a means for maintaining appropriate clinical documentation, and most important, creates a useful framework for successfully proceeding with a suicidal patient. I receive dozens e-mails each year from grateful private practitioners who attest that CAMS has transformed their practice and professional confidence in terms of working with suicidal patients.

Employee Assistance Programs

I am aware of various employee assistance programs (EAPs) that have effectively used CAMS for suicidal employees. Given the fundamentally short-term and assessment-oriented nature of EAP work, the index use CAMS emphasizing the development of a stabilization plan can be well suited to EAP work. As EAP clinicians often have only one to four sessions with an employee-patient, the initial use of CAMS can be a stabilizing and useful start, particularly if an effective referral for the treatment of the patient's suicidal drivers can be achieved. From an ethical standpoint, it is important to disclose within initial informed consent to a potential EAP patient that the *employer* may well be the "client"—not the employee.

Forensic Settings

Some years ago, a psychologist in charge of a state's mental health services for a large population of juvenile offenders across 28 forensic facilities approached me about using CAMS with their suicidal offenders. He told me that the *majority* of youthful offenders in their mental system reported being "suicidal" at some point during their incarcerations. We thus began to employ a modified use of CAMS to great effect within this system (Cardeli, 2015; Holmes, Saghafi, Monahan, Cardeli, & Jobes, 2014; Mohahan, Saghafi, Holmes, Cardeli, & Jobes, 2014; Saghafi, Monahan, Holmes, Cardeli, & Jobes, 2014). Perhaps not surprisingly, one of the challenges we quickly encountered in this effort was that being "suicidal" within this forensic system often meant both increased risk for suicidal—death-oriented—behaviors as well as nonsuicidal self-injury (NSSI) that involved cutting, burning, scratching, head-banging, and the like. Indeed, we observed that the majority of self-destructive behaviors across this sample were of the NSSI variety versus "genuine" suicide risk. Moreover, in such settings there can be obvious "secondary gain" to threatening suicide or engaging in self-harm behaviors that are *perceived* to be suicidal because of the potential instrumental value of malingering in this manner.

Undoubtedly, issues related to suicide risk are remarkably complex in forensic settings. On the one hand, incarceration—whether it be a lockup, jail, or prison—objectively increases the statistical risk of completed suicide considerably (Maris et al., 2000). But on the other hand, the threat of suicide can be instrumentally used as a means of getting oneself out of the general cell block population and into the relative "comfort" of the prison medical ward. Thus clinicians in these settings struggle mightily with discerning "genuine" versus "manipulative" (instrumental) suicidal risk (Cardeli, 2015; Mohahan et al., 2014). Add to this mix the politics of mental health care in forensic settings and the issues of liability should a patient die by suicide and we find ourselves working in one of the most challenging settings imaginable.

While the challenges are considerable, our experience of using CAMS among juvenile offenders has been a net positive (Cardeli, 2015). There are four notable reasons for potentially using CAMS with such populations: (1) there are typically less time pressures, and usually clinicians can work open-endedly with these patients as long as there is some progress; (2) the thorough assessment of risk using the SSF in CAMS may be helpful in discerning genuine versus feigned suicidal risk; (3) CAMS documentation is usually helpful from a liability standpoint; and (4) perhaps most important, incarceration increases suicidal risk; thus it follows that using an evidence-based suicide-specific treatment makes sense for a uniquely at-risk population. That said, recent efforts to use CAMS within adult prison populations have seen mixed results due in part to the discomfort of collaborating and being empathic of a convicted felon. Understandably there are certain aspects of prison culture that compel some clinicians to maintain more of an authoritative "top-down" approach with inmates, whereas other clinicians still seem able to use the approach with a subset of prisoners. My simple observation is that CAMS simply may not be suitable in certain cases or among certain providers and they are certainly free to use other evidence-based treatments for suicide risk instead.

Emergency Departments

Inspired by the work of Barbara Stanley and Greg Brown (see Knox et al., 2012) and their team's use of "SAFE-VET" a one-time suicide-specific intervention focused on safety planning and the use of nondemand telephone follow-up, CAMS Brief Intervention (CAMS-BI) has been on the process-improvement and research drawing board over the last few years. CAMS-BI is a one-session intervention using CAMS first-session procedures with no expectation of continuing care beyond this encounter. In this regard, the patient learns some basic information about his or her suicide risk and develops a CAMS Stabilization Plan with the clinician. Similar to SAFE-VET, an offer is extended for nondemand follow-up contact in a modality that is agreeable to the patient (e.g., caring phone calls, texts, e-mails, letters, tweets, Facebook). In addition, patients so engaged in CAMS-BI may also receive a "Coping Care Package"—an envelope or small box that includes various helpful brochures, hotline numbers, resources, and a copy of *Choosing to Live* by Ellis and Newman (1996), which was written for suicidal people. As with SAFE-VET and other nondemand follow-up oriented interventions (e.g., Jerome Motto's "caring letter" intervention; see Motto & Bostrom, 2001), CAMS-BI would largely target suicidal patients who are *not* interested in ongoing mental health care and the intervention could be used in an emergency department, at discharge from inpatient hospital care, or within psychiatry consultation-liaison services in medical–surgical settings.

Of course, the issue of time is particularly pressing in emergency departments where a doctor or a resident may have only 10–20 minutes to evaluate a patient. Nevertheless, I have a Swiss colleague who routinely uses the SSF to assess emergency department (ED) suicidal patients in about 10–20 minutes using a side-by-side CAMS assessment. He argues that what he potentially loses in time is actually a net gain in relation to the increased cooperation and engagement of the patient. Because ED providers are primarily focused on assessment and disposition, they can do an expedited CAMS-based assessment using Sections A and B and even identifying potential driver problems (Problems #2 and #3) that may be relevant for inpatient or outpatient care. Obviously, stabilization planning and disposition to effective care is the key to not hospitalizing a suicidal patient who presents to the ED. Within such settings, "care transition" is critical, and if the ED practitioner is able to establish a solid stabilization plan and assure a "next-day appointment" with an effective outpatient provider, expensive and potentially stigmatizing inpatient stays may be averted (see Comtois et al., 2011; Jobes, 2016).

Psychiatric Inpatient Settings

For many years, variations of the SSF have been used effectively for assessment of suicidal risk within inpatient psychiatry at the Mayo Clinic (Conrad et al., 2009; Kraft et al., 2010; O'Connor, Jobes, Comtois, et al., 2012; O'Connor, Jobes, Lineberry, & Bostwick, 2010; O'Connor, Jobes, Yeargin, et al., 2012). Over many of these years, the assessment components of the SSF were administered by nursing staff on the inpatient wards and the data were used to meaningfully shape the inpatient treatment plan and inform disposition discharge planning (Lineberry et al., 2006). In more recent years, the SSF has been integrated into an electronic assessment that is routinely used with all Mayo Clinic inpatients at admission across ages (Romanowicz, O'Connor, Schak, Swintak, & Lineberry, 2013).

Beyond the assessment use of the SSF, CAMS has been applied to different inpatient settings for some time. For example, over a decade ago, a team of Swiss inpatient providers (Schilling et al., 2006) treated 45 suicidal inpatients using a German translation of the SSF and an inpatient version of CAMS. These researchers noted dramatic decreases in overall symptom distress and suicidal risk over a 10-day course of inpatient care.

CAMS INTENSIVE INPATIENT CARE

Inspired by the work of Marjan Holloway (Ghahramanlou-Holloway et al., 2012), who developed an intensive suicide-specific inpatient treatment called postadmission cognitive therapy (PACT), we are now exploring the prospect of using an intensive inpatient version of CAMS across a handful of inpatient treatment settings within the United States. So-called "CAMS Intensive Inpatient Care" (CAMS-IIC) is designed to occur over a 3- to 6-day hospital stay. CAMS care is thus compressed into an intensive treatment experience where a suicidal inpatient receives a standard initial CAMS session, at least one interim session, and finally a discharge/disposition session of intensive CAMS-guided care. The goals of the intervention are relatively modest; we aim to provide a thorough assessment of suicidal risk, the identification of patient-defined suicidal drivers, and an optimal discharge/disposition wherein a solid stabilization plan is established before discharge and ideally an outpatient provider is in place to help maintain stabilization and targeted treatment of the patient's suicidal drivers. At a minimum, exposure to CAMS-IIC should help ensure some suicide-specific coping skills within the CAMS Stabilization Plan and a suicide-specific treatment agenda that should helpfully shape post-discharge outpatient care.

THE MENNINGER VERSION OF CAMS

Since the publication of the first edition of this book we have seen extraordinary success using an adapted inpatient version of CAMS at the Menninger Clinic in Houston, Texas. Referred to as CAMS-M (for the Menninger version), this inpatient adaptation of CAMS has proven to be highly successful and has led to a number of publications (Ellis et al., 2010; Ellis, Daza, & Allen, 2012; Ellis, Green., et al., 2012, 2015; Lento, Ellis, Hinnant, & Jobes, 2013). This adapted version of CAMS developed Tom Ellis employs CAMS sometimes twice a week with highly suicidal inpatients over a 50- to 60-day inpatient stay. This being an inpatient setting with longer than usual lengths of stay, the use of CAMS at Menninger has been embellished and elaborated in some unique ways. For example, stabilization planning can be handled readily by skilled nursing staff, while CAMS-trained inpatient psychotherapists can drill into a treatment of a patient's suicidal drivers in an intensive way. While the Menninger length of stay is rather unique, we believe that with serious and chronically suicidal patients (who may have been hospitalized many times), a lengthier inpatient stay can ultimately be justified if it becomes their *last* inpatient admission, if their relationship to suicide fundamentally changes, and if this change is borne out in enduring post-discharge nonsuicidal outcomes (Ellis & Rufino, 2015).

Different CAMS Modalities and Adaptations

Because CAMS is a both a philosophy of care and a flexible suicide-specific clinical framework, we have seen some exciting developments in terms of using CAMS in different treatment modalities; some of these novel adaptations of CAMS are worthy of note.

CAMS-Groups

To date, the use of suicide-specific group therapy has been relatively rare. But since the last edition of this book, a new use of CAMS within a group format has emerged and is now being intensively studied by our team. The first "CAMS-Group" (CAMS-G) used an adapted version of CAMS within a group modality with severely mentally ill suicidal veterans in an outpatient partial treatment program at the Washington, D.C., Veterans Affairs Medical Center (Jennings, 2012). This group approach required an initial first-session use of standard individual CAMS prior to admitting the suicidal veteran into the CAMS-G. Given that members of the group had serious mental health disorders, this particular CAMS-G was somewhat more structured and didactic in nature, but still used both CAMS philosophy and the SSF framework to fundamentally guide the group's suicide-specific treatment process.

A second CAMS-informed group therapy approach was successfully developed for suicidal veterans at the Louisville Veterans Affairs Medical Center (Johnson, 2012; Johnson et al., 2014). In this version, suicidal inpatient veterans were engaged in a standard SSF-based CAMS assessment prior to discharge and admission into the outpatient group. Along with similarly discharged and admitted suicidal veterans, each group session began with an interim SSF assessment and tracking to help shape and inform the suicide-specific group therapy experience. These two early versions of CAMS-G have been unified into a standard CAMS-G format that is now being studied in feasibility pilot studies and ultimately within RCTs. The obvious virtue of a group model is the ability to deliver more suicide-specific care to more patients within a cost-effective treatment modality (Johnson et al., 2014). Moreover, when used as a post-inpatient discharge treatment option we believe that the known risk that follows the post-discharge period can be effectively mitigated by a successful post-discharge care transition. There is also therapeutic potential that may be unique to a group format, such as directly addressing the notion of "perceived burdensomeness" and the value of like-minded suicidal patients sharing effective stabilization techniques and treatments for their suicidal drivers. The use of CAMS-G may well prove to be a landmark innovation for the cost-effective and treatment-effective care of suicidal risk, which is why we are endeavoring to study its potential through clinical research and RCTs.

CAMS with Teenagers and Children

Many providers quiz me about the use of CAMS with teenagers and young children. One of the most glaring shortfalls of the field of suicidology is the remarkably limited literature on suicide under the age of 12 (Anderson, Keyes, & Jobes, 2016). It is almost as if latency-age children neither have suicidal thoughts nor engage in suicidal behaviors, which of course is not the case; on average, 33 children ages 5–11 die each year in the United States (Bridge, Asti, et al., 2015). Until relatively recently I would not recommend the use of CAMS with children under the age of 12. However, new innovative work has now changed my mind, as we have seen clinical success with a highly adapted use of CAMS with young children (ages 5–12) who have been responsive to care (for more information, see Anderson et al., 2016). While this exploratory work is promising, careful and thoughtful empirical research is needed to better understand the potential value (or any concerns) about using CAMS with young suicidal children.

As noted earlier in the chapter, we have more routinely seen the effective use of the SSF with suicidal inpatient teens (Romanowicz et al., 2013) as well as the effective clinical use of CAMS with suicidal incarcerated juvenile offenders (Cardeli, 2015). Generally speaking, we are seeing the effective use of CAMS for many post-pubescent suicidal teenagers. As you are now appreciating, CAMS requires the patient to be the expert of his or her own experience. And with most teenagers that I have known and treated, they are the expert on everything, *especially* themselves! It follows that when CAMS is properly used with suicidal teenagers, they often enthusiastically embrace this signature feature of CAMS philosophy. Thus young people usually find within CAMS-guided care a therapeutic forum within which they can describe and explain *their* intrasubjective suicidal struggle and a treatment of drivers that *they* articulate—which is often a novel experience for many young people.

Some providers feel that terms on the SSF may be too complex or elusive for a child or teenager. To date, the research we have done that pertains precisely to this concern has not proven this to be the case (O'Connor, Brausch, Anderson, & Jobes, 2014; Romanowicz et al., 2013). What may be true, however, is the potential need to pace the approach a bit more slowly. That is, to use the assessment forum created by CAMS engagement as a "teachable moment" in which the provider can describe and help clarify SSF-related constructs to the suicidal teenager. Some teens may initially distrust the adult clinician who gives them both the space and support to elaborate on their suicidality because they are used to adults (e.g., parents, teachers, and coaches) telling them how they feel and what they should be feeling. Invariably when the teenager experientially "gets" what we are trying to do in CAMS related to the phenomenology of their suicidal struggle, the teen can become quite engaged, and trust in the process and clinician often grows exponentially.

A foremost consideration when working with any minors is the need to skillfully engage parents in the treatment process—this is true in general mental health care with minors and it is exceedingly true when dealing with suicidal teens. Frankly, parents are often at the heart of the suicidal teen's troubles, so their engagement can be quite tricky—potentially therapeutic and sometimes disastrous. Within our society, parents are the holders of privilege, so they do have legal rights to information and decision making pertaining to the care of their offspring. As a general matter, we recommend an initial meeting with all parties included (the child-patient and ideally *all* parents or primary caregivers) to sort through issues of communication and mutual support of the treatment plan by all parties (O'Connor, Brausch, et al., 2014). As treatment continues, parents need to be skillfully looped into the process in order to optimize their potential for a pro-therapeutic role within the overall care. We have seen that sometimes describing a bit about CAMS and educating parents to the notion of treating suicidal drivers can be both comforting and helpful in improving parents' understanding of their child's suicidality. While never being alarmist, I speak to parents plainly about the life-or-death nature of suicidal risk—there is no sugarcoating what this situation is about. Many parents—out of fear, embarrassment, or denial—will pointedly dismiss their child's reputed suicidal risk as adolescent melodrama. I mince no words about the perils of minimizing suicidal risk as suicide stubbornly remains a leading cause of death for youth in the United States (and around the world).

A Word about Cultural Considerations

As noted throughout this book, CAMS is used around the world with a broad range of suicidal patients. Particularly in our community-based studies, we have seen CAMS used successfully with diverse samples across cultures (e.g., Comtois et al., 2011; Corona et al., 2013). Indeed, we are currently studying the use of CAMS and the SSF across clinical samples of suicidal patients from the United States, Ireland, Norway, Denmark, Switzerland, and China (Schembari & Jobes, 2015). I know anecdotally that CAMS has been used with virtually every race and creed over the past 20 years with good reported success. I am also aware that many comment on the side-by-side seating being something that may vary from culture to culture. For example, I was presenting video demonstrations of my use of CAMS in a training in Copenhagen, and the clinicians commented on how closely I sat next to the patient; they noted a side-by-side seating that they use but with more physical space between the clinician and patient. Another interesting cultural consideration that I have heard is that members of some cultures may actually *prefer* that the clinician remain in a superior position (i.e., in a more expert and authoritative "doctor" role), rather than what I typically emphasize in standard CAMS-guided care wherein the clinician endeavors to create a more equal and collaborative dynamic.

Recently, we have been working to rigorously translate and scientifically validate a Spanish version of SSF (Bamatter, Barrueco, Oquendo, & Jobes, 2015). Beyond using established translation-back-translation techniques to create a Spanish version, this research effort further developed a set of culture-specific guidelines through expert and community member feedback groups. The result of this process was the development of an appendix to the Spanish version of the SSF emphasizing the following subheadings: Cultural Competence, Cultural Values and Acculturalization, and Cultural Expressions of Distress (Suarez-Balcazar et al., 2011). This kind of culturally sensitive research can thus capitalize on the known virtues of the SSF and CAMS while still contextualizing and enhancing its use with certain populations.

For my part, I believe the evidence and clinical practice show that CAMS can be used effectively across cultures, in part because it is designed and intended to be used with flexibility. Thus cultural accommodation and adaptation are welcome. But I will also readily acknowledge that CAMS simply may not work in every situation, every setting, within every culture, and with every suicidal patient. It is hard to imagine that any one approach to something as complex as suicidal risk would work in every scenario, and that must be true for CAMS as well.

CAMS with Couples and Supportive Others

In a related sense, I have observed how powerful certain aspects of CAMS can be within the presence of a spouse or a significant other. In our clinical trials we routinely embrace the use of "Crisis Support Plans" to create a treatment-supportive role and set of shared expectations that can be negotiated with a spouse, significant other, friend, or family member (Bryan et al., 2011). I remember a case within our Army clinical trial of a seriously depressed Soldier with significant combat-related PTSD and chronic pain. We would periodically have his wife attend sessions in which the SSF was reviewed and his evolving suicidal drivers were presented and explained to her. These were moving and powerful sessions where the spouse was informed about how to not undermine his care, and she further learned about how she could play a significant support role within his stabilization plan and the treatment of his drivers. Hence we see the value of strategic engagement of supportive others within this structured approach as an empowering and valuable way to support CAMS-guided care on a case-by-case basis (i.e., when it seems indicated as a means of serving the patient's best interests).

CAMS and Tele-Health

It may seem odd to talk about using CAMS within a remote treatment arrangement. Yet we have seen the successful use of CAMS as part of our Army process improvement work with a psychologist-provider who does her therapeutic work through tele-health. In this situation, the Soldier-patient who lives some hours away from the military treatment facility has a copy of the SSF that he follows with his provider, who has her copy at the medical center. They see each other onscreen and use the SSF to guide their CAMS sessions. The provider completes the SSF on behalf of the patient, faithfully completing both assessment and treatment-planning sections per the patient's direction. The clinician noted to us how much the patient "enjoyed" this dynamic and that he seemed to relish correcting her when she did not transcribe something exactly as he meant it. This innovative psychologist was convinced that tele-health could be a powerful way to use the CAMS model even though they obviously could not sit next to each other as would be typical in a face-to-face clinical encounter. We plan to explore the feasibility of CAMS within a tele-health treatment modality as part of our ongoing Army process improvement consultation work and in the course of our clinical treatment research in the coming years to meaningfully expand CAMS use beyond the office.

Use of CAMS/SSF by Paraprofessionals

As a suicide-specific clinical intervention, CAMS has been primarily intended for use by licensed mental health providers. We have nevertheless seen successful and increasing use of the assessment aspects of CAMS among paraprofessionals.

PSYCHOLOGICAL TECHNICIANS

In the course of conducting suicide-related process improvement consultations and trainings within the U.S. Military and Veterans Affairs, there have been different hybrid professional/paraprofessional applications of CAMS. For example, within a few military outpatient mental health clinics, we have successfully trained psychological technicians (a.k.a. "psych-techs") in the preliminary use of a CAMS-guided first-session assessment using the SSF. In one such military treatment facility, the licensed mental health providers are required by regulation to conduct extensive intakes of a newly presenting service member patient (sometimes lasting a couple of hours). The exasperated commander who leads one such clinic suggested that we might train her psych-techs to administer Sections A and B of the first-session SSF within a CAMS-inspired initial engagement.

   As an aside, within the U.S. Army, most psych-techs have at least a high school education (sometimes more) and most have fairly limited training and some exposure to mental health care and environments. Many times the tech's role is purely administrative, limited to paperwork and scheduling patients. However, "down-range" in deployed combat environments, techs become known as "docs" and may well be more readily sought out by Soldiers in the field than deployed licensed mental health providers! Given these considerations, from the clinic commander's perspective, while her licensed providers are tied up doing exhaustive intakes, suicidal patients can also get a suicide-specific collaborative SSF assessment provided by well-trained and appropriately supervised psych-techs. Within this adaptation, the psych-techs complete CAMS-oriented first-session assessments and subsequently engage a licensed provider to develop the CAMS Stabilization Plan and the driver-oriented treatment plan (Section C) with the tech present during this portion of the session. Once a patient is engaged in this hybrid manner, the licensed provider can then conduct the CAMS interim treatment work, while also having a tech who is familiar with the case as an added resource for ongoing care and follow-up. In this sense, the tech can be used for increased patient contact (if needed for stabilization) or even well-supervised intervention work with the patient on behalf of the CAMS-based driver-oriented treatment plan (e.g., checking over a patient's therapeutic homework assignment). Again, when techs are engaged within this hybrid model and are subsequently deployed, they now have valuable exposure and experience of working in suicide risk assessment and care that augments their field work when they become the "doc" in theater.

CRISIS CENTERS AND HOTLINES

As noted in the first edition, I have long considered the possible use of the SSF within the CAMS tradition as an approach for assessing suicidal risk within crisis center and hotline work (e.g., Jobes, 2004a). Like the tele-health adaptation, similar adjustments are needed to use CAMS or the SSF in crisis center work. But the potential value of using the SSF as a guide for the hotline worker's assessment of suicidal risk is a natural and easy application of this tool. Moreover, even without being physically in the same space, the overarching philosophy of the CAMS approach can still be effectively applied for a suicidal crisis caller. In my experience, many paraprofessional hotline counselors typically have excellent suicide-specific assessment and counseling skills, often better than some mental health professionals who typically do not receive suicide-specific training in the course of their graduate, medical, or nursing training (Bongar, 2002). Hotline workers know they must have suicide-specific training, because they encounter the issue often and they are well equipped to do so.

Use of CAMS across Licensed Providers

In yet another military treatment facility, we saw the effective use of CAMS for "walk-ins" that were engaged by licensed clinical social workers. The idea here was for the social workers to initially engage a suicidal walk-in Soldier for a few sessions while waiting for a scheduled psychotherapy hour to become available. In this setting we saw that suicidal Soldiers could be well stabilized by two to three sessions of CAMS before being turned over to a new psychotherapy provider when a scheduled therapy hour opened up (Archuleta et al., 2014). We heard anecdotes of suicidal Soldiers who were so engaged, presenting their own cases to their new therapy provider with a sense of pride and accomplishment, providing a full review and analysis of their SSFs to date. In turn, as an expert of CAMS-guided care, the new psychotherapy provider fully appreciated the preliminary stabilization work done by the walk-in provider and was readily able to successfully pick up the Soldier's CAMS-based driver-oriented treatment. I would note that such an approach might not work with every case; for example, a traumatized patient may be understandably reluctant to rehash things with his or her new provider.

Within our clinical research we have explored the potential pairing a case manager with a licensed mental health provider, particularly for complex suicidal cases involving severe mental illness and psychosocial hardships. Indeed, we see in the cognitive therapy for suicide prevention (CT-SP) treatment approach the powerful impact of case managers for complex cases of suicidal patients (Brown, Have, et al., 2005). Moreover, in our own randomized controlled trial at Harborview Hospital with suicidal outpatients (Comtois et al., 2011), we observed the power of case management and that CAMS-trained providers could readily "cover" if a patient's clinician was on leave or sick, and the patient needed to be seen. Because we CAMS clinicians all share an understanding of the model, having a new provider "cover" for the usual provider is not as off-putting as one might expect it to be. Indeed, we again see a sense of pride in the patient introducing his or her case to the appreciative new provider, who understands the CAMS model and can fill in quite well.

Finally along these lines, we have seen CAMS used successfully across services within a large military medical center. At Walter Reed National Military Medical Center, we have engaged in a multi-year process improvement project to train and support adapted uses of CAMS across every part of this flagship medical center for service members in all branches of the U.S. military. To this end, we have trained mental health providers from varying disciplines in the CAMS model (e.g., outpatient providers, inpatient providers, partial day treatment providers, and providers in psychiatry consultation-liaison). The singular goal of this effort has been to have different starting points for the use of CAMS (e.g., in outpatient care, the inpatient unit, the emergency department, or perhaps on a medical-surgical unit) where a suicidal patient may be initially engaged and continued from service to service as indicated. For example, a patient presenting to outpatient care who is too unstable to be handled within outpatient CAMS may require an inpatient stay. But the assessment data from the first-session SSF in the outpatient unit is considered after admission to the inpatient unit as the inpatient's suicidal drivers are further fleshed out in a 5-day hospitalization. Upon discharge, this same patient might be further engaged using CAMS within an intensive outpatient partial program wherein the suicidal drivers of combat-related PTSD and marital infidelity may be effectively treated. Finally, this patient could then be transferred to his or her original outpatient CAMS provider, who can now conclude this line of suicide-specific work that has been effectively delivered and coordinated across three different treatment services within the same medical center. Frankly, the coordinated and sequential use of CAMS across services has been ambitious and challenging to reliably achieve. Such an effort requires strong and sustained leadership as part of a multiyear process improvement effort across services. But we keep on learning.

CAMS FUTURE DEVELOPMENTS

One of the surprising things about writing the second edition of this book has been the experiential realization that this text is no mere retread; it is basically a whole new book. While I have intentionally followed the successful format of the first edition, the many developments, changes, and innovations in the use of CAMS over the past decade have necessitated an almost complete revamping of the book's content. Given both the need and the dynamic evolution of CAMS to date, I have every reason to believe that future developments will continue to move CAMS in novel and exciting directions. What follows are some of my current expectations and speculations about some next steps in the evolution of CAMS.

The Application of Technology

This one is easy. New advances in technology permeate every nook and cranny of our professional and personal lives; thus there is every reason to believe that technological advances and the use of CAMS will continue to evolve, merge, and inevitably take the intervention into new and unforeseen realms of suicide prevention. For example, we have recently seen the power of the "virtual hope box" as a smartphone application for supporting a suicidal person through acute suicidal episodes (Bush et al., 2015). Inspired by the previously mentioned CT-SP intervention work by Beck and colleagues (Wenzel et al., 2009), the virtual hope box app is among the first of an inexorable wave of technological applications that will support, and maybe even displace, standard clinical interventions for suicidal risk.

Along these lines, we have four separate studies under way developing and studying electronic versions of the SSF. For example, since we know from neuroscience research that writing by hand is different than typing (e.g., Longcamp et al., 2008; Longcamp, Boucard, Gilhodes, & Velay, 2006), we feel compelled to carefully study and understand any "E-SSF" that we develop before releasing it for broad-based use. We know that the SSF and/or some CAMS-based computer, tablet, and smartphone applications must and will be developed in the not too distant future. The need to move away from scanning hard copies of SSFs into electronic records is inevitable, but there will not be a precipitous move in this eventual direction until we know more from our empirical research about what exactly happens when the SSF and CAMS are administered electronically.

At this point, there can be little doubt that advances in technology and computing should help improve our ability to understand, predict, and prevent suicidal behaviors in the years to come. We have seen the capacity of Matthew Nock's (Nock et al., 2010) use of the Implicit Associations Test (IAT) for an indirect assessment of suicidal risk through a computer administration that can objectively *predict* future attempt behaviors in a sample of teenage youths who do not realize that they are being assessed for their prospective suicidal behavioral risk within the IAT paradigm. There are other examples of using and applying technology for therapeutic purposes related to suicidal risk (Nock & Dinakar, 2015). The use of therapeutic avatars has been shown in some early feasibility work to be remarkably helpful within medical-surgical treatment environments. For example "Nurse Louise," a virtual medical-surgical nurse avatar, has been shown to effectively provide post-discharge information to medical-surgical patients pending discharge (Berkowitz et al., 2013). What is the prominent virtue of a virtual avatar-clinician? An avatar-clinician can be "built" to not be afraid of a suicidal risk and will neither judge nor shame a suicidal patient. But whether such a technology can deliver a helpful or life-saving form of care remains to be seen through thoughtful and rigorous clinical research. Given the life-or-death implications, societal expectations and demands, and ever-increasing health care costs, it seems inevitable that we will continue to turn to technology for life-saving assessment and treatment. Now funded by an National Institute of Mental Health "Small Business Innovation Research" (SBIR) grant, I am involved with a team of researchers who are developing a "proof of concept" avatar or "relational agent" of an emergency department (ED) intervention using a highly adapted version of CAMS for suicidal patients who come in for ED care (Jobes, 2016).

Innovations in CAMS-Based SSF Assessment

With multiple clinical trials under way, we are now positioned to do exciting assessment research along the lines of expanding previous studies that were limited by small sample sizes. For example, as I noted in Chapter 1, our study of 60 suicidal college students showed that using hierarchical linear modeling (HLM) could be used to *predict* four different reductions of suicidal ideation based on index-session SSF responses (Jobes, Kahn-Greene, et al., 2009). These data were especially compelling because even with a small sample, we saw the predictive validity of a one-time set of ratings from a first-session SSF. Given the promise of these data, we see intriguing potential for using baseline SSF ratings (and other assessment data from the SSF) with much larger clinical samples within our well-powered RCT studies of CAMS, which should provide valuable assessment-based findings in the years ahead.

In a related sense, there is a great deal of interest in using technology to analyze written responses like those obtained on the first-session SSF. For example, our research team (Brancu et al., 2015) used a content analysis software program on SSF qualitative responses obtained from first CAMS sessions with 144 suicidal college students. The software was used to analyze and extract word counts pertaining to "self" versus "relational" SSF qualitative responses within a repeated measures longitudinal design to assess any ability of these constructs to predict the resolution of suicidal ideation and suicidal risk over the course of counseling center care. Using this methodology, we found that suicidal patients with primarily relationally focused word counts were likely to have a quicker suicide risk resolution (six to seven sessions) than those with more self-focused word counts (17–18 sessions). Thus such technology can be used to help us analyze qualitative data in entirely novel ways (Pennebaker, Chung, Ireland, Gonzales, & Booth, 2007), particularly when there is access to "big data" that can lead to linguistic analyses looking for unique patterns of risk within assessment data (e.g., Poulin et al., 2014).

Another major assessment quest is the ongoing search for suicidal typologies or subtypes of suicidal risk. As noted in Chapter 3, we already have reliable stratifications of risk that can help organize suicidal patients into three distinct types: those who are suicidal but attached to living, those who are ambivalently suicidal, and those who are suicidal and markedly attached to dying. This is not a trivial line of investigation. Knowing that we can reliably organize suicidal patients into these three lanes of suicidal motivation is helpful and meaningful in terms of our preliminary studies related to treatment outcomes (Jennings et al., 2012; O'Connor, Jobes, Yeargin, et al., 2012). It is also an important first step to potentially more refined stratifications of risk or suicidal typologies. We intuitively know that suicidal people vary and are not a homogenous population. But within the universe of suicidal people there are undeniable patterns of suicidal states that are worth understanding in much more depth because the treatment implications might be profound. There might one day be a way to sensibly match different treatments and techniques, of different intensities, and doses of care to recognizable types of suicidal states—a compelling treatment prospect that I have been writing about for 20 years (Jobes, 1995a). It is important to note that this treatment-matching notion is not new. In fact, Kovacs and Beck (1977) argued that the focus of treatment might be different for patients at different ends of the WTL–WTD spectrum (e.g., the potential clinical use of problem-solving support for WTL-type patients vs. a more active effort building reasons for living among WTD patients).

CAMS Treatment Research

As noted in Chapter 2 there are four RCTs under way at the time of this writing and a great deal of data-driven CAMS innovations are expected to come from these investigations (Jobes, 2015, 2016; Jobes et al., 2016). For example, we have now developed an adherence scale for CAMS providers called the CAMS Rating Scale (refer to CRS-3 in Appendix F). The CRS has excellent validity and reliability and can be effectively used for both establishing adherence to CAMS as well as fidelity within RCT research (Corona, 2015). If the RCT investigations of CAMS continue to reliably validate CAMS at the highest levels of scientific rigor, a next step will be to conduct dismantling studies to identify the exact mechanisms of change for what makes CAMS effective.

Another exciting treatment research frontier is the potential integration of different treatments. For example, many providers are naturalistically integrating the use of CAMS with DBT. As noted earlier in our Seattle study, the use of CAMS was effective in setting up follow-up DBT care (Comtois et al., 2011). As noted earlier, an RCT of suicidal college students using a SMART design is attempting to rigorously study the differential and sequential impact of using CAMS and DBT (Pistorello & Jobes, 2014). Such research addresses the aforementioned notion of matching different treatments and doses to different suicidal states to achieve optimal outcomes in an efficient and cost-effective manner. As mentioned in Chapter 2, we are pursuing a well-powered replication ($n = 200$) of our earlier RCT conducted at Harborview Medical Center in the Aftercare Focused Study (AFS). This study is funded by the American Foundation for Suicide Prevention and is expressly designed to investigate the known high risk following the immediate postdischarge period for suicidal patients coming out of inpatient care or from emergency departments (Jobes, 2016). Such "care-transition" treatment research is an important new focus in the field of clinical suicidology. There is also an increasing focus on reducing repeat hospitalizations.

CAMS Training Research

During a sabbatical leave some years ago I traveled through a network of eight Veterans Affairs Medical Centers, training a total of 165 mental health providers in the use of CAMS via lecture, PowerPoint slides, and various demonstration videos (Jobes, 2011). While these daylong didactic trainings were uniformly highly rated on posttraining evaluations, fewer than 10 providers were actually using the intervention a year later. Upon reflection, it is my sense that the lack of actually using CAMS was due to both a dearth of reinforcing systemic support and the reality that didactic training alone is often insufficient for most providers to actually *change practice behaviors* (Jobes, 2015, 2016; Pisani et al., 2011).

Regarding systems-level obstacles to clinician behavior change, many evidence-based practices are not implemented because there is little to no behavioral reinforcement for doing so. Indeed, many evidence-based practices can be relatively labor and time intensive. For example, prolonged exposure treatment does not fit neatly into a 45- to 50-minute clinical hour; hence, there is the prospect of seeing fewer patients in a standard 40-hour work week. Consequently, despite a great deal of policy rhetoric promoting the use of evidence-based practices, there is little opportunity to establish their actual use when the clinicians alone are responsible for change (Jobes, Comtois, Brown, & Sung, 2015). Rather, systems of care must change and incentives must be created to induce (or at least make it feasible for) clinicians to actually provide evidence-based practices. Recognition of this the problem underlies why our CAMS team has felt compelled to conduct systems-based process improvement projects that help raise the standard of clinical care related to suicide risk (Archuleta et al., 2014).

Beyond the various systems-level challenges, there are numerous additional barriers to fostering clinician behavior change for adherently using an evidence-based practice such as CAMS that I discussed in Chapter 1. In my considerable experience as a professional trainer, changing clinical practice behaviors (especially among more seasoned clinicians within my own age cohort) has been proven to be a formidable challenge over the years. Clinicians often opt to maintain familiar practices and are very reluctant to try something new. Given all these considerations, as well as what we know to be true from the implementation science literature, we have now embraced a completely different model for adherent training in CAMS. At this point, the literature on professional training of evidence-based practices clearly shows that mere didactic training may not be enough to compel clinicians to change practice behaviors (Barlow, Bullis, Comer, & Ametaj, 2013; Beidas et al., 2012; Karlin et al., 2010). The emerging field of implementation science advocates the value of "integrated" or "blended" training, which involves didactic instruction of key content, plus relevant content-related reading, plus role-playing, plus clinical case consultations. Consequently, my team is now committed to (and we are empirically investigating) a whole new model of CAMS adherence training that involves the following sequential steps of blended training:

1. Establishing a foundation for providers in CAMS-based content.
2. Engaging clinicians in CAMS live role-play training.
3. Engaging clinicians in case consultation discussions of using CAMS.

CAMS foundational training can be done through reading this book and/or engaging in authorized live or Web-based content training in CAMS. Further training in CAMS (including live role-playing and clinical case consultation) can then be done with expert CAMS trainers (for more on authorized CAMS training, see *www.cams-care.com*). In the years ahead we intend to investigate this integrated training model extensively to find both an efficient and cost-effective way to scale up broad-based training in the adherent use of CAMS. I should note that not all adherent CAMS training must be done through this sequence. Since the first edition of this book was published, there have been intrepid clinicians who read the book, copy the SSF, and give the intervention a clinical go with great success. But in my experience, such clinicians are outliers; most providers tend to need a bit more training exposure, role-play practice, and clinical case consultation support.

SUMMARY AND CONCLUSIONS

These are exciting days for working with CAMS in relation to new adaptations and further developments that may lie ahead. After 25 years of hard work, we now see the natural maturing of this suicide-specific assessment and intervention (also refer to Appendix G for "frequently asked questions" about some evolving aspects of the model). There is now compelling use of CAMS across a range of treatment settings as well as adaptation of the approach within different treatment modalities. Future developments related to applying technology, advances in SSF-related assessments, and innovations based on our RCTs will ensure that CAMS will continue to evolve. In addition, improvements in CAMS training is now a major focus of a new integrated/blended model of training to adherence that will be rigorously studied to scale up broad-based access to CAMS training. Finally, as noted in Chapter 1, the fluid and dynamic nature of contemporary and future health care delivery will also compel new adaptations and uses of CAMS that capitalize on its being a suicide-specific, evidence-based, least-restrictive, and a potentially cost-effective way to clinically save lives across a range of settings and suicidal patients. With the maturation of CAMS we now see an approach that has extensive empirical support as an assessment approach. Furthermore, with ongoing clinical trial research we are also seeing the emergence of CAMS as a new driver-oriented clinical intervention with replicated clinical outcomes for effectively treating suicidal risk.

Epilogue

While people have taken their lives throughout recorded history, our more contemporary story begins with how the suicidal "lunatic" was viewed during medieval times. At best, such a person was seen as a deviant. At worst, such a person was thought to be possessed by the devil or evil spirits. In either case, suicidal suffering was clearly not afforded much compassion or anything remotely therapeutic. To be sure, neither prison nor spiritual exorcism offered much relief for someone suffering in this manner.

In the centuries that have followed, there has been a kind of civilized progression in thinking about suicidal people. Importantly, the suicidal lunatic was increasingly seen over time not as a person possessed but rather as a *patient*; someone who was actually mentally ill and therefore in need of compassionate clinical care. However, we do not routinely think of the early asylums of the 16th and 17th centuries as either compassionate or caring environments despite the Age of Enlightenment. Suicidal mentally ill patients were routinely warehoused, shackled, and often "treated" in a barbaric ways. Even in the 20th century, mentally ill patients were wrapped in ice-cold sheets or given insulin treatments to break through psychosis (Kohen, 2004; Sakel, 1935; Tohen, Waternaux, & Oepen, 1994), and the infamous and pervasive use of electroconvulsive therapy (prior to anesthesia and muscle relaxants) resulted in broken bones and even fatalities (Lebensohn, 1999). For years, radical surgical procedures such as lobotomy and cingulotomy were liberally used to dramatically and irreversibly modify the behaviors of the mentally ill (Mashour, Walker, & Martuza, 2005; Valenstein, 1986).

As I write these words in 2016, I can of course reflect on how far we have come in our etiological understanding, diagnosis, and clinical treatments of mental disorders (with clear implications for suicidal patients therein). On the one hand, we have learned so much through our empirical research and our evolving use of technologies to better understand the brain and its inherent disorders. With each passing year, neuroscience, genetics, magnetic imaging, and new research methodologies are helping us unravel the mysteries of the brain and the central nervous system. There can be no doubt that we are in extraordinary period of scientific discovery where new assessments and treatments for suicidal risk are enjoying an unparalleled period of growth and ascendancy (Jobes, 2011, 2014, 2016).

But on the other hand, we are perhaps not as evolved as we would like to think we are when it comes to our contemporary care and the actual *treatment* of the mentally ill, particularly in relation to suicidal risk. In an uncanny similarity to medieval times, too many mentally ill people live on the street in active states of psychosis, hallucinating and responding to voices that exist only in their own minds. Furthermore, prevalence rates of psychiatric disorders for both incarcerated men and women in the United States remain significantly higher than in community cohorts. In the United States there are three times more mentally ill people in prison than in our psychiatric hospitals (Fazel & Seewald, 2012), and mentally ill people are increasingly at risk for the "revolving door" of the forensic settings as a substitute for psychiatric care (Baillargeon, Binswanger, Penn, Williams, & Murray, 2009; Fazel & Yu, 2011; Kinsler & Saxman, 2007).

Given these considerations, it is important to note that in 2014 the American Association of Suicidology ushered into their organizational membership a whole new division of members who self-identify as "Attempt Survivor/Lived Experience." These members are pioneering a whole new perspective on the topic of suicide prevention as they forthrightly acknowledge their own experiences of having suffered through suicidal states and of having made suicide attempts. In my mind, this membership movement harkens back to the late 1970s, when suicide loss "survivors" burst into the field of suicide prevention, becoming a major voice that has fundamentally changed and defined the field ever since (Jobes, Luoma, Hustead, & Mann, 2000).

This new voice is powerful. Members with lived experience are now speaking with conviction and passion about a long-ignored and highly stigmatized experience of what it is like to suffer with suicidal thoughts and behaviors within our modern society and receive "help" within conventional contemporary care. This new voice is demanding to be heard—speaking difficult truths about contemporary mental health care and the treatment of suicidal risk. While there are countless examples of compassionate and effective mental health care, this group is nevertheless speaking to a very different perspective, where care and treatments have been neither compassionate nor effective. In fact, many argue from this unique perspective that their mental health care experiences were coercive, controlling, humiliating, shaming, and even punishing. They are speaking out loudly about negative and iatrogenic clinical experiences suffered in hospitals, agencies, clinics, and offices of psychologists, counselors, psychiatrists, and clinical social workers—the full gamut of mental health professionals and settings.

In one especially poignant example, I actually felt *ashamed* of my profession as I heard the wrenching tale of a survivor of multiple suicide attempts whose life was plagued by suicidal thinking (Yanez, 2015). This brave woman movingly recounted her multiple efforts to seek professional mental health care. She pursued various professional-care paths to find a way through her suicidal nightmare, only to be repeatedly hospitalized and discharged with no real treatment beyond adjustments of her medications. She described one professional who interviewed her on an inpatient unit and never once made eye contact with her. Her earnest and caring outpatient therapist provided "supportive therapy" but was afraid to actually talk to her about her suicidality, avoiding the topic altogether, which made her feel ashamed because the subject was forbidden. After years of suffering and failed treatments her only relief and ultimate recovery came through DBT, a proven and effective treatment for suicidal risk that is used far too rarely within contemporary mental health care for people who have struggled just like her.

Thus while the recent outpouring of scientific efforts to address suicide risk is certainly encouraging, we would be terribly mistaken to believe that we have "solved" the challenge of suicide from a clinical standpoint. In my view, the treatment status quo for suicidal risk is unacceptable; significant changes are needed. Too many lives are being lost that could otherwise be saved through humane assessment and patient-informed care that is tailored to the unique needs of any person who seriously contemplates ending his or her own existence. But as I mentioned in Chapter 1 at the time of this writing, leadership in U.S. health care policy and administration has now boldly asserted the need for "detecting and treating suicidal ideation in all settings" (The Joint Commission, 2016). This is an extraordinary development in the history of clinical suicide prevention with far-reaching implications and it will be interesting to see how this policy directive plays out over the coming years.

After 25 years, CAMS has figuratively passed through the adolescent phase of development and now reached young adulthood. While we are not yet done with our RCTs, the empirical support for CAMS is substantial and continues to grow. CAMS is being used around the world as a compelling clinical approach for suicidal risk. It is a flexible approach that can be modified and adapted to a range of clinical settings and treatment modalities, providing effective care for the spectrum of suicidal states. It is not the only effective method and it does not always work with every patient. But it holds the genuine promise of providing a meaningful answer to the stinging criticisms of our field by offering a compassionate, noncoercive, and healing approach to suicidal risk in a patient-centered way. CAMS will not save every life, but I know that it has saved many. And when lives are clinically saved it is because hope was offered in the face of despair and compassion was rendered versus shame. Critically, offering an opportunity to work collaboratively on one of the most divisive struggles in the human condition is perhaps the best that we can ever offer an anguished soul. And in so doing, we have done right by our fellow traveler in the journey of life.

*   *   *

As a final consideration, it had been some years since I ended my clinical work with Bill that involved using CAMS when he first sought treatment (for the full SSF case example of Bill, see Appendix H). Bill was among the many patients I have seen and treated in 25 years of active clinical practice. As this work goes, we were intensely intimate for a relatively brief period as we battled to save his life during a most precarious moment in his personal journey and struggle. Needless to say, I was delighted 4 years after our mutual termination of therapy, when I came into my practice office early one morning and received the following e-mail from Bill:

Dear Dave,

I know it's been a while, but I wanted to let you know that things are going pretty well on my end. Kathy and I are doing fine, and we are looking forward to retiring in a few years. We now have three amazing grandchildren and the kids are doing great. While my life is not perfect, things overall are darn good. As I reflect on the work that we did together, I have actually come to see that my life is a gift and you helped me preserve that gift at a grave moment in time. My wife has a husband, my kids have a dad, and my grandkids have a grandpa. I now feel blessed to be alive. I would like to simply say thank you for helping to save my life!

Sincerely,
Bill

Suicide Status Form–4 (SSF-4)

*Initial Session, Tracking/Update Interim Session,
Outcome/Disposition Final Session*

CAMS SUICIDE STATUS FORM–4 (SSF-4) INITIAL SESSION

Patient: _____ Clinician: _____ Date: _____ Time: _____

Section A (*Patient*):

Rate and fill out each item according to how you feel <u>right now</u>. Then rank in order of importance 1 to 5
(1 = most important to 5 = least important)

Rank

Rank	
_____	1) RATE PSYCHOLOGICAL PAIN (*hurt, anguish, or misery in your mind, **not** stress, **not** physical pain*): **Low pain: 1 2 3 4 5 :High pain** What I find most painful is: _____
_____	2) RATE STRESS (*your general feeling of being pressured or overwhelmed*): **Low stress: 1 2 3 4 5 :High stress** What I find most stressful is: _____
_____	3) RATE AGITATION (*emotional urgency; feeling that you need to take action; **not** irritation; **not** annoyance*): **Low agitation: 1 2 3 4 5 :High agitation** I most need to take action when: _____
_____	4) RATE HOPELESSNESS (*your expectation that things will not get better no matter what you do*): **Low hopelessness: 1 2 3 4 5 :High hopelessness** I am most hopeless about: _____
_____	5) RATE SELF-HATE (*your general feeling of disliking yourself; having no self-esteem; having no self-respect*): **Low self-hate: 1 2 3 4 5 :High self-hate** What I hate most about myself is: _____
N/A	6) RATE OVERALL RISK OF SUICIDE: **Extremely low risk: 1 2 3 4 5 :Extremely high risk** **(will *not* kill self)** **(will kill self)**

1) How much is being suicidal related to thoughts and feelings about <u>yourself</u>? **Not at all: 1 2 3 4 5 : completely**

2) How much is being suicidal related to thoughts and feeling about <u>others</u>? **Not at all: 1 2 3 4 5 : completely**

Please list your reasons for wanting to live and your reasons for wanting to die. Then rank in order of importance 1 to 5.

Rank	REASONS FOR LIVING	Rank	REASONS FOR DYING

I wish to live to the following extent: Not at all: 0   1   2   3   4   5   6   7   8   : Very much

I wish to die to the following extent: Not at all: 0   1   2   3   4   5   6   7   8   : Very much

The one thing that would help me no longer feel suicidal would be: _____

_____

_____

Section B (*Clinician*):

Y N Suicide ideation   Describe: _____

      • Frequency   _____ per day   _____ per week   _____ per month

      • Duration   _____ seconds   _____ minutes   _____ hours

Y N Suicide plan   When: _____

      Where: _____

      How: _____ Access to means Y N

      How: _____ Access to means Y N

Y N Suicide preparation   Describe: _____

Y N Suicide rehearsal   Describe: _____

Y N History of suicidal behaviors

      • Single attempt   Describe: _____

      • Multiple attempts   Describe: _____

Y N Impulsivity   Describe: _____

Y N Substance abuse   Describe: _____

Y N Significant loss   Describe: _____

Y N Relationship problems   Describe: _____

Y N Burden to others   Describe: _____

Y N Health/pain problems   Describe: _____

Y N Sleep problems   Describe: _____

Y N Legal/financial issues   Describe: _____

Y N Shame   Describe: _____

Section C (*Clinician*):   TREATMENT PLAN

Problem #	Problem Description	Goals and Objectives	Interventions	Duration
1	*Self-Harm Potential*	*Safety and Stability*	*Stabilization Plan Completed* ☐	
2				
3				

YES _____ NO _____   Patient understands and concurs with treatment plan?

YES _____ NO _____   Patient at imminent danger of suicide (hospitalization indicated)?

_____   _____

Patient Signature   Date   Clinican Signature   Date

_____

CAMS STABILIZATION PLAN

Ways to reduce access to lethal means:

1. _____

2. _____

3. _____

Things I can do to cope differently when I am in a suicide crisis (consider crisis card):

1. _____

2. _____

3. _____

4. _____

5. _____

6. **Life or death emergency contact number:** _____

People I can call for help or to decrease my isolation:

1. _____

2. _____

3. _____

Attending treatment as scheduled:

Potential barrier: Solutions I will try:

1. _____

2. _____

Section D (*Clinician Postsession Evaluation*):

MENTAL STATUS EXAM (Circle appropriate items):

ALERTNESS: ALERT   DROWSY   LETHARGIC   STUPOROUS

                              OTHER: _____

ORIENTED TO: PERSON   PLACE   TIME   REASON FOR EVALUATION

MOOD: EUTHYMIC   ELEVATED   DYSPHORIC   AGITATED   ANGRY

AFFECT: FLAT   BLUNTED   CONSTRICTED   APPROPRIATE   LABILE

THOUGHT CONTINUITY: CLEAR & COHERENT   GOAL-DIRECTED   TANGENTIAL   CIRCUMSTANTIAL

                              OTHER: _____

THOUGHT CONTENT: WNL   OBSESSIONS   DELUSIONS   IDEAS OF REFERENCE   BIZARRENESS   MORBIDITY

                              OTHER: _____

ABSTRACTION: WNL   NOTABLY CONCRETE

                              OTHER: _____

SPEECH: WNL   RAPID   SLOW   SLURRED   IMPOVERISHED   INCOHERENT

                              OTHER: _____

MEMORY: GROSSLY INTACT

                              OTHER: _____

REALITY TESTING: WNL

                              OTHER: _____

NOTABLE BEHAVIORAL OBSERVATIONS: _____

DIAGNOSTIC IMPRESSIONS/DIAGNOSIS (DSM/ICD DIAGNOSES):

_____

_____

_____

PATIENT'S OVERALL SUICIDE RISK LEVEL (Check one and explain):

☐ **LOW (WTL/RFL)**   **Explanation:**

☐ **MODERATE (AMB)**   _____

☐ **HIGH (WTD/RFD)**   _____

                                _____

CASE NOTES:

_____

_____

_____

_____

_____

_____

Next Appointment Scheduled: _____ Treatment Modality: _____

_____   _____

Clinican Signature   Date

CAMS SUICIDE STATUS FORM–4 (SSF-4) TRACKING/UPDATE INTERIM SESSION

Patient: _____ Clinician: _____ Date: _____ Time: _____

Section A (*Patient*):

Rate and fill out each item according to how you feel <u>right now</u>.

1) RATE PSYCHOLOGICAL PAIN (*hurt, anguish, or misery in your mind, **not** stress, **not** physical pain*):
Low pain: **1   2   3   4   5**   **:High pain**

2) RATE STRESS (*your general feeling of being pressured or overwhelmed*):
Low stress: **1   2   3   4   5**   **:High stress**

3) RATE AGITATION (*emotional urgency; feeling that you need to take action; **not** irritation; **not** annoyance*):
Low agitation: **1   2   3   4   5**   **:High agitation**

4) RATE HOPELESSNESS (*your expectation that things will not get better no matter what you do*):
Low hopelessness: **1   2   3   4   5**   **:High hopelessness**

5) RATE SELF-HATE (*your general feeling of disliking yourself; having no self-esteem; having no self-respect*):
Low self-hate: **1   2   3   4   5**   **:High self-hate**

6) RATE OVERALL RISK OF SUICIDE:	**Extremely low risk:** (will *not* kill self) **1 2 3 4 5** **:Extremely high risk** (will kill self)

In the past week:

Suicidal Thoughts/Feelings   Y __ N __   Managed Thoughts/Feelings   Y __ N __   Suicidal Behavior   Y __ N __

Section B (*Clinician*):	Resolution of suicidality, if: current overall risk of suicide < 3; in past week: no suicidal behavior and effectively managed suicidal thoughts/feelings ☐ 1st session ☐ 2nd session
	Complete SSF Outcome Form at 3rd <u>consecutive</u> resolution session**

<u>Patient Status:</u>   **TREATMENT PLAN UPDATE**

☐ Discontinued treatment   ☐ No show   ☐ Cancelled   ☐ Hospitalization   ☐ Referred/Other: _____

Problem #	Problem Description	Goals and Objectives	Interventions	Duration
1	*Self-Harm Potential*	*Safety and Stability*	*Stabilization Plan Completed* ☐	
2				
3				

_____   _____   _____   _____
Patient Signature   Date   Clinican Signature   Date

Section C (*Clinician Postsession Evaluation*):

MENTAL STATUS EXAM (Circle appropriate items):

ALERTNESS: ALERT   DROWSY   LETHARGIC   STUPOROUS

OTHER: _____

ORIENTED TO: PERSON   PLACE   TIME   REASON FOR EVALUATION

MOOD: EUTHYMIC   ELEVATED   DYSPHORIC   AGITATED   ANGRY

AFFECT: FLAT   BLUNTED   CONSTRICTED   APPROPRIATE   LABILE

THOUGHT CONTINUITY: CLEAR & COHERENT   GOAL-DIRECTED   TANGENTIAL   CIRCUMSTANTIAL

OTHER: _____

THOUGHT CONTENT: WNL   OBSESSIONS   DELUSIONS   IDEAS OF REFERENCE   BIZARRENESS   MORBIDITY

OTHER: _____

ABSTRACTION: WNL   NOTABLY CONCRETE

OTHER: _____

SPEECH: WNL   RAPID   SLOW   SLURRED   IMPOVERISHED   INCOHERENT

OTHER: _____

MEMORY: GROSSLY INTACT

OTHER: _____

REALITY TESTING: WNL

OTHER: _____

NOTABLE BEHAVIORAL OBSERVATIONS: _____

DIAGNOSTIC IMPRESSIONS/DIAGNOSIS (DSM/ICD DIAGNOSES):

_____

_____

_____

PATIENT'S OVERALL SUICIDE RISK LEVEL (Check one and explain):

☐ **MILD (WTL/RFL)**   **Explanation:**

☐ **MODERATE (AMB)**   _____

☐ **HIGH (WTD/RFD)**   _____

_____

CASE NOTES:

_____

_____

_____

_____

_____

_____

Next Appointment Scheduled: _____ Treatment Modality: _____

_____
Clinican Signature   Date

CAMS SUICIDE STATUS FORM–4 (SSF-4) OUTCOME/DISPOSITION FINAL SESSION

Patient: _____ Clinician: _____ Date: _____ Time: _____

Section A (*Patient*):

Rate and fill out each item according to how you feel <u>right now</u>.

1) RATE PSYCHOLOGICAL PAIN (*hurt, anguish, or misery in your mind, **not** stress, **not** physical pain*): **Low pain:** 1 2 3 4 5 **:High pain**	
2) RATE STRESS (*your general feeling of being pressured or overwhelmed*): **Low stress:** 1 2 3 4 5 **:High stress**	
3) RATE AGITATION (*emotional urgency; feeling that you need to take action; **not** irritation; **not** annoyance*): **Low agitation:** 1 2 3 4 5 **:High agitation**	
4) RATE HOPELESSNESS (*your expectation that things will not get better no matter what you do*): **Low hopelessness:** 1 2 3 4 5 **:High hopelessness**	
5) RATE SELF-HATE (*your general feeling of disliking yourself; having no self-esteem; having no self-respect*): **Low self-hate:** 1 2 3 4 5 **:High self-hate**	
6) RATE OVERALL RISK OF SUICIDE:	**Extremely low risk:** 1 2 3 4 5 **:Extremely high risk** **(will *not* kill self)** **(will kill self)**

In the past week:

Suicidal Thoughts/Feelings Y __ N __   Managed Thoughts/Feelings Y __ N __   Suicidal Behavior Y __ N __

Where there any aspects of your treatment that were particularly helpful to you? If so, please describe these. Be as specific as possible.

What have you learned from your clinical care that could help you if you became suicidal in the future?

Section B (*Clinician*):

<u>Third consecutive session of resolved suicidality:</u>   ___ Yes   ___ No (If no, continue CAMS tracking)

**Resolution of suicidality, if for third consecutive week: current overall risk of suicide < 3; in past week: no suicidal behavior and effectively managed suicidal thoughts/feelings

<u>OUTCOME/DISPOSITION</u> (Check all that apply):

___ Continuing outpatient psychotherapy   ___ Inpatient hospitalization

___ Mutual termination   ___ Patient chooses to discontinue treatment (unilaterally)

___ Referral to: _____

___ Other. Describe: _____

Next Appointment Scheduled (if applicable): _____

_____   _____
Patient Signature   Date   Clinican Signature   Date
_____

Section C (*Clinician Postsession Evaluation*):

MENTAL STATUS EXAM (Circle appropriate items):

ALERTNESS:	ALERT DROWSY LETHARGIC STUPOROUS
	OTHER: _____
ORIENTED TO:	PERSON PLACE TIME REASON FOR EVALUATION
MOOD:	EUTHYMIC ELEVATED DYSPHORIC AGITATED ANGRY
AFFECT:	FLAT BLUNTED CONSTRICTED APPROPRIATE LABILE
THOUGHT CONTINUITY:	CLEAR & COHERENT GOAL-DIRECTED TANGENTIAL CIRCUMSTANTIAL
	OTHER: _____
THOUGHT CONTENT:	WNL OBSESSIONS DELUSIONS IDEAS OF REFERENCE BIZARRENESS MORBIDITY
	OTHER: _____
ABSTRACTION:	WNL NOTABLY CONCRETE
	OTHER: _____
SPEECH:	WNL RAPID SLOW SLURRED IMPOVERISHED INCOHERENT
	OTHER: _____
MEMORY:	GROSSLY INTACT
	OTHER: _____
REALITY TESTING:	WNL
	OTHER: _____
NOTABLE BEHAVIORAL OBSERVATIONS:	_____

DIAGNOSTIC IMPRESSIONS/DIAGNOSIS (DSM/ICD DIAGNOSES):

_____

_____

_____

PATIENT'S OVERALL SUICIDE RISK LEVEL (Check one and explain):

☐ **LOW (WTL/RFL)**   **Explanation:**

☐ **MODERATE (AMB)**   _____

☐ **HIGH (WTD/RFD)**   _____

_____

CASE NOTES:

_____

_____

_____

_____

_____

_____

_____

_____

Clinican Signature   Date

_____

Coding Manual for
the SSF Core Assessment Scales

Qualitative Assessment

SSF CODING MANUAL:
A CATEGORIZATION OF SSF CORE ASSESSMENT QUALITATIVE VARIABLES—PAIN, STRESS, AGITATION, HOPELESSNESS, AND SELF-HATE

OVERVIEW

This coding manual will serve as a guide for examining open-ended, qualitative responses provided by suicidal outpatients on an assessment instrument called the Suicide Status Form (SSF; Jobes et al., 1997). The SSF is a suicide risk assessment instrument used in treatment settings around the world. It consists of six self-report items that measure a patient's suicide risk. Specifically, the SSF includes ratings of five valid, reliable, and theoretically based items (on 5-point, low-to-high Likert scales) thought to underlie suicidal behavior (Jobes et al., 1997). These include: Psychological Pain, Stress, Agitation, Hopelessness, and Self-Hate. In addition, a sixth item examines a patient's overall behavioral suicide risk. The patient is also given the opportunity to provide written open-ended responses that explain the five constructs. The following coding procedure specifically focuses on these qualitative responses and provides a way to categorize a patient's responses to the five stem cues following each SSF Core Assessment.

GENERAL GUIDELINES FOR CODING

Coders will receive five separate stacks of responses on index cards. These five stacks will represent each of the coding constructs: Pain, Stress, Agitation, Hopelessness, and Self-Hate. First, coders will go through an initial sort of the cards for each construct (one construct at a time), placing responses under the appropriate coding category. After this initial sort of each of the five main constructs, a second sort will be allowed so that coders can review their initial coding decisions and revise them as needed before making their final coding choices. In order for researchers to understand the decision-making process, we ask that coders discuss their rationale for coding decisions.

The categories within each construct should be considered mutually exclusive of one another. Therefore, each response should be placed in *one* category. While some interpretation may be required when deciding on the best category for a given response, generally, coders should take the response "at face value" without giving too much thought into the motivations or situation that may surround the response.

For each response, coders are also asked to rate their confidence in the code they have assigned. A confidence rating of 1 indicates a low confidence level, 2 indicates a medium confidence level, and 3 indicates a high confidence level.

SPECIFIC GUIDELINES FOR CODING

We ask that you please feel free to use the manual as needed because certain decision rules specific to each category are included in the manual.

If two types of responses are mentioned in a single response, place it in the category of the *first* response identified. For example, if the response says "my job and my depression" then place the first response, "my job," in its proper category, but if the response reads, "my depression and my job" then place "my depression" in its proper category.

Please note that some of the constructs may have one or more categories in common. It is important, however, that each construct's category is reviewed carefully, as ones that may be very similar in definition may also have critical nuances specific to that item that will affect coding decisions. For example, more than one construct has a "Future" category; however, these definitions are not the same, so please be mindful of critical differences that may affect your decisions.

WHAT ARE THE CODINGS USED FOR?

Coding the SSF Core Assessment variables will enable those involved in this line of research to identify common categories into which these responses might fall. Theoretical, research, and clinical implications of these qualitative data can guide researchers and clinicians to more accurately assess a person's suicidal risk as well as possibly tailor a patient's treatment to address his or her idiosyncratic experiences and needs.

PAIN (PSYCHACHE)

The Psychological Pain variable in the SSF (Jobes et al., 1997) is based on Shneidman's (1993) construct of "psychache." Shneidman purported that the most basic ingredient of suicide is psychache. Psychache is intrinsically psychological and it refers to the hurt, anguish, soreness, aching, and psychological pain of the mind. Psychache is a necessary force in leading a person into a suicidal crisis. Suicide occurs when the psychache is deemed intolerable or unbearable to a person, so suicide is a combined movement toward cessation and a movement away from this intolerable emotion. More specifically, this psychological pain arises out of the frustration of one's vital psychological needs (e.g., affiliation, nurturance, and understanding), whereas these vital needs are ones whose frustration cannot be tolerated. Suicide then can become a direct means of ending one's pain.

There is a somewhat elusive and ill-defined quality of psychache (Shneidman, 1993). Attempts to describe psychological pain have resulted in definitions of intolerable emotions (Murray, 1938); aloneness (Adler & Buie, 1979; Maltsberger, 1988); anxiety, self-contempt, and rage (Maltsberger, 1988); and a more global distress (Derogatis & Savitz, 1999). These may be important contributors to psychache, but Shneidman (1993) argues that they do not capture the inherent complexity and multidetermined nature of psychache. Therefore, the stem phrase **"What I find most painful is. . ."** was added to the Psychological Pain item on the SSF to further elucidate to both patients and clinicians the true phenomenology and the idiosyncratic quality of a suicidal person's psychological pain.

Coding Categories (Total of 7)

1. Self

This category refers to responses that are specific to one's self, or when a reference to one's self is clearly inferred. These can be statements about feelings or qualities about the self. These tend to include descriptions of enduring traits, core attributes, or harsh self-critiques or external descriptors about the self.

Examples:
"I am such a loser."
"I can't do anything right."
"Being overweight."

2. Relational

This category refers to responses that make references to specific relationship problems or issues with children, spouse, partner, parents, friends, significant others, or any other social interaction. Any response that speaks to being hurt by others or hurting others goes here; specific references about being alone or isolated also go here.

Examples:
"My family is so messed up."
"Loneliness."
"Having no friends."

3. Role/Responsibilities

This category refers to responsibilities or obligations related to common adult role expectations including the role of the worker, homemaker, or student. Responses may be specific examples of a role or responsibility or may be an expression of feeling inefficient in these roles. Responses such as academic concerns, financial burdens, or job concerns are included here. Specific future-oriented statements regarding career are also included. Statements that refer to lack of direction or purpose should be placed in the Helpless category.

Examples:
"Have no idea what kind of job I want to get after school."
"I can't decide on a job."
"I suck at being a parent."
"My house is a mess."

4. Global/General

This category refers to nonspecific, broad statements that are completely inclusive and therefore vague. These responses indicate a general, all-encompassing, or overarching sense of being overwhelmed and/or unable to cope.

Examples:
"Seems like everything."
"Life in general."
"The world is a total pain."

5. Helpless

This category refers to implied or specific references to feeling out of control, trapped, or lost. References to feeling directionless are also in included in this category. General statements about hopelessness about one's inability to cope, function, or achieve in the future should be placed here.

Examples:
"I am so out of control."
"I feel so trapped."
"I will fail no matter how hard I try."

6. Unpleasant Internal States

This category refers to specific, discrete descriptions of hurting, distress, suffering, emotional pain, and other negative emotions in the mood spectrum. They are symptom-oriented responses, and are more state-like than trait-like. These responses are free of intrasubjective self-references (e.g., "I hate myself because I always worry.") and are not global (e.g., "Everything makes me sad.").

Examples:
"Depression."
"My nervousness."
"This misery."

7. Unsure/Unable to Articulate

This category refers to responses in which the person is uncertain or unable to respond. It may include responses that seem purposely evasive, avoidant, or apathetic.

Examples:
"Don't know."
"Not sure."
"Who cares?"

STRESS (PRESS)

The Stress variable in the SSF (Jobes et al., 1997) is based on Shneidman's (1993) construct of "press," which was developed from Murray's (1938) work on the theory of press. Press refers to those aspects of the inner and outer world or environment that move, touch, impinge upon, and significantly psychologically affect an individual. Stress or press can then be a facilitating force driving some individuals toward a suicidal crisis, particularly when one experiences multiple sources of stress repeated over long periods of time. Presses can be either positive or negative and include what are termed *beta presses*—an individual's perception of a specific aspect of the environment—or *alpha presses*—the objective or real aspects of the environment. Presses can facilitate or impede the efforts of an individual to reach a given goal; in other words, the press of an object is thought of in terms of what it can do *to* or *for* the person. By understanding presses, we can know more about what a person may do if we have a picture of his or her motives or directional tendencies combined with a sense of the way in which he or she views or interprets the environment. Thus, the stem phrase **"What I find most stressful is . . ."** was added to the Stress item on the SSF to identify and describe suicidal patient's self-reports about the most meaningfully descriptive categories of stresses.

Coding Categories (Total of 8)

1. Relational

This category refers to responses that make references to specific relationship problems or issues with children, spouse, partner, parents, friends, significant others, or any other social interaction. Any response that speaks to being hurt by others or hurting others goes here; specific references about being alone or isolated also go here.

Examples:
"Making my family proud about my new job."
"My girlfriend is pulling away from me."
"I don't have any friends here and I feel like an outsider."

2. Self

This category refers to responses that are specific to one's self, or when a reference to one's self is clearly inferred. These can be statements about feelings or qualities about the self. These tend to include descriptions of enduring traits, core attributes, or harsh self-critiques or external descriptors about the self.

Examples:
"I'm not a good person."
"I am unable to lose 10 pounds."
"I'm weak and too emotional."

3. Role/Responsibilities

This category refers to responsibilities or obligations related to common adult role expectations including the roles of the worker, homemaker, or student. Responses may be specific examples of a role or responsibility or may be an expression of feeling inefficient in these roles. Responses such as academic concerns, financial burdens, or job concerns are included here. Specific future-oriented statements regarding career are also included. Statements that refer to lack of direction or purpose should be placed in the Helpless category.

Examples:
"Having no idea what kind of job I want to get after school."
"I can't deal with thinking about my future."
"I can't handle being at home all day with the kids."

4. Unpleasant Internal States

This category refers to specific, discrete descriptions of hurting, distress, suffering, emotional pain, and other negative emotions in the mood spectrum. They are symptom-oriented responses, and are more state-like than trait-like. These responses are free of intrasubjective self-references (e.g., "I hate myself because I always worry.") and are not global (e.g., "Everything makes me sad.").

Examples:
"I'm worried and nervous all the time."
"This pain is too much."
"I am sick of being depressed."

5. Global/General

This category refers to nonspecific, broad statements that are completely inclusive and therefore vague. These responses indicate a general, all-encompassing, or overarching sense of being overwhelmed and/or unable to cope.

Examples:
"The world around me."
"Life."
"Everything."

6. Situation-Specific

This category pertains to situation-specific responses (i.e., responses that speak to a certain place or time). Any reference made about a specific situation or circumstance, or any references made to a certain place, time, or events go here as well. (Note: A mention of a specific person would be better placed in the Relational category.)

Examples:
"When I come home to my empty apartment at night."
"First thing when I wake up."
"Whenever I hear a song by our favorite band."

7. Helpless

This category refers to implied or specific references to feeling out of control, lost, or trapped. References to feeling directionless are also in included in this category. General statements about hopelessness about one's inability to cope, function, or achieve in the future should be placed here. (If the statement refers to a role or responsibility [e.g., "My career"], place it in the Role/Responsibilities category.)

Examples:
"Feeling so lost that I don't know where to go."
"I have no idea where I'm going."
"I will never amount to anything no matter what I do."

8. Unsure/Unable to Articulate

This category refers to responses in which the person is uncertain or unable to respond. It may include responses that seem purposely evasive, avoidant, or apathetic.

Examples:
"I don't know."
"I'm not saying."
"Who knows?"

AGITATION (PERTURBATION)

The Agitation SSF variable is based on Shneidman's (1993) construct of "perturbation." Perturbation is a Shneidman neologism that refers to a general term meaning the state of being upset or perturbed. In relation to suicide, perturbation includes (1) perceptual constriction, and (2) a penchant for precipitous self-harm or inimical action. Constriction refers to the reduction of an individual's perceptual and cognitive range. At its worst, constriction includes a narrow way of thinking, tunnel vision, and focusing on only a few options, with death and escape becoming the only solution to the problems of psychache and frustrated needs. A penchant for action refers to impulsivity, or a strong tendency to get things over with and come to quick resolution while having little patience and low tolerance for stressful situations. At its worst, there is a clear tendency toward precipitous and potentially impulsive self-destructive actions.

There is no other term in the suicidology literature that quite captures what Shneidman intended to describe by the term *perturbation*. Terms such as *anxiety, turmoil, impulsiveness, irritation,* or *annoyance* do not capture the cognitive and affective complexity inherent in the perturbation construct. Perhaps because of this, the construct can be elusive and difficult for both clinicians and patients to understand. In Luoma's (1999) study of SSF constructs, perturbation was one of the most difficult notions for undergraduates to grasp; their conceptual understanding tended to focus on negative emotions. This focus on negative emotions misses both the cognitively oriented perceptual constriction and the more affectivity oriented urgency or impulsiveness. Thus, building off this work the revised agitation SSF item was specifically defined as "emotional urgency; feeling that you need to take action; **not** irritation; **not** annoyance." Again, the revised definition only speaks to the emotional urgency side of the definition and does not speak to perceptual constriction per se. Finally, the stem used on the SSF form also includes a temporal component. Open-ended responses will therefore tend to be situation specific, because subjects are responding to the prompt, **"I need to take action when . . ."**

Coding Categories (Total of 9)

1. Compelled to Act

This category deals with a person's explicit desire to urgently change something in his or her life, a recognized need for a quick solution, a need to take action. Embedded in this category is an awareness of the lack of change (being stuck) and the need to do something decisive.

Examples:
"I just want to fix things now."
"I'm not doing anything."
"Something needs to be done to end this state I'm in."

2. Global/General

This category refers to nonspecific, broad statements that are completely inclusive and therefore vague. These responses indicate a general, all-encompassing, or overarching sense of being overwhelmed and/or unable to cope.

Examples:
"I feel utterly swamped."
"Everything comes down on me."
"My head is jumbled with all that I have to deal with."

3. Helpless

This category refers to explicit or implied statements regarding feeling out of control, lost, or unable to change things. References to feeling a loss of direction and not knowing about the future are also included in this category. References to constricted thinking, a lack of options, a narrow view of things as well as general statements about one's inability to cope, function, and achieve in the future should also be placed here.

Examples:
"Things are out of control."
"There is nothing I can do to make it better."
"I have no options, nothing will change."

4. Unsure/Unable to Articulate

This category refers to responses in which the person is uncertain or unable to respond. It may include responses that seem purposely evasive, avoidant, or apathetic.

Examples:
"Don't know."
"Unsure."
"Wouldn't you like to know?"

5. Situation-Specific

This category pertains to situation-specific responses (i.e., responses that speak to a certain place or time). Any reference made about a specific situation, circumstance, or any references made to a certain place, time, or events go here as well. (Note: A mention of a specific person would be better placed in the Relational category.)

Examples:
"I come home to my empty apartment at night."
"First thing when I wake up."
"I hear a song by our favorite band."

6. Unpleasant Internal States

This category refers to specific, discrete descriptions of hurting, distress, suffering, emotional pain, and other negative emotions in the mood spectrum. They are symptom-oriented responses, and are more state-like than trait-like. These responses are free of intrasubjective self-references (e.g., "I hate myself because I always worry.") and are not global (e.g., "Everything makes me sad.").

Examples:
"I feel anxious."
"I fall apart after I get angry."
"The depression is more than I can stand."

7. Self

This category refers to responses that are specific to one's self, or when a reference to one's self is clearly inferred. These can be statements about feelings or qualities about the self. These tend to include descriptions of enduring traits, core attributes, harsh self-critiques, or external descriptors about the self.

Examples:
"I see what a loser I am."
"I get particularly pathetic."
"I am such a mess, no one will love me."

8. Relational

This category refers to responses that make references to specific relationship problems or issues with children, spouse, partner, parents, friends, significant others, or any other social interaction. Any response that speaks to being hurt by others or hurting others goes here; specific references about being alone or isolated also go here.

Examples:
"Jim yells at me."
"I think about how I have no one who loves me in a romantic way."
"I disappoint my dad."

9. Role/Responsibilities

This category refers to responsibilities or obligations related to common adult role expectations, including the roles of the worker, homemaker, or student. Responses may be specific examples of a role or responsibility or an expression of feeling inefficient in these roles. Responses such as academic concerns, financial burdens, or job concerns are included here. Specific future-oriented statements regarding career are also included. Statements that refer to lack of direction or purpose should be placed in the Helpless category.

Examples:
"I think about how I have no idea what kind of job I want to get after school."
"I think about my finances."
"I see how I suck at being a parent."

HOPELESSNESS

Hopelessness is a cognitive style rather than an emotional state; this distinction that makes hopelessness different from depression. Beck and colleagues (1979) refer to hopelessness as a set of beliefs an individual has that his or her situation will not improve regardless of what that individual does to change the situation. This set of beliefs can be focused on anything in an individual's life. It is theorized that individuals who believe their situation will never improve "give up" on life and lack desire to endure a situation they believe will never get better.

Hopelessness has been consistently found to be an important component of suicide risk and can be specifically addressed and modified in treatment (Brown, Beck, Steer, & Grisham, 2000). Hopelessness has also been proposed to be a construct that has different levels of conviction. For example, individuals who *think* their situation will not improve are at a lower risk for suicide than individuals who truly *believe* their situation will never get better.

Most measures of hopelessness tend to assess the global sense of the construct; however, more recent studies have emerged that are beginning to assess related constructs and components of hopelessness. For example, perfectionism is proposed to be a contributing factor to suicide risk. The theory is that individuals who set and maintain unrealistically high standards and expectations are at risk of suicide due to the fact that their standards are set so high that, in reality, they cannot achieve them. The individuals adopt a hopeless attitude because they will never be able to attain the personal or social expectations placed on them.

Other research suggests that hopeless individuals are unable to generate positive thoughts about the future or can only foresee negative events happening. These various theories and related constructs all have one common theme within hopelessness: The individual does not believe a situation will improve regardless of what is done. Little work has been published on the specific areas that individuals find hopeless. Therefore, the stem used on the SSF form also includes a temporal component. Open-ended responses will therefore tend to be situation specific, because subjects are responding to the prompt **"I am most hopeless about . . ."**

Coding Categories (Total of 7)

1. General/Global

This category refers to nonspecific, broad statements that are completely inclusive and therefore vague. These responses indicate a general, all-encompassing, or overarching sense of being overwhelmed and/or unable to cope.

> **Examples:**
> "Life."
> "Everything."
> "Things in general."

2. Future

This category refers to broad statements or inferences about an individual's future. These statements can be *specific* or *nonspecific* statements about the future. Any global statements about the future would be placed in this category along with specific statement about any specific dreams, skills, events, or experiences (except career or school; see Role/Responsibilities) with a *clear reference to the future*.

> **Examples:**
> "The future."
> "Achieving my dreams."
> "Reaching my goals."

3. Relational

This category refers to responses that make references to specific relationship problems or issues with children, spouse, partner, parents, friends, significant others, or any other social interaction. Any response that speaks to being hurt by others or hurting others goes here; specific references about being alone or isolated also go here.

Examples:
"People at work."
"My relationship with my boyfriend."
"Everybody."

4. Role/Responsibilities

This category refers to responsibilities or obligations related to common adult role expectations, including the role of the worker, homemaker, or student. Responses may be specific examples of a role or responsibility or may be an expression of feeling inefficient in these roles. Responses such as academic concerns, financial burdens, or job concerns are included here. These responses can be broad references in the present about getting things done. Specific future-oriented statements regarding career are also included.

Examples:
"Achieving my career ambitions."
"Getting done with school."
"Money."

5. Self

This category refers to responses that are specific to one's self, or when a reference to one's self is clearly inferred. These can be statements about feelings or qualities about the self. These tend to include descriptions of enduring traits, core attributes, or harsh self-critiques or external descriptors about the self. Statements about gaining control of one's behavior, thoughts, or feelings would be included in this category.

Examples:
"Understanding myself."
"Being too fat."
"I'm bad at dealing with my emotions."

6. Unpleasant Internal States

This category refers to specific, discrete descriptions of hurting, distress, suffering, emotional pain, and other negative emotions in the mood spectrum. They are symptom-oriented responses, and are more state-like than trait-like. These responses are free of intrasubjective self-references (e.g., "I hate myself because I always worry.") and are not global (e.g., "Everything makes me sad.").

Examples:
"My anxiety will never go away."
"How I fall apart after I get angry."
"I am afraid I will always be depressed."

7. Unsure/Unable to Articulate

This category refers to responses in which the person is uncertain or unable to respond. It may include responses that seem purposely evasive, avoidant, or apathetic.

Examples:
"Don't know."
"Not sure."
"Who cares?"

SELF-HATE

Self-hate can be conceptualized as the negative affect that proceeds from an increase in self-awareness (Baumeister, 1990). The individual experiences an event that falls short of personal standards and/or expectations. Consequently, when internal attributions are made to explain that event, one begins to hate the self and seeks to diminish this state through cognitive deconstruction. The deconstruction lowers thought processes and inhibitions, making a suicide attempt more likely.

Typically individuals have a preferred view of the self, which is supported and maintained by various psychological mechanisms. When these views are challenged (especially in the context of therapy) the patient may witness the "dreaded sense of self" as opposed to the former "ideal self." Such a transition often leads to self-hate and can act as a trigger for a suicide attempt (Baumeister, 1990).

Finally, self-hate can be conceptualized as a cycle. The idea is that an individual engages in self-detrimental actions due to self-hate. The negative consequences of such actions lead to an increase in self-hate, which may become a cycle. The individual may then either downgrade achievements to confirm to an initial view of the self (high achievement self-hate) or strive less in order to justify potential failures. Therefore, the stem **"What I hate most about myself is . . ."** is included to further elucidate a suicidal person's experience of self-hate.

Coding Categories (Total of 7)

1. Helpless

This category refers to explicit or implied statements regarding feeling out of control, lost, or unable to change things. References to feeling a loss of direction and not knowing about the future are also included in this category. References to constricted thinking, a lack of options, a narrow view of things as well as general statements about ones inability to cope, function, and achieve in the future should also be placed here.

Examples:
"I'm not able to talk about my problem."
"I have no way of stopping my depression."
"I have nowhere to go from here."

2. Internal Descriptors

This category refers to statements about an individual's lack of positive qualities or the presence of negative qualities in him- or herself. These can also be statements about feelings about the self and tend to include harsh self-critiques about inner descriptors of the self.

Examples:
"I'm a coward."
"I'm not intelligent."
"I'm a mess all the time."

3. External Descriptors

This category refers to statements about how an individual dislikes some external, outer aspect of him- or herself such as his or her personal appearance, body, or behaviors he or she is engaging in.

Examples:
"I always look angry."
"I'm ugly."
"My body."

4. Relational

This category refers to responses that make references to specific relationship problems or issues with children, spouse, partner, parents, friends, significant others, or any other social interaction. Any response that speaks to being hurt by others or hurting others goes here; specific references about being alone or isolated go here as well.

Examples:
"Hurting my parents."
"My girlfriend broke up with me."
"I can't fit in here at school."

5. Global/General

This category refers to nonspecific, broad statements that are completely inclusive and therefore vague. These responses indicate a general, all-encompassing, or overarching sense of being dissatisfied with life in general and/or overwhelmed.

Examples:
"Everything about me."
"Myself."
"My entire life."

6. Role/Responsibilities

This category refers to statements about responsibilities or obligations related to common adult role expectations including the role of the worker, homemaker, or student. Responses may be specific examples of a role or responsibility or may be an expression of feeling inefficient in these roles. Responses such as academic concerns, financial burdens, or job concerns are included here. Specific future-oriented statements regarding career are also included. Statements that refer to lack of direction or purpose should be placed in the Helpless category.

Examples:
"I can't make enough money."
"I can't decide on a job."
"I suck at being a parent."

7. Unsure/Unable to Articulate

This category refers to responses in which the person is uncertain or unable to respond. It may include responses that seem purposely evasive, avoidant, or apathetic.

Examples:
"Don't know."
"Can't say."
"You tell me."

Coding Manual for SSF Reasons for Living versus Reasons for Dying

SSF CODING MANUAL:
THE CATEGORIZATION OF REASONS FOR LIVING AND REASONS FOR DYING

OVERVIEW

Past empirical and theoretical work in the area of suicidology has focused primarily on two separate and diametrically opposite areas: risk factors and motivations for suicide (Reasons for Dying), and life-sustaining beliefs (Reasons for Living). These two bodies of research have provided rich and useful insight into the motivations for suicide. However, to more fully understand an individual's suicidal motivation requires a more comprehensive, balanced consideration: what sustains one's life versus what makes one want to give up? Perhaps examining both reasons for living *and* reasons for dying together may enable us to better understand the significance of both sides of the suicidal equation.

WHY REASONS FOR LIVING AND DYING?

Linehan and colleagues (1983) believed that suicidal individuals lacked life-oriented beliefs that would keep them from completing suicide. They developed the Reasons for Living Inventory to measure how important these beliefs are for not dying by suicide. Six factors were identified as sets of reasons for living: Survival and Coping, Responsibility to Family, Child-Related Concerns, Fear of Suicide, Fear of Social Disapproval, and Moral Objections. However, the information gleaned from the Reasons for Living Inventory only contributes to one side of the equation. It is also important to understand an individual's motivation to die by suicide and what factors exist in place of the beliefs for living. This is why it is important to ask for reasons for dying as well. This line of thinking led to the development of the RFL versus RFD assessment in order to formally study the full suicidal equation. In an effort to better understand the suicidal mind, individuals who expressed feelings of suicidality were asked to list their RFL and their RFD. The individuals were asked to organize each list in order of importance.

Superordinate Categories

Jobes and Mann (1999) showed that the RFL and RFD can be organized into meaningfully different reliable coding categories. One purpose of the current coding process is to further organize the categories into larger, more inclusive superordinate categories: hopefulness for self, others, and future, and hopelessness for self, others, and future.

Hopefulness and Hopelessness for Self, Others, and the Future

According to Beck's (1967) cognitive theory of depression, depressed individuals express a negative view of themselves, their world, and their future—the "cognitive triad." These negative views are often translated into feelings and expressions of hopelessness or negative expectations. Beck (1986) discussed that feelings of hopelessness are one of the single best predictors of suicidality as well as an excellent indicator of current suicidal intent. In contrast to hopelessness as a risk factor for suicidality, hopefulness can be considered a protective factor against it. Range and Penton (1994) found that RFL are positively correlated with hope and negatively correlated with hopelessness.

Self and Other

Bakan (1966) used the terms *agency* and *communion* to indicate the poles of a continuum for human experience. Agency signifies the desire for individuation, self-protection, and self-direction. Communion signifies the desire for personal relationships, attachment and intimacy. Each individual falls somewhere on this continuum. This notion of agency and communion can be built on when attempting to understand the suicidal individual. Jobes (1995) described this continuum using the terms *intrapsychic* (self) and *interpsychic* (relational). The intrapsychic pole of the continuum would be defined by a concentration on internal, subjective, phenomenological issues. The suicidal individual who would be described as being intrapsychic would focus primarily on issues pertaining to the self rather than to others. At the opposite end of the continuum, the interpsychic pole would be understood as a concentration on external, relational issues. In this case, the suicidal individual would focus predominantly on others and interpersonal relationships rather than on the self.

Connecting Categories to Superordinate Categories

To determine which categories would fit into each of the superordinate categories, an addendum to the coding manual would need to be developed and tested for interrater reliability. However, theory and common sense can be applied to make assumptions about which superordinate category each category would fall in. Based on the literature on motivations for suicide and life-sustaining beliefs, RFL should be placed in the overarching category of Hopefulness, and RFD should be placed in Hopelessness. The RFL categories Enjoyable Things, Beliefs, and Self would fall under the heading of Hopefulness about the Self. The RFL categories Family, Friends, Responsibility to Others, and Burdening Others would fall under the heading of Hopefulness about Others. The remaining RFL categories Hopefulness for the Future and Plans and Goals would fall under the heading of Hopefulness for the Future. Likewise, the RFD categories of Loneliness, General Descriptors of Self, and the Escape categories would fall under the heading of Hopelessness about the Self. The RFD categories of Others (Relationships) and Unburdening Others would fall under the category of Hopelessness about Others. The RFD category of Hopelessness would clearly fall under the heading of Hopelessness about the Future.

GENERAL GUIDELINES FOR CODING

Coders will be given actual responses from the lists made by the suicidal patients on RFL and RFD. Patients typically listed up to five responses for each list. Each response is provided in its own line of a coding sheet. There are two separate sets of coding sheets, one for RFL and one for RFD. Each set of responses should be coded independently of one the other. The categories within a set should be considered as mutually exclusive of one another. Therefore, each reason should only be placed into *one* category and subsequently given *one* code. When coding a reason, although some interpretation may be necessary, the coder should generally take the response at face value and do as little guesswork as possible into the motivations and/or circumstances that might surround the reason.

Specific Guidelines for Coding

The category labels are located at the top of the columns on the right side of the coding sheets. The coders are given the collection of responses for that set. Coders are to make a determination about which category the response should be placed into and put a checkmark in the appropriate category column. Before proceeding to the next response, the coder should rate from 1 to 5 the confidence of his or her choice in the Confidence Rating column. The rating is made on a scale from 1 to 5, 1 being "not confident at all" and 5 being "highly confident." Once the response has been placed in a category and the confidence rating has been completed, the coder should then move to the next response. After completing these tasks for one set of responses, the coder should repeat the process for the other set of responses.

WHAT ARE THE CODINGS USED FOR?

There are two purposes for coding the RFL/RFD assessment responses. The first is to identify common categories into which these reasons might fall. The second is to use these categorized responses to develop types of suicidal individuals that can potentially inform treatment outcomes.

Reasons for Living Coding Categories

1. Family

This category deals with any references to family such as marriage or children.

> **Examples:**
> "My parents."
> "My parents love me."
> "My husband."

2. Friends

This category refers to any mention of friends including specific names (e.g., John or Cindy). References to a boyfriend or girlfriend should also be placed in this category. If the response indicates that the person referred to is a family member, then place in the family category.

Note: If both family and friends are mentioned in the same response, place it in the category of the first group that is identified. For example, if the response says "family and friends," then place this response in the family category, but if the response reads "friends and family," place it in the friends category.

3. Responsibility to Others

This category deals with responses that have to do with responsibilities and obligations owed to other people.

> **Examples:**
> "Working in the bookstore."
> "I don't want to disappoint people."
> "I have to teach my students."

4. Burdening Others

This category refers to statements regarding concerns, fears, or anxieties around troubling or burdening others (family, friends, other specifically identified individuals) with the aftermath of their suicide.

> **Examples:**
> "Family guilt," or "I don't want to upset anyone."
> "My parents would be really upset if I died."
> "Father Brian would be very upset if I killed myself."

5. Plans and Goals

This category deals with statements referring to future-oriented plans. The statements may express a desire to see something through or to deal with things that are left to be completed. These are typically self-oriented statements. However, they should be placed in this category when referring to goals or future plans. These statements contain a sense of action. More general "self" referencing statements should be placed in the Self category, category 9.

> **Examples:**
> "I want to finish school," or "I want to travel to Europe."
> "I want to have children someday."
> "There is still so much that I want to do with my life."

6. Hopefulness for the Future

This category refers to future-oriented statements that deal with vague abstract yearnings. The statements express a hopeful attitude or refer to a curiosity of how things are going to turn out, but are more passive than those statements falling in the category of Plans and Goals, category 5.

Examples:
"My dreams."
"I think things will work out," or "I hope I will stop feeling bad."
"I want to find out what is going to happen."

7. Enjoyable Things

This category refers to activities or objects that are merely mentioned or are referred to as something that is enjoyed. These references also include objects of value like a pet or a possession.

Examples:
"Chinese food."
"Playing the piano," or "Music."
"Going to the movies."

8. Beliefs

This category deals with responses referring to religion, personal beliefs, or ethics. These responses may include but are not limited to references to God or another religious figure. If the statement refers to a specified religious figure in the context of burdening this individual, then this statement should be place in the Burdening Others category, category 3.

Examples:
"It is a sin," or "I want to be able to go to heaven."

9. Self

This category deals with references specific to the self or when the reference to self is clearly inferred. These include references to feelings or qualities about the self. The responses can also be references to owing oneself something. These are not future-oriented statements. If the statements make references to the future, they should be placed in either the Plans and Goals or Hopefulness for the Future categories (category 5 or 6).

Examples:
"Myself."
"I don't want to let myself down."
"I'm not that kind of person."

Reasons for Dying Coding Categories

1. Others (Relationships)

This category deals with references to other people, both explicitly and inferred.

Examples:
"To see my mother in heaven."
"Retribution."

2. Unburdening Others

This category refers to suicide as a solution for ending the hardship that the individual believes he or she causes other people.

Examples:
"To stop hurting others."
"To not cause anyone else stress."
"Relieve the financial burden on my family."

3. Loneliness

This category refers to statements about loneliness.

Examples:
"I don't want to be lonely anymore."
"I don't have anyone."
"I have no one to talk to."

4. Hopelessness

This category refers to statements about hopelessness about the future.

Examples:
"Things may never get better," or "I don't think things will work out."
"I'm afraid I'll never reach my goals," or "I'm never going to amount to anything."
"I'm depressed that things will never change."

5. General Descriptors of Self

This category deals with feelings about the self as well as general references to the self.

Examples:
"Myself."
"I'm not worth anything."
"I will always feel this way."

Note: The next several categories deal with the issue of escape. Escape refers to a statement dealing with a need or desire to get away from or end something. The "something" could be a feeling, an obligation, or an event.

6. Escape—In General

This category refers to general statement about escape as well as references to a general attitude of giving up.

Examples:
"I want to find peace," or ""I can't take it anymore."
"Escape," or "There would be less stress."
"I need a rest," or "To end my life." or "Life sucks."

7. Escape—The Past

This category deals with statements generally referring to the past or getting away from past experiences and feelings.

Examples:
"My childhood was not fun," or "I would like to start over."
"I want to break from my past."

8. Escape—The Pain

This category refers to specific statements about psychological pain and the desire to stop the pain.

Examples:
"I don't want to feel pain anymore."
"No more misery."
"I want to stop the hurt, the ache."

9. Escape—Responsibilities

This category deals with statements making references to getting out of responsibilities.

Examples:
"I don't want to be responsible anymore."
"To not be responsible."
"I hate working in the bookstore."

Coding Manual
for the SSF One-Thing Response

SSF CODING MANUAL:
THE ONE-THING RESPONSE

OVERVIEW

The Suicide Status Form (SSF; Jobes, 2012) is a suicide risk assessment instrument that attempts to measure a client's suicidality from both a quantitative and qualitative standpoint. This coding manual will be used to analyze qualitative data derived from a specific assessment construct of the SSF, namely, the "One-Thing" Response. In this assessment suicidal patients are prompted to provide a written answer to the following question: **"The one thing that will help me no longer feel suicidal is . . ."** This manual employs three conceptual dimensions (Orientation; Reality Testing; Clinical Utility) in an attempt to reliably group various written open-ended responses to the "One-Thing" assessment.

The purpose of the coding task is to further test and refine the SSF to establish it as a valid and reliable suicide risk assessment instrument. In particular, the codings for the "One-Thing" Response will help clinicians and researchers understand an important facet of a patient's suicidality, namely, the one thing that may make a difference in terms of potential suicide risk.

GENERAL GUIDELINES FOR CODING

Step 1

Coders will receive a pack of index cards. Each card depicts one client's answer to the "One-Thing" prompt. The coders will be asked to make an <u>initial</u> sort and rate each response according to the three conceptual dimensions:

1. Orientation (Self vs. Relational vs. Not Codable)
2. Reality Testing (Realistic vs. Unrealistic vs. Not Codable)
3. Clinical Utility (Clinically Relevant Information vs. No Clinically Relevant Information vs. Not Codable)

The three choices for each coding dimension are mutually exclusive; hence, a response cannot be both "self" and "others." Each response should be coded in terms of these three coding dimensions and should thus have three coding responses.

Example:

"I want to have a better relationship with my peers."

1. Orientation (Relational)
2. Reality Testing (Realistic)
3. Clinical Utility (Clinically Relevant Information)

Step 2

After the initial sort, a <u>second</u> sort will be performed to make sure that the coders are comfortable with their choices. In order that we may better understand the decision-making process, the coders should discuss the rationale behind their specific coding. In addition, the coders should rate their confidence in the coding they have made for each particular response. The confidence levels are as follows:

1 = indicates a low level of confidence
2 = indicates a medium level of confidence
3 = indicates a high level of confidence

CODING DEFINITIONS AND EXAMPLES

Coding Dimension One: The Orientation of the Person's Response

Self

This category refers to anything about <u>the self</u>: It can be something that the person does/does not, feels/feels not, thinks/thinks not, or descriptions that are self-referential.

Examples:

"To like myself better."
"To be less depressed."
"To no longer have these sad feelings."
"Obtain a better grade in class."
"Find more interests and be more confident."
"Go away for a while."

Relational

This category refers to anything about <u>relationships or others</u>: It can be any social relationship (family, coworkers, romantic, etc.) and it can be either an existing relationship, an old relationship, or lack of a relationship.

Examples:

"To have Jim love me again."
"To have someone who I can talk to who understands me."
"Somehow having more/better friends."
"Relief from memories of parental abuse."
"Seeing my mom again who died."
"Problems with boyfriend."

Not Codable

In this category, there is no content to the answer or no answer at all: <u>It does not</u> receive further coding on the other two dimensions.

Examples:

"Don't know."
"How should I know?"
"Who cares?"
"I'm no longer suicidal."

Coding Dimension Two: The Reality Testing of the Person's Response

Realistic

This category refers to any item that can theoretically be obtained or that has a high probability of being achieved.

Examples:

"To have good friends."
"To have someone to talk to."
"To feel confident."
"Date more often with nice men."
"To pass my exams."
"To one day have a great family."

Unrealistic

This category refers to any item that is theoretically impossible, or not likely to be obtained/achieved.

Examples:

"To be free of all stress."
"Not to have been raped—undo the past."
"No thinking, no feeling, no worrying about things."
"A modern-day miracle."

Not Codable

There is no content to the answer or no answer at all; <u>it does not</u> receive further coding on the other two dimensions.

Examples:

"Don't know."
"How should I know?"
"Who cares?"
"I'm no longer suicidal."

Coding Dimension Three: The Clinical Utility of the Person's Response

Clinically Relevant Information

This category refers to any comments that identify new information related to a starting point for therapy or the use of a specific therapeutic technique. In other words, does the response guide or shape possible clinical interventions?

Examples:

"Do better in school." (academic skills)
"To rebuild a relationship with Mary." (social skills)
"To date more often." (social skills)
"To have good friends." (social skills)
"To not have been abused." (abuse issues)
"Less stress." (progressive relaxation)

No Clinically Relevant Information

This category refers to any item that is vague or requests the help of resolving suicidality, or is not addressable by clinical intervention.

Examples:

"To be reborn."
"To win a million dollars."
"To marry Madonna."

Not Codable

In this category there is no content to the answer or no answer at all: <u>It does not</u> receive further coding on the other two dimensions.

Examples:

"Don't know."
"How should I know?"
"Who cares?"
"I'm no longer suicidal."

SPECIFIC GUIDELINES AND DECISION RULES FOR CODING

The coders should use the manual as needed during the coding process. This section is designed to provide coding guidance and certain decision rules for uncertain codings. At least three possible coding dilemmas may arise in relation to coding "One-Thing" Responses.

Dilemma 1: Multiple Responses

Might occur in any of the three dimensions.

Example:

"To not be so stressed, to have more dates, for this semester to be over."

1. Orientation   (Self)
2. Reality Testing   (Realistic)
3. Clinical Utility (Clinically Relevant Direction)

If two or more answers are identified, a decision rule is to use the <u>first response</u> in a string of responses. In this case, the answer is "to not be so stressed."

Dilemma 2: Specificity versus Broad Concept

Occurs only in the Reality Testing Dimension. The coders should take these statements at face value without any attempt to philosophize about the details of the statement. For example, it could be that a client has a restraining order against them. In the second example, it could be that the client has nowhere to live or has no means to live in California. In the third example, the client might not be able to find another job. All this does not matter for the present purpose. The task is to rate whether a given response is obtainable in <u>a rather broad manner</u>. If a statement has any chance of being fulfilled it is to be coded as realistic. All of the foregoing examples would be realistic.

Examples:

> "To get back with my boyfriend Jim."
> "To go back home to California."
> "To get another job, a more fulfilling one."

Dilemma 3: Unrealistic but Clinically Relevant

Occurs only in the Clinical Utility Dimension.

Example:

> "To be free of all stress."

This would be coded as "unrealistic" insofar as it is simply not possible. However, it has clinical utility (Clinically Relevant Information) because it tells us that the client has a difficulty with stress and possibly in dealing with stress. Thus, a Reality Testing "Unrealistic" rating <u>does not</u> necessarily imply a clinical utility "No Clinically Relevant Information" rating. In other words, simply because a response is unrealistic does not mean that it is not clinically useful.

THE SSF "ONE-THING" CODING SHEET

Patient ID	Orientation	Reality Testing	Clinical Utility
	Self _____ Relational _____ Not Codable _____ C.L. 1 2 3	Realistic _____ Unrealistic _____ Not Codable _____ C.L. 1 2 3	Provides Clinically Relevant Info _____ Provides No Clinically Relevant Info _____ Not Codable _____ C.L. 1 2 3
	Self _____ Relational _____ Not Codable _____ C.L. 1 2 3	Realistic _____ Unrealistic _____ Not Codable _____ C.L. 1 2 3	Provides Clinically Relevant Info _____ Provides No Clinically Relevant Info _____ Not Codable _____ C.L. 1 2 3
	Self _____ Relational _____ Not Codable _____ C.L. 1 2 3	Realistic _____ Unrealistic _____ Not Codable _____ C.L. 1 2 3	Provides Clinically Relevant Info _____ Provides No Clinically Relevant Info _____ Not Codable _____ C.L. 1 2 3
	Self _____ Relational _____ Not Codable _____ C.L. 1 2 3	Realistic _____ Unrealistic _____ Not Codable _____ C.L. 1 2 3	Provides Clinically Relevant Info _____ Provides No Clinically Relevant Info _____ Not Codable _____ C.L. 1 2 3
	Self _____ Relational _____ Not Codable _____ C.L. 1 2 3	Realistic _____ Unrealistic _____ Not Codable _____ C.L. 1 2 3	Provides Clinically Relevant Info _____ Provides No Clinically Relevant Info _____ Not Codable _____ C.L. 1 2 3
	Self _____ Relational _____ Not Codable _____ C.L. 1 2 3	Realistic _____ Unrealistic _____ Not Codable _____ C.L. 1 2 3	Provides Clinically Relevant Info _____ Provides No Clinically Relevant Info _____ Not Codable _____ C.L. 1 2 3
	Self _____ Relational _____ Not Codable _____ C.L. 1 2 3	Realistic _____ Unrealistic _____ Not Codable _____ C.L. 1 2 3	Provides Clinically Relevant Info _____ Provides No Clinically Relevant Info _____ Not Codable _____ C.L. 1 2 3
	Self _____ Relational _____ Not Codable _____ C.L. 1 2 3	Realistic _____ Unrealistic _____ Not Codable _____ C.L. 1 2 3	Provides Clinically Relevant Info _____ Provides No Clinically Relevant Info _____ Not Codable _____ C.L. 1 2 3
	Self _____ Relational _____ Not Codable _____ C.L. 1 2 3	Realistic _____ Unrealistic _____ Not Codable _____ C.L. 1 2 3	Provides Clinically Relevant Info _____ Provides No Clinically Relevant Info _____ Not Codable _____ C.L. 1 2 3
	Self _____ Relational _____ Not Codable _____ C.L. 1 2 3	Realistic _____ Unrealistic _____ Not Codable _____ C.L. 1 2 3	Provides Clinically Relevant Info _____ Provides No Clinically Relevant Info _____ Not Codable _____ C.L. 1 2 3

CAMS Therapeutic Worksheet

Understanding Your Suicidality

CAMS THERAPEUTIC WORKSHEET: UNDERSTANDING YOUR SUICIDALITY

Date of Session: _____   Session #: _____

I. PERSONAL STORY OF SUICIDALITY

Why are you suicidal? How do you understand your suicidality? How do you understand your relationship to suicide? What is your personal story?

_____

_____

_____

_____

_____

II. DRIVERS OF SUICIDALITY

Problem #2: _____

Problem #3: _____

Now let us examine the factors underlying your suicidality, or what we refer to as "drivers." Please only complete those sections that have relevance toward your own experience of suicidality. Your answers may overlap with the information you provided on the Suicide Status Form in the first therapy session. However, new information may also be added over the course of treatment in order to most accurately reflect your personal experience of suicidality.

What are the "direct drivers" that lead me to feeling suicidal?

Specific *thoughts* (e.g., "It would be easier on everyone if I were dead.")

_____

_____

_____

Specific *feelings* (e.g., "I just feel so much shame.")

_____

_____

_____

Specific *behaviors* (e.g., "When I waste time all day long.")

_____

_____

_____

Specific *themes* (e.g., patterns in relationships or self-concept)

_____

_____

_____

What are the "indirect drivers" that lead me to feel suicidal?

Indirect drivers: Underlying factors that contribute, but do not necessarily lead to, acute suicidal ideation, feelings, and behaviors (e.g., homelessness, depression, substance abuse, PTSD, isolation).

_____

_____

_____

III. SUICIDAL CONCEPTUALIZATION

Suicide as an Option

↑

Describe *bridges* and *barriers* to going to the next level

↑

Direct Drivers (transpose information here)

↑

Describe *bridges* and *barriers* to going to the next level

↑

Indirect Drivers (transpose information here)

APPENDIX F

CAMS Rating Scale (CRS.3)

CAMS RATING SCALE (CRS.3)

Clinician: _____ Patient Initials: _____ Date of Session: _____

ID#: _____ Rater: _____ Date of Rating: _____

Session #: _____ ( ) Videotape ( ) Audiotape ( ) Live observation

( ) Adherence ( ) Spot-check

Directions: The CAMS framework entails several key components, which are reflected in the organized subsections of the CRS. For each session, assess the clinician on a 7-point scale from 0 to 6 and record the rating on the line next to each item number. At the end of each subsection, you may provide written feedback related to the scores.

N/A	0	1	2	3	4	5	6
N/A	Poor	Barely	Mediocre	Satisfactory	Good	Very Good	Excellent

PART I: CAMS Therapeutic Philosophy

Collaboration

1. _____ **The clinician expressed empathy with the patient's suicidal wish.**

   0 = The clinician had a judgmental, controlling attitude toward the suicidal patient.

   2 = The clinician acknowledged the suicidal wish in a neutral fashion.

   4 = The clinician acknowledged a nonjudgmental understanding of the suicidal patient.

   6 = The clinician communicated a deep appreciation for why and how the patient is suicidal.

2. _____ **All assessments were conducted interactively with substantial input from both clinician and patient.**

   0 = The clinician dominated the assessment, talked over/interrupted the patient.

   2 = The clinician somewhat engaged the patient in the assessment process.

   4 = The clinician effectively engaged the patient in an interactive assessment.

   6 = The clinician and patient engaged in a highly interactive assessment with substantial shared input.

3. _____ **The treatment plan was designed and modified interactively with substantial input from both clinician and patient.**

   0 = The clinician did not engage the patient in interactive treatment planning (e.g., did not use side-by-side seating; told the patient what treatment would entail in a directive manner).

   2 = The clinician somewhat engaged in interactive treatment planning but mostly ignored patient's input.

   4 = The clinician consistently sought patient's input to design/modify the treatment plan.

   6 = The clinician substantially engaged patient in highly interactive treatment planning.

4. _____ **All interventions (in-session) were selected and modified interactively with substantial input and participation from both clinician and patient.**

   0 = The clinician did not seek or ignored patient's input on treatment interventions.

   2 = The clinician somewhat sought input from patient on treatment interventions.

   4 = The clinician consistently sought and used patient input to interactively select and modify interventions.

   6 = The clinician sought substantial input from the patient to interactively select and modify interventions.

Any additional comments, suggestions, and feedback for the clinician's improvement with regard to collaboration:

_____

_____

_____

Suicide Focus

5. _____ **The clinician clarified the CAMS agenda to focus on factors related to the suicidal wish any time it appeared necessary; when factors arose that were not directly or indirectly leading to suicidal thoughts/behaviors for this patient, they were acknowledged as important, but not the focus of the current work**

    0 = The clinician completely ignored the CAMS agenda and the session focused on factors that are not related to suicidality.

    2 = The clinician somewhat acknowledged the CAMS agenda but did not consistently redirect discussion back to suicide drivers.

    4 = The clinician clarified the CAMS agenda and constructively redirected the patient back to suicidal drivers.

    6 = The clinician reliably clarified the CAMS agenda and skillfully redirected focus back to suicidal drivers.

Any additional comments, suggestions, and feedback for the clinician's improvement with regard to suicide focus:

_____

_____

_____

PART II: CAMS Clinical Session Framework

Assess for Risk

6. _____ **The dyad followed the framework for initiating and completing the SSF assessment at the beginning of the session.**
*Initial session: The dyad completed sections A and B of the SSF
**Subsequent sessions: The dyad completed section A of the SSF

    0 = The dyad did not complete the SSF assessment at any point during the session.

    2 = The dyad completed the SSF assessment, though it was not initiated and completed at the beginning of the session.

    4 = The SSF was initiated at the beginning of the session, though it may not have been completed in a timely fashion.

    6 = The SSF assessment was initiated and completed at the beginning of the session (initial session: the SSF was initiated within 5–10 minutes; subsequent sessions: the SSF was initiated at the beginning of the session).

Any additional comments, suggestions, and feedback for the clinician's improvement with regard to risk assessment:

_____

_____

_____

Treatment Planning

7. _____ **The dyad developed and/or updated a stabilization plan (e.g., safety plan [SP] or crisis response plan [CRP], or CAMS Stabilization Plan [CSP]), which includes regularly attending therapy sessions, addressing barriers to care, means restriction, decreasing isolation, and use of a coping card.**

    0 = The stabilization plan was not developed/updated during the session.

    2 = The stabilization plan was developed/updated, but contained options that are not likely to be feasible/effective for the patient when experiencing a suicidal crisis.

    4 = The stabilization plan reflected the options that are likely to work, though the discussion regarding the stabilization plan could be fleshed out with greater detail to increase the likelihood of being effective.

    6 = The stabilization plan contained useful, patient-specific coping options, which were discussed in detail and revisited/amended as needed in follow-up sessions.

8. _____ **The treatment plan identified and targeted the most relevant direct and/or indirect drivers of suicidal thought and behaviors as determined by the dyad.**
*Direct Drivers: Specific *thoughts* (e.g., "It would be easier on everyone if I were dead"), *feelings* (e.g., "I just feel so much shame"), and *behaviors* (e.g., interpersonal conflict with partner).
**Indirect drivers: Underlying factors that contribute, but do not necessarily lead to acute suicidal ideation (e.g., homelessness, depression, substance abuse, PTSD, isolation).

0 = The treatment plan did not target the most relevant drivers of suicidal thoughts/behaviors.

2 = The treatment plan targeted several drivers of suicidality, but did not place sufficient emphasis on the relevant drivers for the patient.

4 = The treatment plan reflected several of the most relevant drivers for the patient.

6 = The treatment plan targeted the most relevant drivers that significantly contribute to the patient's suicidal thoughts and/or behaviors.

9. _____ **The treatment plan established the use of suicide-specific, problem-focused interventions to target and treat the drivers of the patient's suicidal thoughts/behaviors.**
* Suicide-specific interventions may include: Removing access to means, addressing suicide-promoting beliefs, and decreasing interpersonal isolation; anything that addresses the thoughts, feelings, and behaviors that are most linked to the patient's suicidal thoughts/behaviors.

0 = The treatment plan did not reflect the use of suicide-specific interventions to address the drivers.

2 = The treatment plan reflected the use of some suicide-specific interventions related to common drivers, but were not sufficiently tailored to the patient's drivers.

4 = The treatment plan reflected the use of suicide-specific interventions, but more effort is needed to fine-tune these interventions to better address the idiosyncratic nature of the patient's drivers.

6 = The treatment plan reflected the use of suicide-specific interventions that were well tailored to patient-specific themes and cues of suicidality that have been well established as drivers.

Any additional comments, suggestions, and feedback for the clinician's improvement with regard to treatment planning:

_____

_____

_____

Intervention

10. _____ **The session included the use of suicide-specific, problem-focused interventions to target and treat the drivers of suicidality.**
*Suicide-specific interventions may include: Removing access to means, addressing suicide-promoting beliefs, and increasing interpersonal connectedness; anything that addresses the thoughts, feelings, and behaviors that are most linked to the patient's suicidality.
**If incorporating the CAMS Therapeutic Worksheet (CTW), it should be used appropriately and referenced in subsequent sessions thereafter as necessary.

0 = The in-session therapeutic approaches did not reflect the use of suicide-specific interventions to address the drivers.

2 = The in-session therapeutic approaches were related to the drivers, although they were not explicitly linked to the manner in which the driver is leading the patient to consider suicide as an option for solving problems.

4 = The in-session therapeutic approaches reflected the use of suicide-specific interventions, although they could be more fine-tuned to better address the idiosyncratic nature of the patient's drivers.

6 = The in-session therapeutic approaches reflected the use of well-tailored, suicide-specific interventions that are directly linked to the idiosyncratic nature of the patient's suicidal drivers.

11. _____ **The session included a discussion about hope, reasons for living, plans, goals, purpose, and meaning.**

0 = The in-session therapeutic approaches did not address hope, reasons for living, plans, goals, purpose, and meaning.

2 = The in-session therapeutic approaches included a brief discussion of hope, reasons for living, plans, goals, and meaning, but did not sufficiently engage the patient in the discussion of these constructs.

4 = The in-session therapeutic approaches included a discussion of hope, reasons for living, plans, goals, and meaning, but the clinician did not sufficiently incorporate this discussion into establishing treatment goals.

6 = The in-session therapeutic approaches included a collaborative discussion about hope, reasons for living, plans, goals, and meaning, and these constructs were well incorporated into establishing treatment goals.

Any additional comments, suggestions, and feedback for the clinician's improvement with regard to intervention:

_____

_____

_____

PART III: CAMS Overall Rating

12. _____ How would you rate the clinician's overall adherence to the CAMS framework?

0 = The session did not include collaboration or focus on drivers of suicidality, and the assessment/treatment protocol was not followed.

2 = The clinician managed the session adequately, but the content of the session only rarely reflected the essential elements of CAMS.

4 = The clinician focused on suicidal drivers and completed the assessment/treatment approaches, although the session was unfocused or noncollaborative for short periods of time.

6 = The clinician attended to all aspects of CAMS, with consistent collaboration and focus on drivers throughout the session, as well as meaningful use and completion of the assessment/treatment protocol.

13. _____ How receptive was the patient to this model of treatment?

0 = The patient was completely unwilling to engage in the CAMS session that focused on suicide drivers.

2 = The patient was somewhat receptive to CAMS, but displayed frequent attempts to sway the conversation toward another subject and/or was hesitant to collaborate with the clinician regarding assessment and treatment of suicidal drivers.

4 = The patient was willing to engage in the CAMS model, but required several prompts to stay on task.

6 = The patient was completely engaged throughout the session, with a desire to discuss and address his or her own suicidality through the CAMS model.

14. _____ How comfortable did the clinician seem?

0 = The clinician was not comfortable discussing the patient's suicidality using the CAMS model.

2 = The clinician completed most necessary components of the CAMS clinical framework, but displayed no spontaneity in the session, as marked by a lack of follow-up questions, engagement, and discussions regarding CAMS-relevant information provided by the patient.

4 = The clinician displayed comfort implementing the CAMS model throughout the session, showing only a few instances where he/she was unsure how to engage the patient further when completing aspects of the CAMS clinical framework.

6 = The clinician displayed complete comfort throughout the session, showing a mastery of the CAMS philosophy and clinical framework; there were creative uses of the approach and a willingness to take calculated risks and engage fully with the patient regarding his or her suicidality.

Any additional comments, suggestions, and feedback for the clinician's improvement:

_____

_____

_____

Frequently Asked
Questions about CAMS

FAQs ABOUT CAMS

Question: There is so much paperwork with CAMS, is it okay to use just parts of the SSF and not necessarily all the forms?

Answer Yes, there is a lot of paperwork, but most of it is completed in session with the patient. Also remember that extensive and thorough documentation of assessment and treatment is the most protective thing you can have in cases of malpractice liability. Having said that, I know that many clinicians use only certain portions of the SSF. For example, some clinicians use only the assessment portions (A and B) of the first two pages of the index-session SSF; others do not like to use the HIPAA pages, preferring the use of other documentation. Throughout this book, I have endeavored to emphasize the flexible and adaptable nature of CAMS and the SSF. In this sense, I am genuinely interested in clinicians using any or all of the materials as they see fit. Obviously from my own bias, however, using CAMS as I have outlined it in this book makes the most sense from both a research, treatment, and liability standpoint. I will also add that in more recent years, I have felt less inclined to say "anything goes" and still call the process "CAMS"—if you want the full support and potential protectiveness that CAMS offers from liability, you should use the full SSF and not parts.

Question: Can I continue to track ongoing suicidal risk in a case even though the patient technically meets the criteria for resolution?

Answer Yes, of course. I know a number of clinicians who decide to persist for additional interim CAMS sessions even though CAMS resolution criteria are technically met. In some cases, the provider needs a bit more time to ensure that the patient is truly "out of the woods" in terms of his or her attachment to suicide. This practice decision is up to the clinician's discretion.

Question: How hard should I push to get other people in the patient's life involved in support of CAMS stabilization planning and driver-oriented treatment?

Answer As with all clinical decision making, it depends on the case. But I tend to be very preoccupied with the importance of trying to engage supportive others. Of course, this must be done with a signed release by the patient if he or she is an adult. Some patients are very reluctant to get others involved; other patients seem quite comfortable with the concept. It is perhaps more important to have at least considered the potential value of engaging significant others. In other words, if you ultimately judge that it is not in the patient's best interest to engage others, it is still important to document your clinical decision making about this professional judgment. With kids, parental involvement is typically a must—how much or how little depends on your judgment as to what is in the child's best interest.

Question: When is a patient too young for CAMS?

Answer The youngest patient I have used this approach with was 12. However, CAMS has been used with children as young as 5 years old (Anderson et al., 2016). In such cases, the clinician may need to take a much more active and directive role in explaining the SSF constructs in language that the child can appreciate and understand. The same holds for patients with cognitive limitations. As long as one can be patient with the process and work to clarify SSF constructs in a more deliberate manner, there is no reason that CAMS cannot be used with a broad range of suicidal patients.

Question: What if the patient refuses to let you take an adjacent seat?

Answer There are certain cases in which physical boundary issues may necessarily prohibit the adjacent seating arrangement recommended in CAMS. A patient's refusal to have you switch seats must be understood and respected and you should never force the issue. In such cases, CAMS can proceed in a face-to-face manner, passing the clipboard back and forth at the transition points. I am very sensitive to the therapeutic value of adjacent seating and the potential for discomfort. We must always respect and honor the patient's wishes on this matter while still advocating for the value of collaboration and not venturing into an adversarial dynamic.

Question: I have a case that I have worked with for some years. We are totally stuck, and the issue of suicide has been contentious in our work. Can I really introduce CAMS at this point with any hope of it being helpful?

Answer Yes, you can. I have had three long-term cases in which a significant overhaul of the treatment plan was absolutely necessary, particularly in relation to the issue of suicide. I would suggest introducing the idea of needing to reexamine the treatment from top to bottom. In this regard, you can propose a new approach (CAMS), which might actually give the two of you a fresh start and the potential to grapple with the issue of suicide differently than you have previously. I often receive feedback from clinicians who have learned CAMS using it with just such cases. They typically report back to me that the patient was intrigued and engaged by CAMS. Moreover, these long-term patients often express appreciation for the clinician's effort to "reboot" the treatment.

Question: CAMS just takes too much time; how am I supposed to work this approach into my busy clinical schedule?

Answer It is true that CAMS may take a bit more time, particularly when you are first learning to use it. But with familiarity and repeated use, the pacing gets easier and quicker. Many evidence-based treatments tend to take a bit longer to administer. Given the life-or-death suicidal presentation, I would argue this extra time is well spent if it helps to save a life.

Question: I like CAMS, but we must use electronic records where I work. What do I do about the SSF being a hard-copy form?

Answer The answer for now is to scan the SSF into your electronic records or perhaps maintain a separate file of your SSF documentation as a "Psychotherapy Note" (under the Privacy Rule designation of HIPAA) and referencing your use of CAMS in your electronic medical record documentation. We are currently working hard in our ongoing clinical research to develop an "E-SSF," but we know an electronic version is not equivalent to the hard copy, so until the requisite research is done validating an E-SSF, we advocate the use of the hard copy.

Question: Can I use CAMS with psychotic patients?

Answer: I used to say that CAMS may not be effective with disordered thinking. But in recent years I have seen many clinicians use CAMS successfully with patients with severe mental illness/psychosis. Give it a try, if it does not work, move on to some other approach.

Complete CAMS
Case Example of Bill

CAMS SUICIDE STATUS FORM–4 (SSF-4) INITIAL SESSION

Patient: _Bill_____ Clinician: _____DJ_____ Date: _____ Time: _____

Section A (*Patient*):

Rank

Rate and fill out each item according to how you feel <u>right now</u>. Then rank in order of importance 1 to 5 (1 = most important to 5 = least important)

Rank	
_3_	1) RATE PSYCHOLOGICAL PAIN (*hurt, anguish, or misery in your mind, **not** stress, **not** physical pain*): **Low pain:** 1 2 3 4 **(5)** :High pain What I find most painful is: _my life, my marriage_
_4_	2) RATE STRESS (*your general feeling of being pressured or overwhelmed*): **Low stress:** 1 2 3 **(4)** 5 :High stress What I find most stressful is: _everything_
_5_	3) RATE AGITATION (*emotional urgency; feeling that you need to take action; **not** irritation; **not** annoyance*): **Low agitation:** 1 2 **(3)** 4 5 :High agitation I most need to take action when: _I fight with my wife_
_1_	4) RATE HOPELESSNESS (*your expectation that things will not get better no matter what you do*): **Low hopelessness:** 1 2 3 4 **(5)** :High hopelessness I am most hopeless about: _feeling trapped_
_2_	5) RATE SELF-HATE (*your general feeling of disliking yourself; having no self-esteem; having no self-respect*): **Low self-hate:** 1 2 3 4 **(5)** :High self-hate What I hate most about myself is: _I'm a loser_
N/A	6) RATE OVERALL RISK OF SUICIDE: **Extremely low risk:** 1 2 **(3)** 4 5 :**Extremely high risk** **(will *not* kill self)** **(will kill self)**

1) How much is being suicidal related to thoughts and feelings about <u>yourself</u>? **Not at all:** 1 2 3 4 **(5)**: completely

2) How much is being suicidal related to thoughts and feeling about <u>others</u>? **Not at all:** 1 2 3 4 **(5)**: completely

Please list your reasons for wanting to live and your reasons for wanting to die. Then rank in order of importance 1 to 5.

Rank	REASONS FOR LIVING	Rank	REASONS FOR DYING
1	wife	3	wife and kids
2	kids	1	trapped/escape
		2	loser
		4	miserable

I wish to live to the following extent: **Not at all:** 0 1 **(2)** 3 4 5 6 7 8 : Very much

I wish to die to the following extent: **Not at all:** 0 1 2 3 4 5 **(6)** 7 8 : Very much

The one thing that would help me no longer feel suicidal would be: _to be free—not trapped_

(Y) N Suicide ideation   Describe: *most nights, before bedtime*
- Frequency   *2–3* per day   _____ per week   _____ per month
- Duration   _____ seconds   *30* minutes   *2* hours

(Y) N Suicide plan   When: *evenings, late at night*
Where: *in his study at home*
How: *gunshot to forehead*   Access to means (Y) N
How: _____   Access to means Y N

(Y) N Suicide preparation   Describe: *has drafted suicide notes*

(Y) N Suicide rehearsal   Describe: *has put gun to his head*

Y (N) History of suicidal behaviors
- Single attempt   Describe: *n/a*
- Multiple attempts   Describe: *n/a*

Y (N) Impulsivity   Describe: *"no one would say I'm impulsive"*

(Y) N Substance abuse   Describe: *binge drinking – has been sober before*

Y (N) Significant loss   Describe: *n/a*

(Y) N Relationship problems   Describe: *withdrawing from others/marital problems*

(Y) N Burden to others   Describe: *"they will be better off without me"*

Y (N) Health/pain problems   Describe: *n/a*

(Y) N Sleep problems   Describe: *bouts of insomnia – history of sleep issues*

(Y) N Legal/financial issues   Describe: *no legal – financial stress*

(Y) N Shame   Describe: *loser – "I'm a failure"*

TREATMENT PLAN

Problem #	Problem Description	Goals and Objectives	Interventions	Duration
1	*Self-Harm Potential*	*Safety and Stability*	*Stabilization Plan Completed* ☑	*3 mo.*
2	*failing marriage*	*save marriage improve communication*	*couples therapy, insight, CBT, BA therapy*	*3 mo.*
3	*hopeless*	*↑ hope*	*Hope Kit, read "Choosing to Live"*	*3 mo.*

YES __✔__ NO _____   Patient understands and concurs with treatment plan?

YES _____ NO __✔__   Patient at imminent danger of suicide (hospitalization indicated)?

_____   _____
Patient Signature   Date   Clinican Signature   Date

CAMS STABILIZATION PLAN

Ways to reduce access to lethal means:

1. *give guns to my brother — will leave voicemail by 9:00 P.M.*

2. *decrease my drinking/consider AA?*

3. _____

Things I can do to cope differently when I am in a suicide crisis (consider crisis card):

1. *take dog for a walk*

2. *watch ESPN*

3. *go out and shoot some hoops*

4. *do some journaling*

5. *try to talk to my wife or kids*

6. **Life or death emergency contact number:** *555-123-4567   DJ cell*
Lifeline 800-273-TALK

People I can call for help or to decrease my isolation:

1. *my brother*

2. *my neighbor Fred*

3. _____

Attending treatment as scheduled:

Potential barrier:	Solutions I will try:
1. *I'll come*	*(not applicable)*
2.	

Section D (Clinician Postsession Evaluation):

<u>MENTAL STATUS EXAM</u> (Circle appropriate items):

ALERTNESS: (ALERT) DROWSY LETHARGIC STUPOROUS

OTHER: _____

ORIENTED TO: (PERSON) (PLACE) (TIME) (REASON FOR EVALUATION)

MOOD: (EUTHYMIC) ELEVATED DYSPHORIC AGITATED ANGRY

AFFECT: FLAT BLUNTED CONSTRICTED (APPROPRIATE) LABILE

THOUGHT CONTINUITY: (CLEAR & COHERENT) GOAL-DIRECTED TANGENTIAL CIRCUMSTANTIAL

OTHER: _____

THOUGHT CONTENT: (WNL) OBSESSIONS DELUSIONS IDEAS OF REFERENCE BIZARRENESS MORBIDITY

OTHER: _____

ABSTRACTION: (WNL) NOTABLY CONCRETE

OTHER: _____

SPEECH: (WNL) RAPID SLOW SLURRED IMPOVERISHED INCOHERENT

OTHER: _____

MEMORY: (GROSSLY INTACT)

OTHER: _____

REALITY TESTING: (WNL)

OTHER: _____

NOTABLE BEHAVIORAL OBSERVATIONS: *generally cooperative, testy around gun issue*

<u>DIAGNOSTIC IMPRESSIONS/DIAGNOSIS (DSM/ICD DIAGNOSES):</u>

deferred
R/O major depression, generalized anxiety
monitor alcohol use and insomnia

<u>PATIENT'S OVERALL SUICIDE RISK LEVEL</u> (Check one and explain):

☐ **LOW (WTL/RFL)**   **Explanation:**
☑ **MODERATE (AMB)**   *Fairly high risk, but is on board with CAMS treatment,*
☐ **HIGH (WTD/RFD)**   *giving gun to his brother decreases his risk*

<u>CASE NOTES:</u>

Bill is a 50-year-old white male who complains of marital distress and hopelessness. Poor mental health compliance. He is depressed and is drinking. He is willing to give up his gun and give CAMS a go. Explore the use of couples therapy, possible Rx, CBT, Behavioral Activation.

Next Appointment Scheduled: _____ Treatment Modality: _____

_____
Clinican Signature   Date

CAMS SUICIDE STATUS FORM–4 (SSF-4) TRACKING/UPDATE INTERIM SESSION (2)

Patient: *Bill*_____ Clinician: *DJ*_____ Date: _____ Time: _____

Section A (*Patient*):

Rate and fill out each item according to how you feel <u>right now</u>.

1) RATE PSYCHOLOGICAL PAIN (*hurt, anguish, or misery in your mind, **not** stress, **not** physical pain*):   **Low pain:** 1   2   3 **(4)** 5 :High pain
2) RATE STRESS (*your general feeling of being pressured or overwhelmed*):   **Low stress:** 1   2   3 **(4)** 5 :High stress
3) RATE AGITATION (*emotional urgency; feeling that you need to take action; **not** irritation; **not** annoyance*):   **Low agitation:** 1 **(2)** 3   4   5 :High agitation
4) RATE HOPELESSNESS (*your expectation that things will not get better no matter what you do*):   **Low hopelessness:** 1   2   3 **(4)** 5 :High hopelessness
5) RATE SELF-HATE (*your general feeling of disliking yourself; having no self-esteem; having no self-respect*):   **Low self-hate:** 1   2   3 **(4)** 5 :High self-hate
6) RATE OVERALL RISK   **Extremely low risk:** 1 **(2)** 3   4   5 :**Extremely high risk**   OF SUICIDE: **(will *not* kill self)**   **(will kill self)**

In the past week:
Suicidal Thoughts/Feelings Y ✔ N __   Managed Thoughts/Feelings   Y ✔ N __   Suicidal Behavior   Y __ N ✔

Section B (*Clinician*):	Resolution of suicidality, if: current overall risk of suicide < 3; in past week: no suicidal behavior and effectively managed suicidal thoughts/feelings ☑ 1st session ☐ 2nd session
	Complete SSF Outcome Form at 3rd <u>consecutive</u> resolution session

<u>Patient Status:</u>   **TREATMENT PLAN UPDATE**   *Rx consultation*

☐ Discontinued treatment   ☐ No show   ☐ Cancelled   ☐ Hospitalization   ☑ Referred/Other: *couples therapy*

Problem #	Problem Description	Goals and Objectives	Interventions	Duration
1	*Self-Harm Potential*	*Safety and Stability*	*Stabilization Plan Completed* ☑	*3 mo.*
2	*marital problems*	*save marriage improve communication*	*referred to couples therapy*	*3 mo.*
3	*hopeless*	*↑ hope*	*read about Hope Kit – read "Choosing to Live"*	*3 mo.*

_____   _____   _____   _____
Patient Signature   Date   Clinican Signature   Date

Section C (*Clinician Postsession Evaluation*):

MENTAL STATUS EXAM (Circle appropriate items):

ALERTNESS: (ALERT) DROWSY LETHARGIC STUPOROUS

               OTHER: _____

ORIENTED TO: (PERSON) (PLACE) (TIME) (REASON FOR EVALUATION)

MOOD: (EUTHYMIC) ELEVATED DYSPHORIC AGITATED ANGRY

AFFECT: FLAT BLUNTED CONSTRICTED (APPROPRIATE) LABILE

THOUGHT CONTINUITY: (CLEAR & COHERENT) GOAL-DIRECTED TANGENTIAL CIRCUMSTANTIAL

               OTHER: _____

THOUGHT CONTENT: (WNL) OBSESSIONS DELUSIONS IDEAS OF REFERENCE BIZARRENESS MORBIDITY

               OTHER: _____

ABSTRACTION: (WNL) NOTABLY CONCRETE

               OTHER: _____

SPEECH: (WNL) RAPID SLOW SLURRED IMPOVERISHED INCOHERENT

               OTHER: _____

MEMORY: (GROSSLY INTACT)

               OTHER: _____

REALITY TESTING: (WNL)

               OTHER: _____

NOTABLE BEHAVIORAL OBSERVATIONS: *doing better overall – calmer*

DIAGNOSTIC IMPRESSIONS/DIAGNOSIS (DSM/ICD DIAGNOSES):

major depressive disorder – recurrent

ETOH abuse

PATIENT'S OVERALL SUICIDE RISK LEVEL (Check one and explain):

☐ **MILD (WTL/RFL)**   **Explanation:**

☑ **MODERATE (AMB)**   *seems brighter and more hopeful with the prospect of*

☐ **HIGH (WTD/RFD)**   *couples therapy*

CASE NOTES:

Bill is improved overall – he reports not drinking and attending AA meetings – he has used coping skills in stabalization plan and his sleep is a little better – he is willing to take a referral for medication consultation.

Next Appointment Scheduled: _____ Treatment Modality: *CAMS + couples + Rx referral*

_____
Clinican Signature   Date

CAMS SUICIDE STATUS FORM–4 (SSF-4) TRACKING/UPDATE INTERIM SESSION (3)

Patient: *Bill*   Clinician: *DJ*   Date: _____ Time: _____

Section A (*Patient*):

Rate and fill out each item according to how you feel <u>right now</u>.

1) RATE PSYCHOLOGICAL PAIN (*hurt, anguish, or misery in your mind, **not** stress, **not** physical pain*):   **Low pain:**   1   2   (**3**)   4   5   **:High pain**
2) RATE STRESS (*your general feeling of being pressured or overwhelmed*):   **Low stress:**   1   (**2**)   3   4   5   **:High stress**
3) RATE AGITATION (*emotional urgency; feeling that you need to take action; **not** irritation; **not** annoyance*):   **Low agitation:**   1   (**2**)   3   4   5   **:High agitation**
4) RATE HOPELESSNESS (*your expectation that things will not get better no matter what you do*):   **Low hopelessness:**   1   2   (**3**)   4   5   **:High hopelessness**
5) RATE SELF-HATE (*your general feeling of disliking yourself; having no self-esteem; having no self-respect*):   **Low self-hate:**   1   2   (**3**)   4   5   **:High self-hate**
6) RATE OVERALL RISK   **Extremely low risk:** (**1**)   2   3   4   5   **:Extremely high risk**   OF SUICIDE: **(will *not* kill self)**   **(will kill self)**

In the past week:

Suicidal Thoughts/Feelings   Y ✔ N __   Managed Thoughts/Feelings   Y ✔ N __   Suicidal Behavior   Y __ N ✔

Section B (*Clinician*):	Resolution of suicidality, if: current overall risk of suicide < 3; in past week: no suicidal behavior and effectively managed suicidal thoughts/feelings ☐ 1st session ☑ 2nd session
	Complete SSF Outcome Form at 3rd <u>consecutive</u> resolution session

<u>Patient Status:</u>   **TREATMENT PLAN UPDATE**

☐ Discontinued treatment   ☐ No show   ☐ Cancelled   ☐ Hospitalization   ☑ Referred/Other: *couples therapy*

Problem #	Problem Description	Goals and Objectives	Interventions	Duration
1	*Self-Harm Potential*	*Safety and Stability*	*Stabilization Plan Completed* ☑	*3 mo.*
2	*marital distress*	*work on marital communication*	*couples therapy CBT/insight psychotherapy*	*3 mo.*
3	*hopeless*	↑ *hope*	*virtual Hope Kit on phone Choosing to Live*	*3 mo.*

_____   _____

Patient Signature   Date   Clinican Signature   Date

Section C (*Clinician Postsession Evaluation*):

MENTAL STATUS EXAM (Circle appropriate items):

ALERTNESS: (ALERT) DROWSY LETHARGIC STUPOROUS

OTHER: _____

ORIENTED TO: (PERSON) (PLACE) (TIME) (REASON FOR EVALUATION)

MOOD: (EUTHYMIC) ELEVATED DYSPHORIC AGITATED ANGRY

AFFECT: FLAT BLUNTED CONSTRICTED (APPROPRIATE) LABILE

THOUGHT CONTINUITY: (CLEAR & COHERENT) GOAL-DIRECTED TANGENTIAL CIRCUMSTANTIAL

OTHER: _____

THOUGHT CONTENT: (WNL) OBSESSIONS DELUSIONS IDEAS OF REFERENCE BIZARRENESS MORBIDITY

OTHER: _____

ABSTRACTION: (WNL) NOTABLY CONCRETE

OTHER: _____

SPEECH: (WNL) RAPID SLOW SLURRED IMPOVERISHED INCOHERENT

OTHER: _____

MEMORY: (GROSSLY INTACT)

OTHER: _____

REALITY TESTING: (WNL)

OTHER: _____

NOTABLE BEHAVIORAL OBSERVATIONS: *continues to improve*

DIAGNOSTIC IMPRESSIONS/DIAGNOSIS (DSM/ICD DIAGNOSES):

major depressive disorder – recurrent
ETOH abuse – reports being sober 3 weeks

PATIENT'S OVERALL SUICIDE RISK LEVEL (Check one and explain):

☑ **MILD (WTL/RFL)**   **Explanation:**
☐ **MODERATE (AMB)**   *following CAMS well – excited about couples therapy – is*
☐ **HIGH (WTD/RFD)**   *starting SSRI Rx*

CASE NOTES:

Bill is doing notably better – attending AA meetings and has an AA sponsor, is
pleased with couples therapy, is working on hopelessness, will develop virtual Hope Kit
on his phone, and is reading Choosing to Live as well as journaling every night.

Next Appointment Scheduled: _____ Treatment Modality: *Rx + couples therapy*

_____
Clinician Signature   Date

CAMS SUICIDE STATUS FORM–4 (SSF-4) TRACKING/UPDATE INTERIM SESSION (4)

Patient: *Bill*   Clinician: *DJ*   Date: _____ Time: _____

Section A (*Patient*):

Rate and fill out each item according to how you feel <u>right now</u>.

1) RATE PSYCHOLOGICAL PAIN (*hurt, anguish, or misery in your mind, **not** stress, **not** physical pain*):
Low pain: 1   2   3   4   **(5)**   :High pain

2) RATE STRESS (*your general feeling of being pressured or overwhelmed*):
Low stress: 1   2   3   4   **(5)**   :High stress

3) RATE AGITATION (*emotional urgency; feeling that you need to take action; **not** irritation; **not** annoyance*):
Low agitation: 1   2   3   **(4)**   5   :High agitation

4) RATE HOPELESSNESS (*your expectation that things will not get better no matter what you do*):
Low hopelessness: 1   2   3   4   **(5)**   :High hopelessness

5) RATE SELF-HATE (*your general feeling of disliking yourself; having no self-esteem; having no self-respect*):
Low self-hate: 1   2   3   4   **(5)**   :High self-hate

6) RATE OVERALL RISK OF SUICIDE:	**Extremely low risk:** (**will *not* kill self**) 1 2 **(3)** 4 5 :**Extremely high risk** (**will kill self**)

In the past week:
Suicidal Thoughts/Feelings Y ✔ N ___   Managed Thoughts/Feelings Y ___ N ✔   Suicidal Behavior Y ✔ N ___

Section B (*Clinician*):

Resolution of suicidality, if: current overall risk of suicide < 3; in past week: no suicidal behavior and effectively managed suicidal thoughts/feelings ☐ 1st session ☐ 2nd session

Complete **SSF Outcome Form at 3rd <u>consecutive</u> resolution session**

<u>Patient Status:</u>   **TREATMENT PLAN UPDATE**   *Rx + couples*

☐ Discontinued treatment   ☐ No show   ☐ Cancelled   ☐ Hospitalization   ☑ Referred/Other: *therapy*

Problem #	Problem Description	Goals and Objectives	Interventions	Duration
1	Self-Harm Potential	Safety and Stability	*revised* Stabilization Plan Completed ☑	3 mo.
2	betrayal and trust with wife	deal with betrayal ↑ trust with wife	couples therapy insight-oriented psychotherapy	3 mo.
3	hopeless + self-esteem	↑ hope improve self-esteem	CBT homework insight-oriented psychotherapy	3 mo.

_____   _____   _____   _____
Patient Signature   Date   Clinican Signature   Date

MENTAL STATUS EXAM (Circle appropriate items):

ALERTNESS:　　　　　　　　(ALERT) DROWSY　LETHARGIC　STUPOROUS

OTHER: _____

ORIENTED TO:　　　　　　　(PERSON) (PLACE) (TIME) (REASON FOR EVALUATION)

MOOD:　　　　　　　　　　EUTHYMIC　ELEVATED　DYSPHORIC　(AGITATED)　ANGRY

AFFECT:　　　　　　　　　FLAT　BLUNTED　CONSTRICTED　APPROPRIATE　(LABILE)

THOUGHT CONTINUITY:　　　(CLEAR & COHERENT)　GOAL-DIRECTED　TANGENTIAL　CIRCUMSTANTIAL

OTHER: _____

THOUGHT CONTENT:　　　　(WNL)　OBSESSIONS　DELUSIONS　IDEAS OF REFERENCE　BIZARRENESS　MORBIDITY

OTHER: _____

ABSTRACTION:　　　　　　(WNL)　NOTABLY CONCRETE

OTHER: _____

SPEECH:　　　　　　　　　WNL　(RAPID)　SLOW　SLURRED　IMPOVERISHED　INCOHERENT

OTHER: _____

MEMORY:　　　　　　　　　(GROSSLY INTACT)

OTHER: _____

REALITY TESTING:　　　　　(WNL)

OTHER: _____

NOTABLE BEHAVIORAL OBSERVATIONS: *crisis session — Bill very upset*

DIAGNOSTIC IMPRESSIONS/DIAGNOSIS (DSM/ICD DIAGNOSES):

major depressive disorder

ETOH abuse

PATIENT'S OVERALL SUICIDE RISK LEVEL (Check one and explain):

☐ **MILD (WTL/RFL)**　　　　**Explanation:**

☐ **MODERATE (AMB)**　　　*major disclosure in couples therapy about betrayal of wife in*

☑ **HIGH (WTD/RFD)**　　　*affair and fathering a daughter who lives in Canada*

CASE NOTES:

Difficult session. Bill "dropped a bomb" in couples therapy about 20+-year-old affair
that resulted in the birth of a daughter — mother and daughter live in Canada — wife
very upset but willing to work in couples therapy — found him researching drugs on
Internet — Bill called me as per CAMS Stabilization Plan.

Next Appointment Scheduled: _____　Treatment Modality: *R/O hospitalization*
　　　　　　　　　　　　　　　　　　　　　　　　　　　　　　　　　　　　Rx + couples therapy

_____
Clinican Signature　　　　　　　　　　Date

CAMS SUICIDE STATUS FORM–4 (SSF-4) TRACKING/UPDATE INTERIM SESSION (5)

Patient: *Bill* _____ Clinician: *DJ* _____ Date: _____ Time: _____

Section A (*Patient*):

Rate and fill out each item according to how you feel <u>right now</u>.

1) RATE PSYCHOLOGICAL PAIN (*hurt, anguish, or misery in your mind, **not** stress, **not** physical pain*):   **Low pain:**   1   2   ③   4   5   :High pain
2) RATE STRESS (*your general feeling of being pressured or overwhelmed*):   **Low stress:**   1   2   ③   4   5   :High stress
3) RATE AGITATION (*emotional urgency; feeling that you need to take action; **not** irritation; **not** annoyance*):   **Low agitation:**   1   2   ③   4   5   :High agitation
4) RATE HOPELESSNESS (*your expectation that things will not get better no matter what you do*):   **Low hopelessness:**   1   2   3   ④   5   :High hopelessness
5) RATE SELF-HATE (*your general feeling of disliking yourself; having no self-esteem; having no self-respect*):   **Low self-hate:**   1   2   3   ④   5   :High self-hate
6) RATE OVERALL RISK OF SUICIDE: **Extremely low risk:**   1   2   ③   4   5   :Extremely high risk   **(will *not* kill self)**   **(will kill self)**

In the past week:

Suicidal Thoughts/Feelings Y ✔ N __   Managed Thoughts/Feelings Y __ N ✔   Suicidal Behavior Y __ N ✔

Section B (*Clinician*):

Resolution of suicidality, if: current overall risk of suicide < 3; in past week: no suicidal behavior and effectively managed suicidal thoughts/feelings ☐ 1st session ☐ 2nd session

Complete **SSF Outcome Form at 3rd <u>consecutive</u> resolution session**

Patient Status: **TREATMENT PLAN UPDATE**   *Rx + couples*

☐ Discontinued treatment ☐ No show ☐ Cancelled ☐ Hospitalization ☑ Referred/Other: *therapy*

Problem #	Problem Description	Goals and Objectives	Interventions	Duration
1	*Self-Harm Potential*	*Safety and Stability*	*Stabilization Plan Completed* ☑	*3 mo.*
2	*trust with wife*	*improve trust*	*"date night"* *6-month* *behavioral contract*	*3 mo.*
3	*sense of self*	*improve self-esteem*	*historical work* *+ CBT*	*3 mo.*

_____ _____   _____ _____
Patient Signature   Date   Clinican Signature   Date

Section C (*Clinician Postsession Evaluation*):

MENTAL STATUS EXAM (Circle appropriate items):

ALERTNESS: (ALERT) DROWSY LETHARGIC STUPOROUS

OTHER: _____

ORIENTED TO: (PERSON) (PLACE) (TIME) (REASON FOR EVALUATION)

MOOD: (EUTHYMIC) ELEVATED DYSPHORIC AGITATED ANGRY

AFFECT: FLAT BLUNTED CONSTRICTED (APPROPRIATE) LABILE

THOUGHT CONTINUITY: (CLEAR & COHERENT) GOAL-DIRECTED TANGENTIAL CIRCUMSTANTIAL

OTHER: _____

THOUGHT CONTENT: (WNL) OBSESSIONS DELUSIONS IDEAS OF REFERENCE BIZARRENESS MORBIDITY

OTHER: _____

ABSTRACTION: (WNL) NOTABLY CONCRETE

OTHER: _____

SPEECH: (WNL) RAPID SLOW SLURRED IMPOVERISHED INCOHERENT

OTHER: _____

MEMORY: (GROSSLY INTACT)

OTHER: _____

REALITY TESTING: (WNL)

OTHER: _____

NOTABLE BEHAVIORAL OBSERVATIONS: *calmer, no longer in crisis*

DIAGNOSTIC IMPRESSIONS/DIAGNOSIS (DSM/ICD DIAGNOSES):

major depressive disorder
ETOH abuse

PATIENT'S OVERALL SUICIDE RISK LEVEL (Check one and explain):

☐ **MILD (WTL/RFL)**   **Explanation:**

☑ **MODERATE (AMB)**   *doing better than last session – working hard in couples*

☐ **HIGH (WTD/RFD)**   *therapy on issue of marital betrayal*

CASE NOTES:

Bill and wife appear to be committed to working things out in couples therapy – are
using 6-month behavioral contract to rebuild trust. Bill is relieved she knows his
"secret" and that she is willing to give him 6 months to prove himself to her – working
on self-esteem directly as new problem/driver.

Next Appointment Scheduled: _____ Treatment Modality: *Rx + couples therapy*

_____
Clinican Signature   Date

CAMS SUICIDE STATUS FORM–4 (SSF-4) TRACKING/UPDATE INTERIM SESSION (6)

Patient: _Bill_____ Clinician: _DJ_____ Date: _____ Time: _____

Section A (*Patient*):

Rate and fill out each item according to how you feel <u>right now</u>.

1) RATE PSYCHOLOGICAL PAIN (*hurt, anguish, or misery in your mind, **not** stress, **not** physical pain*):   **Low pain:** 1 (2) 3 4 5 :High pain
2) RATE STRESS (*your general feeling of being pressured or overwhelmed*):   **Low stress:** 1 (2) 3 4 5 :High stress
3) RATE AGITATION (*emotional urgency; feeling that you need to take action; **not** irritation; **not** annoyance*):   **Low agitation:** (1) 2 3 4 5 :High agitation
4) RATE HOPELESSNESS (*your expectation that things will not get better no matter what you do*):   **Low hopelessness:** 1 2 (3) 4 5 :High hopelessness
5) RATE SELF-HATE (*your general feeling of disliking yourself; having no self-esteem; having no self-respect*):   **Low self-hate:** 1 2 (3) 4 5 :High self-hate
6) RATE OVERALL RISK OF SUICIDE: **Extremely low risk:** 1 (2) 3 4 5 :**Extremely high risk**   **(will *not* kill self)**   **(will kill self)**

In the past week:

Suicidal Thoughts/Feelings Y ✔ N __   Managed Thoughts/Feelings Y ✔ N __   Suicidal Behavior Y __ N ✔

Section B (*Clinician*):

Resolution of suicidality, if: current overall risk of suicide < 3; in past week: no suicidal behavior and effectively managed suicidal thoughts/feelings ☑ 1st session ☐ 2nd session

Complete **SSF Outcome Form at 3rd <u>consecutive</u> resolution session**

<u>Patient Status:</u>   **TREATMENT PLAN UPDATE**   *Rx + couples*

☐ Discontinued treatment ☐ No show ☐ Cancelled ☐ Hospitalization ☑ Referred/Other: _*therapy*_____

Problem #	Problem Description	Goals and Objectives	Interventions	Duration
1	*Self-Harm Potential*	*Safety and Stability*	*Stabilization Plan Completed* ☑	*3 mo.*
2	*trust with wife*	*improve trust*	*6-month contract couples therapy insight-oriented work*	*3 mo.*
3	*sense of self*	*improve self-love and compassion*	*journaling CBT homework*	*3 mo.*

_____   _____   _____   _____
Patient Signature   Date   Clinican Signature   Date

Section C (*Clinician Postsession Evaluation*):

MENTAL STATUS EXAM (Circle appropriate items):

ALERTNESS: (ALERT) DROWSY LETHARGIC STUPOROUS

OTHER: _____

ORIENTED TO: (PERSON) (PLACE) (TIME) (REASON FOR EVALUATION)

MOOD: (EUTHYMIC) ELEVATED DYSPHORIC AGITATED ANGRY

AFFECT: FLAT BLUNTED CONSTRICTED APPROPRIATE LABILE

THOUGHT CONTINUITY: (CLEAR & COHERENT) GOAL-DIRECTED TANGENTIAL CIRCUMSTANTIAL

OTHER: _____

THOUGHT CONTENT: (WNL) OBSESSIONS DELUSIONS IDEAS OF REFERENCE BIZARRENESS MORBIDITY

OTHER: _____

ABSTRACTION: (WNL) NOTABLY CONCRETE

OTHER: _____

SPEECH: (WNL) RAPID SLOW SLURRED IMPOVERISHED INCOHERENT

OTHER: _____

MEMORY: (GROSSLY INTACT)

OTHER: _____

REALITY TESTING: (WNL)

OTHER: _____

NOTABLE BEHAVIORAL OBSERVATIONS: *guardedly hopeful / brighter affect*

DIAGNOSTIC IMPRESSIONS/DIAGNOSIS (DSM/ICD DIAGNOSES):

major depressive disorder

ETOH abuse

_____

PATIENT'S OVERALL SUICIDE RISK LEVEL (Check one and explain):

☑ **MILD (WTL/RFL)**   **Explanation:**

☐ **MODERATE (AMB)**   *feels like he has "second chance" with his wife – only a*

☐ **HIGH (WTD/RFD)**   *passing thought of suicide in last week*

_____

CASE NOTES:

Bill is doing better – feels like maybe his marriage can maybe be saved. His affect is brighter, he is working with AA sponsor and attending meetings. Bill likes journaling and finds behavioral contract very helpful as a means to win back the trust of his wife. He seems cautiously hopeful.

_____

_____

Next Appointment Scheduled: _____ Treatment Modality: _____

_____

Clinican Signature   Date

235

CAMS SUICIDE STATUS FORM–4 (SSF-4) TRACKING/UPDATE INTERIM SESSION (7)

Patient: *Bill* _____ Clinician: *DJ* _____ Date: _____ Time: _____

Section A (*Patient*):

Rate and fill out each item according to how you feel <u>right now</u>.

1) RATE PSYCHOLOGICAL PAIN (*hurt, anguish, or misery in your mind, **not** stress, **not** physical pain*):   **Low pain:**   1   **(2)**   3   4   5   :High pain
2) RATE STRESS (*your general feeling of being pressured or overwhelmed*):   **Low stress:**   **(1)**   2   3   4   5   :High stress
3) RATE AGITATION (*emotional urgency; feeling that you need to take action; **not** irritation; **not** annoyance*):   **Low agitation:**   **(1)**   2   3   4   5   :High agitation
4) RATE HOPELESSNESS (*your expectation that things will not get better no matter what you do*):   **Low hopelessness:**   1   **(2)**   3   4   5   :High hopelessness
5) RATE SELF-HATE (*your general feeling of disliking yourself; having no self-esteem; having no self-respect*):   **Low self-hate:**   1   **(2)**   3   4   5   :High self-hate
6) RATE OVERALL RISK   **Extremely low risk:**   **(1)**   2   3   4   5   :Extremely high risk   OF SUICIDE: **(will *not* kill self)**   **(will kill self)**

In the past week:

Suicidal Thoughts/Feelings   Y __   N ✔   Managed Thoughts/Feelings   Y ✔   N __   Suicidal Behavior   Y __   N ✔

Section B (*Clinician*):	Resolution of suicidality, if: current overall risk of suicide < 3; in past week: no suicidal behavior and effectively managed suicidal thoughts/feelings ☐ 1st session ☑ 2nd session

                                 Complete SSF Outcome Form at 3rd <u>consecutive</u> resolution session**

<u>Patient Status:</u>   **TREATMENT PLAN UPDATE**   *Rx + couples*

☐ Discontinued treatment   ☐ No show   ☐ Cancelled   ☐ Hospitalization   ☑ Referred/Other: *therapy* _____

Problem #	Problem Description	Goals and Objectives	Interventions	Duration
1	*Self-Harm Potential*	*Safety and Stability*	*Stabilization Plan Completed* ☑	*3 mo.*
2	*trust in marriage*	*be trustworthy*	*couples therapy insight psychotherapy*	*3 mo.*
3	*self-regard*	*self-love and compassion*	*journaling insight psychotherapy*	*3 mo.*

Patient Signature   Date   Clinican Signature   Date

Section C (*Clinician Postsession Evaluation*):

MENTAL STATUS EXAM (Circle appropriate items):

ALERTNESS: (ALERT) DROWSY LETHARGIC STUPOROUS

OTHER: _____

ORIENTED TO: (PERSON) (PLACE) (TIME) (REASON FOR EVALUATION)

MOOD: (EUTHYMIC) ELEVATED DYSPHORIC AGITATED ANGRY

AFFECT: FLAT BLUNTED CONSTRICTED (APPROPRIATE) LABILE

THOUGHT CONTINUITY: (CLEAR & COHERENT) GOAL-DIRECTED TANGENTIAL CIRCUMSTANTIAL

OTHER: _____

THOUGHT CONTENT: (WNL) OBSESSIONS DELUSIONS IDEAS OF REFERENCE BIZARRENESS MORBIDITY

OTHER: _____

ABSTRACTION: (WNL) NOTABLY CONCRETE

OTHER: _____

SPEECH: (WNL) RAPID SLOW SLURRED IMPOVERISHED INCOHERENT

OTHER: _____

MEMORY: (GROSSLY INTACT)

OTHER: _____

REALITY TESTING: (WNL)

OTHER: _____

NOTABLE BEHAVIORAL OBSERVATIONS: *doing much better overall*

DIAGNOSTIC IMPRESSIONS/DIAGNOSIS (DSM/ICD DIAGNOSES):

major depressive disorder

ETOH abuse

PATIENT'S OVERALL SUICIDE RISK LEVEL (Check one and explain):

☑ **MILD (WTL/RFL)** **Explanation:**
☐ **MODERATE (AMB)** *Bill seems to have turned a corner. Couples therapy is going*
☐ **HIGH (WTD/RFD)** *well and "date nights" are a success!*

CASE NOTES:

Bill is doing much better – AA sponsor is a huge support and Rx seems to help as well.
Sleep is better and morale much improved. He feels like he may redeem himself to his
wife. Is following couples contract to the letter. Possible resolution of CAMS next
session.

Next Appointment Scheduled: _____ Treatment Modality: *Rx + couples therapy*

_____
Clinican Signature   Date

CAMS SUICIDE STATUS FORM–4 (SSF-4) OUTCOME/DISPOSITION FINAL SESSION (8)

Patient: *Bill* _____ Clinician: *DJ* _____ Date: _____ Time: _____

Section A (*Patient*):

Rate and fill out each item according to how you feel <u>right now</u>.

1) RATE PSYCHOLOGICAL PAIN (*hurt, anguish, or misery in your mind, **not** stress, **not** physical pain*):   **Low pain:**   1 **(2)** 3 4 5 :High pain
2) RATE STRESS (*your general feeling of being pressured or overwhelmed*):   **Low stress:** **(1)** 2 3 4 5 :High stress
3) RATE AGITATION (*emotional urgency; feeling that you need to take action; **not** irritation; **not** annoyance*):   **Low agitation:** **(1)** 2 3 4 5 :High agitation
4) RATE HOPELESSNESS (*your expectation that things will not get better no matter what you do*):   **Low hopelessness:** **(1)** 2 3 4 5 :High hopelessness
5) RATE SELF-HATE (*your general feeling of disliking yourself; having no self-esteem; having no self-respect*):   **Low self-hate:** 1 **(2)** 3 4 5 :High self-hate
6) RATE OVERALL RISK OF SUICIDE: **Extremely low risk:** **(1)** 2 3 4 5 :Extremely high risk   (will *not* kill self)   (will kill self)

In the past week:

Suicidal Thoughts/Feelings Y ___ N ✔   Managed Thoughts/Feelings Y ✔ N ___   Suicidal Behavior Y ___ N ✔

Where there any aspects of your treatment that were particularly helpful to you? If so, please describe these. Be as specific as possible.

Stabilization plan — 6-month couples contract has really helped

What have you learned from your clinical care that could help you if you became suicidal in the future?

talk to wife, use my virtual hope box, contact therapist

Section B (*Clinician*):

<u>Third consecutive session of resolved suicidality:</u> ✔ Yes ___ No (If no, continue CAMS tracking)

**Resolution of suicidality, if for third consecutive week: current overall risk of suicide < 3; in past week: no suicidal behavior and effectively managed suicidal thoughts/feelings

<u>OUTCOME/DISPOSITION</u> (Check all that apply):

✔ Continuing outpatient psychotherapy   ___ Inpatient hospitalization

___ Mutual termination   ___ Patient chooses to discontinue treatment (unilaterally)

___ Referral to: _____

✔ Other. Describe: *will continue AA, couples therapy, + Rx* _____

Next Appointment Scheduled (if applicable): _____

Patient Signature   Date   Clinican Signature   Date

Section C (*Clinician Postsession Evaluation*):

MENTAL STATUS EXAM (Circle appropriate items):

ALERTNESS: (ALERT) DROWSY   LETHARGIC   STUPOROUS

OTHER: _____

ORIENTED TO: (PERSON) (PLACE) (TIME) (REASON FOR EVALUATION)

MOOD: (EUTHYMIC) ELEVATED   DYSPHORIC   AGITATED   ANGRY

AFFECT: FLAT   BLUNTED   CONSTRICTED   APPROPRIATE   LABILE

THOUGHT CONTINUITY: (CLEAR & COHERENT) GOAL-DIRECTED   TANGENTIAL   CIRCUMSTANTIAL

OTHER: _____

THOUGHT CONTENT: (WNL) OBSESSIONS   DELUSIONS   IDEAS OF REFERENCE   BIZARRENESS   MORBIDITY

OTHER: _____

ABSTRACTION: (WNL) NOTABLY CONCRETE

OTHER: _____

SPEECH: (WNL) RAPID   SLOW   SLURRED   IMPOVERISHED   INCOHERENT

OTHER: _____

MEMORY: (GROSSLY INTACT)

OTHER: _____

REALITY TESTING: (WNL)

OTHER: _____

NOTABLE BEHAVIORAL OBSERVATIONS: *the best I've seen Bill — seems happy*

DIAGNOSTIC IMPRESSIONS/DIAGNOSIS (DSM/ICD DIAGNOSES):

major depressive disorder
ETOH abuse
_____

PATIENT'S OVERALL SUICIDE RISK LEVEL (Check one and explain):

☑ **LOW (WTL/RFL)**   **Explanation:**
☐ **MODERATE (AMB)**   *meets criteria for CAMS resolution*
☐ **HIGH (WTD/RFD)**   _____
                           _____

CASE NOTES:

Bill is ready to resolve CAMS care and move beyond suicide-focused treatment. Couples therapy is hard but is going well. AA and sponsor are making a difference and he is working the 12 steps. Rx seems helpful too. Will continue 1x/week psychotherapy + couples work + Rx.

_____   _____
Clinican Signature   Date

References

Adler, G., & Buie, D. H., Jr. (1979). Aloneness and borderline psychopathology: The possible relevance of child development issues. *International Journal of Psychoanalysis, 60,* 83–96.

Ajdacic-Gross, V., Ring, M., Gadola, E., Lauber, C., Bopp, M., Gutzwiller, F., et al. (2008). Suicide after bereavement: An overlooked problem. *Psychological Medicine, 38,* 673–676.

Allen, J. G., Fonagy, P., & Bateman, A. W. (2008). *Mentalizing in clinical practice.* Arlington, VA: American Psychiatric Publishing.

American Psychiatric Association. (2013). *Diagnostic and statistical manual of mental disorders* (5th ed.). Arlington, VA: Author.

Anderson, A. R., Keyes, G. M., & Jobes, D. A. (2016). Understanding and treating suicidal risk in children. *Practice Innovations* [Epub ahead of print].

Andreasson, K., Krogh, K., Rosenbaum, B., Gluud, C., Jobes, D., & Nordentoft (2014). The DiaS trial: Dialectical behaviour therapy vs. collaborative assessment and management of suicidality on self-harm in patients with a recent suicide attempt and borderline personality disorder traits, study protocol for a randomized controlled trial. *Trials Journal, 15,* 194.

Andreasson, K., Krogh, J., Wenneberg, C., Jessen, H. K. L., Krakauer, K., Gluud, C., et al. (2016). Effectiveness of dialectical behavior therapy versus collaborative assessment and management of suicidality for reduction of self-harm in adults with borderline personality traits and disorder—A randomized observer-blinded clinical trial. *Depression and Anxiety* [Epub ahead of print].

Andreasson, K., Krogh, J., Wenneberg, C., Jessen, H. K., Krakauer, K., Gluud, C., et al. (2015, June). *Dialectical behavior therapy vs. CAMS for patients with borderline personality traits and suicide attempt—A randomized clinical trial.* Paper presented at the Congress of the International Association for Suicide Prevention, Montreal, Quebec, Canada.

Anestis, M. D., Soberay, K. A., Gutierrez, P. M., Hernández, T. D., & Joiner, T. E. (2014). Reconsidering the link between impulsivity and suicidal behavior. *Personality and Social Psychology Review, 18,* 366–386.

Apil, S. R., Hoencamp, E., Judith Haffmans, P. M., & Spinhoven, P. (2012). A stepped care relapse prevention program for depression in older people: A randomized controlled trial. *International Journal of Geriatric Psychiatry, 27,* 583–591.

Archuleta, D., Jobes, D. A., Pujol, L., Jennings, K., Crumlish, J., Lento, R. M., et al. (2014). Raising the clinical standard of care for suicidal Soldiers: An Army process improvement initiative. *U.S. Army Medical Department Journal, Oct.–Dec.*, 55–66.

Arkov, K., Rosenbaum, B., Christiansen, L., Jonsson, H., & Munchow, M. (2008). Treatment of suicidal patients: The collaborative assessment and management of suicidality. *Ugeskr Laeger, 170*, 149–153.

Baillargeon, J., Binswanger, I. A., Penn, J. V., Williams, B. A., & Murray, O. J. (2009). Psychiatric disorders and repeat incarcerations: The revolving prison door. *American Journal of Psychiatry, 166*, 103–109.

Bakan, D. (1966). *The duality of human existence.* Chicago: Rand McNally.

Ballard, E. D., Horowitz, L. H., Jobes, D. A., Wagner, B. M., Pao, M., & Teach, S. J. (2013). Association of positive responses to suicide screening questions with hospital admission and repeat emergency department visits in children and adolescents. *Pediatric Emergency Care, 29*, 1–7.

Bamatter, W., Barrueco, S., Oquendo, M., & Jobes, D. A. (2015). *Translation and validation of the SSF-IV into Spanish.* Unpublished manuscript.

Barlow, D. H., Bullis, J. R., Comer, J. S., & Ametaj, A. A. (2013). Evidence-based psychological treatments: An update and a way forward. *Annual Review of Clinical Psychology, 9*, 1–27.

Bateman, A., & Fonagy, P. (2006). *Mentalization-based treatment for borderline personality disorder: A practical guide.* New York: Oxford University Press.

Bateman, A., & Fonagy, P. (2009). Randomized controlled trial of outpatient mentalization-based treatment versus structured clinical management for borderline personality disorder. *American Journal of Psychiatry, 166*, 1355–1364.

Baumeister, R. F. (1990). Suicide as escape from self. *Psychological Review, 97*, 90–113.

Beck, A. T. (1967). *Depression: Clinical, experimental, and theoretical aspects.* New York: Harper & Row.

Beck, A. T. (1986). Hopelessness as a predictor of eventual suicide. *Annals of New York Academy of Sciences, 487*, 90–96.

Beck, A. T., Rush, A. J., Shaw, B. F., & Emery, G. (1979). *Cognitive therapy of depression.* New York: Guilford Press.

Beck, A. T., & Steer, R. A. (1991). *Manual for Beck Scale for Suicide Ideation.* San Antonio, TX: Psychological Corporation.

Beck, A. T., & Steer, R. A. (1993). *Manual for Beck Hopelessness Scale.* San Antonio, TX: Psychological Corporation.

Beck, A. T., Steer, R. A., Kovacs, M., & Garrison, B. (1985). Hopelessness and eventual suicide: A 10-year prospective study of patients hospitalized with suicidal ideation. *American Journal of Psychiatry, 142*, 559–563.

Beidas, R. S., Edmunds, J. M., Marcus, S. C., & Kendall, P. C. (2012). Training and consultation to promote implementation of an empirically supported treatment: A randomized trial. *Psychiatric Services, 63*, 660–665.

Bender, E. (2014, October 10). Psychiatrists can minimize malpractice-suit anxiety. *Psychiatric News.* Retrieved from *http://psychnews.psychiatryonline.org/doi/full/10.1176/pn.38.16.0011.*

Bennett, K. M., Vaslef, S. N., Shapiro, M. L., Brooks, K. R., & Scarborough, J. E. (2009). Does intent matter?: The medical and societal burden of self-inflicted injury. *Journal of Trauma, 67*, 841–847.

Berkowitz, R., Fang, Z., Helfand, B., Jones, R., Schreiber, R., & Paasche-Orlow, M. (2013). Project Re-Engineered Discharge (RED) lowers hospital readmissions of patients discharged from a skilled nursing facility. *Journal of the American Medical Directors Association, 14*, 736–740.

Berman, A. L., & Jobes, D. A. (1991). *Adolescent suicide: Assessment and intervention.* Washington, DC: American Psychological Association.

Berman, A. L., Jobes, D. A., & Silverman, M. M. (2006). *Adolescent suicide: Assessment and intervention* (2nd ed.). Washington, DC: American Psychological Association.

Bonanno, G. A., & Castonguay, L. G. (1994). On balancing approaches to psychotherapy: Prescriptive patterns of attention, motivation, and personality. *Psychotherapy: Theory, Research, Practice, Training, 31,* 571–587.

Bongar, B. (2002). *The suicidal patient: Clinical and legal standards of care* (2nd ed.). Washington, DC: American Psychological Association.

Borges, G., & Rosovsky, H. (1996). Suicide attempts and alcohol consumption in an emergency room sample. *Journal of Studies on Alcohol and Drugs, 57,* 543–558.

Bostwick, J. M., & Pankratz, V. S. (2000). Affective disorders and suicide risk: A reexamination. *American Journal of Psychiatry, 157,* 1925–1932.

Boudreaux, E. D., & Horowitz, L. M. (2014). Suicide risk screening and assessment: Designing instruments with dissemination in mind. *American Journal of Preventive Medincine, 47,* S163–S169.

Brancu, M., Jobes, D. A., Wanger, B., Greene, J., & Fratto, T. (2015, July 28). Are there linguistic markers of suicidal writing that can predict the course of treatment?: A repeated measures longitudinal analysis. *Archives of Suicide Research* [Epub ahead of print].

Brent, D. A., Perper, J. A., Moritz, G., Baugher, M., Roth, C., Balach, L., et al. (1993). Stressful life events, psychopathology, and adolescent suicide: A case control study. *Suicide and Life-Threatening Behavior, 23,* 179–187.

Bridge, J. A., Asti, L., Horowitz, L. M., Greenhouse, J. B., Fontanella, C. A., Sheftall, A. H., et al. (2015). Suicide trends among elementary school-aged children in the United States from 1993 to 2012. *Journal of the American Medical Association Pediatrics, 169,* 673–677.

Bridge, J. A., Reynolds, B., McBee-Strayer, S. M., Sheftall, A. H., Ackerman, J., Stevens, J., et al. (2015). Impulsive aggression, delay discounting, and adolescent suicide attempts: Effects of current psychotropic medication use and family history of suicidal behavior. *Journal of Child and Adolescent Psychopharmacology, 25,* 114–123.

Britton, P. C., Conner, K. R., & Maisto, S. A. (2012). An open trial of motivational interviewing to address suicidal ideation with hospitalized veterans. *Journal of Clinical Psychology, 68,* 961–971.

Britton, P. C., Patrick, H., Wenzel, A., & Williams, G. C. (2011). Integrating motivational interviewing and self-determination theory with cognitive behavioral therapy to prevent suicide. *Cognitive and Behavioral Practice, 18,* 16–27.

Britton, P. C., Williams, G. C., & Conner, K. R. (2008). Self-determination theory, motivational interviewing, and the treatment of clients with acute suicidal ideation. *Journal of Clinical Psychology, 64,* 52–66.

Bromet, E., Andrade, L. H., Hwang, I., Sampson, N. A., Alonso, J., de Girolamo, G., et al. (2011). Cross-national epidemiology of DSM-IV major depressive episode. *BMC Medicine, 9,* 1–17.

Brown, G. K. (2001). *A review of suicide assessment measures for intervention research with adults and older adults.* Bethesda, MD: National Institute of Mental Health. Available at *http://ruralccp.org/lyra-data/storage/asset/brown-nd-27cb.pdf.*

Brown, G. K., Beck, A. T., Steer, R. A., & Grisham, J. R. (2000). Risk factors for suicide in psychiatric outpatients: A 20-year prospective study. *Journal of Consulting and Clinical Psychology, 68,* 371–377.

Brown, G. K., Have, T. T., Henriques, G. R., Xie, S. X., Hollander, J. E., & Beck, A. T. (2005) Cognitive therapy for the prevention of suicide attempts. *Journal of the American Medical Association, 294,* 563–570.

Brown, G. K., Steer, R. A., Henriques, G. R., & Beck, A. T. (2005). The internal struggle between the wish to die and the wish to live: A risk factor for suicide. *American Journal of Psychiatry, 162,* 1977–1979.

Brown, M. Z., & Chapman, A. L. (2007). Stopping self-harm once and for all: Relapse prevention in dialectical behavior therapy. In K. A. Witkiewitz & G. A. Marlatt (Eds.), *Therapist's guide to evidence-based relapse prevention* (pp. 191–213). Burlington, MA: Elsevier.

Bryan, C. J., Blount, T., Kanzler, K. A., Morrow, C. E., Corso, K. A., Corso, M. A., et al. (2014). Reliability and normative data for the Behavioral Health Measure (BHM) in primary care behavioral health settings. *Family, Systems, and Health, 32,* 89–100.

Bryan, C. J., Corso, K., Rudd, M., & Cordero, L. (2008). Improving identification of suicidal patients in primary care through routine screening. *Primary Care and Community Psychiatry, 13,* 143–147.

Bryan, C. J., Jennings, K. W., Jobes, D. A., & Bradley, J. C. (2012). Understanding and preventing military suicide. *Archives of Suicide Research, 16,* 95–110.

Bryan, C. J., Morrow, C. E., Etienne, N., & Ray-Sannerud, B. (2013). Guilt, shame, and suicidal ideation in a military outpatient clinical sample. *Depression and Anxiety, 30,* 55–60.

Bryan, C. J., & Rudd, M. D. (2006). Advances in the assessment of suicide risk. *Journal of Clinical Psychology, 62,* 185–200.

Bryan, C. J., & Rudd, M. D. (2010). *Managing suicide risk in primary care.* New York: Springer.

Bryan, C. J., Stone, S. L., & Rudd, M. D. (2011). A practical, evidence-based approach for means-restriction counseling with suicidal patients. *Professional Psychology: Research and Practice, 42,* 339–346.

Bush, N. E., Dobscha, S. K., Crumpton, R., Denneson, L. M., Hoffman, J. E., Crain, A., et al. (2015). A virtual hope box smartphone app as an accessory to therapy: Proof-of-concept in a clinical sample of veterans. *Suicide and Life-Threatening Behavior, 24,* 1–9.

Capron, D. W., Fitch, K., Medley, A., Blagg, C., Mallott, M., & Joiner, T. (2012). Role of anxiety sensitivity subfactors in suicidal ideation and suicide attempt history. *Depression and Anxiety, 29,* 195–201.

Cardeli, E. (2015). *Characteristics and functions of suicide attempts versus nonsuicidal self-injury in juvenile confinement.* Unpublished doctoral dissertation, The Catholic University of America, Washington, DC.

Cavanagh, J. T. O., Carson, A. J., Sharpe, M., & Lawrie, S. M. (2003). Psychological autopsy studies of suicide: A systematic review. *Psychological Medicine, 33,* 395–405.

Centers for Disease Control and Prevention, National Center for Injury Prevention and Control. (2010). Web-based Injury Statistics Query and Reporting System (WISQARS). Retrieved from *www.cdc.gov/injury/wisqars/index.html.*

Centers for Disease Control and Prevention, National Center for Injury Prevention and Control. (2014). CDC data and statistics fatal injury report for 2011. Retrieved from *www.cdc.gov/injury/wisqars/fatal_injury_reports.html.*

Chiles, J. A., & Strosahl, K. D. (1995). *The suicidal patient: Principles of assessment, treatment, and case management.* Washington, DC: American Psychiatric Association.

Claassen C. A., & Larkin, G. L. (2005). Occult suicidality in an emergency department population. *British Journal of Psychiatry, 186,* 352–353.

Collins, L. M., Murphy, S. A., & Strecher, V. (2007). The multiphase optimization strategy (MOST) and the sequential multiple assignment randomized trial (SMART): New methods for more potent eHealth interventions. *American Journal of Preventive Medicine, 32,* S112–S118.

Comtois, K. A., Jobes, D. A., O'Connor, S., Atkins, D. C., Janis, K., Chessen, C., et al. (2011). Collaborative assessment and management of suicidality (CAMS): Feasibility trial for next-day appointment services. *Depression and Anxiety, 28,* 963–972.

Conrad, A. K., Jacoby, A. M., Jobes, D. A., Lineberry, T., Jobes, D., Shea, C., et al. (2009). A pychometric investigation of the suicide status form with suicidal inpatients. *Suicide and Life-Threatening Behavior, 39,* 307–320.

Conwell, Y., Duberstein, P. R., Cox, C., Herrmann, J., Forbes, N., & Caine, E. D. (1998). Age differences in behaviors leading to completed suicide. *American Journal of Geriatric Psychiatry, 6,* 122–126.

Coombs, D. W., Miller, H. L., Alarcon, R., Herlihy, C., Lee, J. M., & Morrison, D. P. (1992). Presuicide attempt communications between parasuicides and consulted caregivers. *Suicide and Life-Threatening Behavior, 22,* 289–302.

Coope, C., Donovan, J., Wilson, C., Barnes, M., Metcalfe, C., Hollingworth, W., et al. (2015).

Characteristics of people dying by suicide after job loss, financial difficulties and other economic stressors during a period of recession (2010–2011): A review of coroners' records. *Journal of Affective Disorders, 183,* 98–105.

Corona, C. (2015, April). *The psychometric properties of the CAMS Rating Scale: A preliminary evaluation.* Paper presented at the annual conference of the American Association of Suicidology, Atlanta, GA.

Corona, C., & Jobes, D. A. (2013, April). *The role of response style in suicide risk assessment and treatment.* Paper presented at the annual conference of the American Association of Suicidology, Austin, TX.

Corona, C. D., Jobes, D. A., Nielsen, A. C., Pedersen, C. M., Jennings, K. W., Lento, R. M., et al. (2013). Assessing and treating different suicidal states in a Danish outpatient sample. *Archives of Suicide Research, 17,* 302–312.

Crowley, K. J., Arnkoff, D. B., Glass, C. R., & Jobes, D. A. (2014, April). Collaborative assessment and management of suicidality (CAMS): Adherence to a flexible clinical framework. In C. Corona (Chair), *The collaborative assessment and management of suicidality: Perspectives from the Catholic University suicide prevention lab.* Symposium presented at the annual conference of the American Association of Suicidology, Los Angeles, CA.

Crumlish, J. A. (1996). *Therapist responses to difficult patient presentations.* Unpublished doctoral dissertation, The Catholic University of America, Washington, DC.

Daniel, S. S., & Goldston, D. B. (2012). Hopelessness and lack of connectedness to others as risk factors for suicidal behavior across the lifespan: Implications for cognitive-behavioral treatment. *Cognitive and Behavioral Practice, 19,* 288–300.

Dawes, R. M., Faust, D., & Meehl, P. E. (1989). Clinical versus actuarial judgment. *Science, 243,* 1668–1674.

Derogatis, L. R., Lipman, R. S., Rickels, K., Uhlenhuth, E. H., & Covi, L. (1974). The Hopkins Symptom Checklist (HSCL): A self-report symptom inventory. *Behavioral Science, 19,* 1–15.

Derogatis, L. R., Rickels, K., & Rock, A. (1976). The SCL-90 and the MMPI: A step in the validation of a new self-report scale. *British Journal of Psychiatry, 128,* 280–289.

Derogatis, L. R., & Savitz, K. L. (1999). The SCL-90-R, Brief Symptom Inventory, and Matching Clinical Rating Scales. In M. E. Maruish (Ed.), *The use of psychological testing for treatment planning and outcomes assessment* (pp. 679–724). Mahwah, NJ: Erlbaum.

Dimidjian, S., Goodman, S. H., Felder, J. N., Gallop, R., Brown, A. P., & Beck, A. (2014). An open trial of mindfulness-based cognitive therapy for the prevention of perinatal depressive relapse/recurrence. *Archives of Women's Mental Health, 18,* 85–94.

Dimidjian, S., Hollon, S. D., Dobson, K. S., Schmaling, K. B., Kohlenberg, R. J, Addis, M. E., et al. (2006). Randomized trial of behavioral activation, cognitive therapy, and antidepressant medication in the acute treatment of adults with major depression. *Journal of Consulting and Clinical Psychology, 74,* 658–670.

Dozois, D. J. A., Mikail, S., Alden, L. E., Bieling, P. J., Bourgon, G., Clark, D. A., et al. (2014). The CPA presidential task force on evidence-based practice of psychological treatments. *Canadian Psychology, 55,* 153–160.

Drapeau, C. W., & McIntosh, J. L. (for the American Association of Suicidology). (2014, October 18). *U.S.A. suicide 2012: Official final data.* Washington, DC: American Association of Suicidology. Retrieved from *www.suicidology.org.*

Drozd, J. F., Jobes, D. A., & Luoma, J. B. (2000). The collaborative assessment and management of suicidality in Air Force mental health clinics. *The Air Force Psychologist, 18,* 6–11.

Ducasse, D., René, E., Béziat, S., Guillaume, S., Courtet, P., & Olié, E. (2014). Acceptance and commitment therapy for management of suicidal patients: A pilot study. *Psychotherapy and Psychosomatics, 83,* 374–376.

Durkheim, E. (1951). *Suicide: A study in sociology* (J. A. Spaulding & G. Simpson, Trans.). Glencoe, IL: Free Press. (Original work published 1897)

Eddins, C. L., & Jobes, D. A. (1994). Do you see what I see?: Patient and clinician perceptions of underlying dimensions of suicidality. *Suicide and Life-Threatening Behavior, 24*, 170–173.

Eisenberg, M. E., & Resnick, M. D. (2006). Suicidality among gay, lesbian and bisexual youth: The role of protective factors. *Journal of Adolescent Health, 39*, 662–668.

Elkin, I., Shea, M., Watkins, J. T., Imber, S. D., Sotsky, S. M., Collins, J. F., et al. (1989). National Institute of Mental Health Treatment of Depression Collaborative Research Program: General effectiveness of treatments. *Archives of General Psychiatry, 46*, 971–982.

Ellis, T. E. (2004). Collaboration and a self-help orientation in therapy with suicidal clients. *Journal of Contemporary Psychotherapy, 34*, 41–57.

Ellis, T. E., Allen, J. G., Woodson, H., Frueh, B. C., & Jobes, D. A. (2010). Implementing an evidence-based approach to working with suicidal inpatients. *Bulletin of the Menninger Clinic, 73*, 339–354.

Ellis, T. E., Daza, P., & Allen, J. G. (2012). Collaborative assessment and management of suicidality at Menninger (CAMS-M): An inpatient adaptation and implementation. *Bulletin of the Menninger Clinic, 76*, 147–171.

Ellis, T. E., Green, K. L., Allen, J. G., Jobes, D. A., & Nadorff, M. R. (2012). Use of the collaborative assessment and management of suicidality in an inpatient setting: Results of a pilot study. *Psychotherapy, 49*, 72–80.

Ellis, T. E., & Newman, C. F. (1996). *Choosing to live: How to defeat suicide through cognitive therapy.* Oakland, CA: New Harbinger.

Ellis, T. E., & Patel, A. B. (2012). Client suicide: What now? *Cognitive and Behavioral Practice, 19*, 277–287.

Ellis, T. E., & Rufino, K. A. (2015, April). *CAMS in a psychiatric inpatient setting: Outcomes and follow-up.* Paper presented at the annual conference of the American Association of Suicidology, Atlanta, GA.

Ellis, T. E., Rufino, K. A., Allen, J. G., Fowler, J. C., & Jobes, D. A. (2015). Impact of a suicide-specific intervention within inpatient psychiatric care: The collaborative assessment and management of suicidality. *Suicide and Life-Threatening Behavior* [Epub ahead of print].

Esposito-Smythers, C., & Spirito, A. (2004). Adolescent substance use and suicidal behavior: A review with implications for treatment research. *Alcoholism: Clinical and Experimental Research, 28*, 77S–88S.

Familoni, J., & Rasmusson, A. (2012, May). *Randomized controlled study: Tailored evaluation and treatment for PTSD progression and suicide prevention by application of thermal imaging.* Presentation at Suicide Prevention Research Interim Progress Report meeting, Military Operational Medicine Research Program, Ft. Detrick, MD.

Fazaa, N., & Page, S. (2003). Dependency and self-criticism as predictors of suicidal behavior. *Suicide and Life-Threatening Behavior, 33*, 172–185.

Fazaa, N., & Page, S. (2005). Two distinct personality configurations: Understanding the therapeutic context with suicidal individuals. *Journal of Contemporary Psychotherapy, 35*, 331–346.

Fazel, S., & Seewald, K. (2012). Severe mental illness in 33,588 prisoners worldwide:Systematic review and meta-regression analysis. *British Journal of Psychiatry, 200*, 364–373.

Fazel, S., & Yu, R. (2011). Psychotic disorders and repeat offending: Systematic review and meta-analysis. *Schizophrenia Bulletin, 37*, 800–810.

Fergusson, D., Doucette, S., Glass, K. C., Shapiro, S., Healy, D., Hebert, P., et al. (2005). Association between suicide attempts and selective serotonin reuptake inhibitors: Systematic review of randomised controlled trials. *British Medical Journal, 330*, 396.

Figueroa, R., Harman, J., & Engberg, J. (2004). Use of claims data to examine the impact of length of inpatient psychiatric stay on readmission rate. *Psychiatric Services, 55*, 560–565.

Florentine, J. B., & Crane, C. (2010). Suicide prevention by limiting access to methods: A review of theory and practice. *Social Science and Medicine, 70*, 1626–1632.

Foa, E. B. (2010). Dissemination of evidence-based psychological treatments for posttraumatic stress disorder in the Veterans Health Administration. *Journal of Traumatic Stress, 23*, 663–673.

Foa, E., Hembree, E., & Rothbaum, B. O. (2007). *Prolonged exposure therapy for PTSD: Emotional processing of traumatic experiences therapist guide*. New York: Oxford University Press.

Fratto, T., Jobes, D. A., Pentiuc, D., Rice, R., & Tendick, V. (2004). *The SSF One-Thing Assessment for Suicidal Risk*. Unpublished manuscript, The Catholic University of America, Washington, DC.

Freud, S. (1961). *Civilization and its discontents* (J. Strachey, Trans.). New York: Norton. (Original work published 1930)

Garfield, S. L. (1994). Research on client variables in psychotherapy. In A. E. Bergin & S. L. Garfield (Eds.), *Handbook of psychotherapy and behavior change* (4th ed., pp. 190–228). New York: Wiley.

Gay, P. (1989). *The Freud reader*. New York: Norton.

Ghahramanlou-Holloway, M., Cox, D. W., & Greene, F. N. (2012). Post-admission cognitive therapy: A brief intervention for psychiatric inpatients admitted after a suicide attempt. *Cognitive and Behavioral Practice, 19*, 233–244

Gibbons, R. D., Brown, C. H., Hur, K., Davis, J. M., & Mann, J. J. (2012). Suicidal thoughts and behavior with antidepressant treatment: Reanalysis of the randomized placebo-controlled studies of fluoxetine and venlafaxine. *Archives of General Psychiatry, 69*, 580–587

Giner, L., Blasco-Fontecilla, H., Perez-Rodriguez, M. M., Garcia-Nieto, R., Giner, J., Guija, J. A., et al. (2013). Personality disorders and health problems distinguish suicide attempters from completers in a direct comparison. *Journal of Affective Disorders, 151*, 474–483.

Glashouwer, K. A., de Jong, P. J., Penninx, B. W., Kerkhof, A. J., van Dyck, R., & Ormel, J. (2010). Do automatic self-associations relate to suicidal ideation? *Journal of Psychopathology and Behavioral Assessment, 32*, 428–437

Gleeson, J. F., Cotton, S. M., Alvarez-Jimenez, M., Wade, D., Gee, D., Crisp, K., et al. (2011). A randomized controlled trial of relapse prevention therapy for first-episode psychosis patients: Outcome at 30-month follow-up. *Schizophrenia Bulletin, 39*, 436–448.

Goldstein, J. (1993). Psychiatry. In W. F. Bynum & R. Porter (Eds.), *Companion encyclopedia of the history of medicine* (Vol. 2, pp. 1350–1372). New York: Routledge.

Goldstein, T. R., Bridge, J. A., & Brent, D. A. (2008). Sleep disturbance preceding completed suicide in adolescents. *Journal of Consulting and Clinical Psychology, 76*, 84–91.

Goldston, D. B. (2003). *Measuring suicidal behavior and risk in children and adolescents*. Washington, DC: American Psychological Association.

Goodman, M. (2012, May). *Affective startle and suicide risk*. Presentation at Suicide Prevention Research Interim Progress Report meeting, Military Operational Medicine Research Program, Ft. Detrick, MD.

Goodman, M. (2015, May). *High-risk suicidal behavior in veterans: Assessment and predictors and efficacy of dialectical behavior therapy*. Presentation at the Suicide Prevention Research Interim Progress Report meeting, Military Operational Medicine Research Program, Ft. Detrick, MD.

Gould, M. S. (2013, June). *Follow-up contact by crisis center workers*. Presentation at the National Lifeline Standards Training and Practice Steering Committee Meeting, Rockville, MD.

Gould, M. S., Kalafat, J., Harris-Munfakh, J. L., & Kleinman, M. (2007). An evaluation of crisis hotline outcomes part 2: Suicidal callers. *Suicide and Life-Threatening Behavior, 37*, 338–352.

Gould, M. S., Munfakh, J. L., Kleinman, M., & Lake, A. M. (2012). National suicide prevention lifeline: Enhancing mental health care for suicidal individuals and other people in crisis. *Suicide and Life-Threatening Behavior, 42*, 22–35.

Gunnell, D., Saperia, J., & Ashby, D. (2005). Selective serotonin reuptake inhibitors (SSRIs) and suicide in adults: Meta-analysis of drug company data from placebo controlled, randomized controlled trials submitted to the MHRA's safety review. *British Medical Journal, 330*, 385.

Gysin-Maillart, A., Schwab, S., Soravia, L., Megert, M., & Michel, K. (2016). A novel brief therapy for patients who attempt suicide: A 24-month follow-up randomized controlled study of the attempted suicide short intervention program. *PLoS Medicine* [Epub ahead of print].

Harris, K. M., McLean, J. P., Sheffield, J., & Jobes, D. A. (2010). The internal suicide debate hypothesis: Exploring the life versus death struggle. *Suicide and Life Threatening Behavior, 40*, 181–192.

Harris, R. (2009). *ACT made simple: An easy to read primer on acceptance and commitment therapy.* Oakland, CA: New Harbinger.

Harrison, D. P., Stritzke, W. G., Fay, N., Ellison, T. M., & Hudaib, A. R. (2014). Probing the implicit suicidal mind: Does the Death/Suicide Implicit Association Test reveal a desire to die, or a diminished desire to live? *Psychological Assessment, 26,* 831–840.

Hashmi, S., & Kapoor, R. (2010). Degree of proof necessary to establish proximate causation of suicide. *Journal of the American Academy of Psychiatry and the Law, 38,* 130–132.

Hawton, K. (2007). Restricting access to methods of suicide: Rationale and evaluation of this approach to suicide prevention. *Crisis: Journal of Crisis Intervention and Suicide Prevention, 28,* 4–9.

Hayes, S. C., Strosahl, K. D., & Wilson, K. G. (2011). *Acceptance and commitment therapy: The process and practice of mindful change* (2nd ed.). New York: Guilford Press.

Hendin, H., Haas, A. P., Maltsberger, J. T., Szanto, K., & Rabinowicz, H. (2004). Factors contributing to therapists' distress after the suicide of a patient. *American Journal of Psychiatry, 161,* 1442–1446.

Henriques, G., Beck, A. T., & Brown, G. K. (2003). Cognitive therapy for adolescent and young adult suicide attempters. *American Behavioral Scientist, 46,* 1258–1268.

Higgins, E. T. (1999). When do self-discrepancies have specific relations to emotions?: The second-generation question of Tangney, Niedenthal, Covert, and Barlow (1998). *Journal of Personality and Social Psychology, 77,* 1313–1317.

Higgins, E. T., Roney, C. J. R., Crowe, E., & Hymes C. (1994). Ideal versus ought predilections for approach and avoidance: Distinct self-regulatory systems. *Journal of Personality and Social Psychology, 66,* 276–286.

Holmes, J., Saghafi, S., Monahan, M., Cardeli, E., & Jobes, D. (2014, April). *Self-hate and suicide: An analysis of incarcerated youth.* Paper presented at the 47th annual conference of the American Association of Suicidology, Los Angeles, CA.

Hooley, J. M., Franklin, J. C., & Nock, M. K. (2014). Chronic pain and suicide: Understanding the association. *Current Pain and Headache Reports, 18,* 1–6.

Horowitz, L. M., Bridge, J. A., Pao, M., & Boudreaux, E. D. (2014). Screening youth for suicide risk in medical settings: Time to ask questions. *American Journal of Preventive Medicine, 47,* S170–S174.

Horowitz, L. M., Snyder, D., Ludi, E., Rosenstein, D. L., Kohn-Godbout, J., Lee, L., et al. (2013). Ask suicide-screening questions to everyone in medical settings: The asQ'em quality improvement project. *Psychosomatics, 54,* 239–247.

Horvath, A. O., & Symonds, B. D. (1991). Relationship between working alliance and outcome in psychotherapy: A meta-analyisis. *Journal of Counseling Psychology, 38,* 139–149.

Hufford, M. R. (2001). Alcohol and suicidal behavior. *Clinical Psychology Review, 21,* 797–811.

Huijbers, M. J., Spijker, J., Donders, A. R. T., van Schaik, D. J., van Oppen, P., Ruhé, H. G., et al. (2012). Preventing relapse in recurrent depression using mindfulness-based cognitive therapy, antidepressant medication or the combination: Trial design and protocol of the MOMENT study. *BMC Psychiatry, 12,* 125.

Hunsley, J. (2015). Translating evidence-based assessment principles and components into clinical practice settings. *Cognitive and Behavioral Practice, 22,* 101–109.

Jacobson, N. S., Martell, C. R., & Dimidjian, S. (2001). Behavioral activation treatment for depression. *Clinical Psychology: Science and Practice, 8,* 255–270.

Jacoby, A. M. (2003). *Negative countertransference in psychotherapy with suicidal patients.* Unpublished doctoral dissertation, The Catholic University of America, Washington, DC.

Jennings, K. (2015). *Investigating the internal struggle hypothesis of suicide: Differential assessments of suicidal states using reasons for living and reasons for dying qualitative responses.* Unpublished doctoral dissertation, The Catholic University of America, Washington, DC.

Jennings, K., Jobes, D., O'Connor, S., & Comtois, K. (2012, April). *Suicide Status Form (SSF) macrocoded typologies of treatment-engaged suicidal patients and associated clinical implications.* Paper presented at the annual conference of the American Association of Suicidology, Baltimore, MD.

Jennings, K. W. (2012, June). *CAMS in a group format*. Presentation at the annual DOD/VA Suicide Prevention Conference, Washington, DC.

Jobes, D. A. (1995a). The challenge and promise of clinical suicidology. *Suicide and Life-Threatening Behavior, 25*, 437–449.

Jobes, D. A. (1995b). Psychodynamic treatment of adolescent suicide attempters. In J. Zimmerman & G. M. Asnis (Eds.), *Treatment approaches with suicidal adolescents* (pp. 137–154). New York: Wiley.

Jobes, D. A. (2000). Collaborating to prevent suicide: A clinical-research perspective. *Suicide and Life-Threatening Behavior, 30*, 8–17.

Jobes, D. A. (2001, April). *Quantitative/qualitative assessment of suicidality*. Paper presented at the annual conference of the American Association of Suicidology, Atlanta, GA.

Jobes, D. A. (2003). Understanding suicide in the 21st century. *Preventing Suicide: The National Journal, 2*, 2–4.

Jobes, D. A. (2004a, April). *Crisis center use of the SSF*. Workshop presentation at the annual conference of the American Association of Suicidology, Miami, FL.

Jobes, D. A. (2004b, October). *The psychology of suicide: Research on what suicidal patients have to say*. Keynote address at the 3rd annual Military Suicide Prevention Conference, Crystal City, VA.

Jobes, D. A. (2005). *Assessing and treating suicidal college students*. Unpublished research grant proposal.

Jobes, D. A. (2006). *Managing suicidal risk: A collaborative approach*. New York: Guilford Press.

Jobes, D. A. (2011). Suicidal blackmail: Ethical and risk management issues in contemporary clinical care. In W. B. Johnson & G. P. Koocher (Eds.), *Ethical conundrums, quandaries, and predicaments in mental health practice: A casebook from the files of experts* (pp. 33–40). New York: Oxford University Press.

Jobes, D. A. (2012). The collaborative assessment and management of suicidality (CAMS): An evolving evidence-based clinical approach to suicidal risk. *Suicide and Life-Threatening Behavior, 42*, 640–653.

Jobes, D. A. (2013a, September). *Innovations in suicide risk assessment and crisis intervention*. Invited plenary address to the Congress of the International Association for Suicide Prevention, Oslo, Norway.

Jobes, D. A. (2013b, September). *A randomized trial of the collaborative assessment and management of suicidality vs. enhanced care as usual for suicidal Soldiers*. Panel presentation at the Congress of the International Association for Suicide Prevention, Oslo, Norway.

Jobes, D. A. (2013c). Reflections on suicide among Soldiers. *Psychiatry, 76*, 126–131.

Jobes, D. A. (2014, August). *Active duty military and veterans suicide risk: Perspectives from a collaborative clinical approach*. Panel presentation at the annual convention of the American Psychological Association, Washington, DC.

Jobes, D. A. (2015, June). *CAMS as an intervention for suicide risk*. Plenary presentation at the Congress of the International Association for Suicide Prevention, Montreal, Quebec, Canada.

Jobes, D. A. (2016, April). *Changing clinical care to save lives*. Linehan Award Presentation at the 49th annual conference of the American Association of Suicidology, Chicago, IL.

Jobes, D. A., & Berman, A. L. (1993). Suicide and malpractice liability: Assessing and revising policies, procedures, and practice in outpatient settings. *Professional Psychology: Research and Practice, 24*, 91–99.

Jobes, D. A., & Bostwick, J. M. (2006, April). *Perturbed suicidality: Research and treatment*. Research presentation at the annual conference of the American Association of Suicidology, Seattle, WA.

Jobes, D. A., & Bowers, M. (2015). Treating suicidal risk in a post-healthcare reform era. *Journal of Aggression, Conflict and Peace Research, 7*, 167–178.

Jobes, D. A., Bryan, C. J., & Neal-Walden, T. A. (2009). Conducting suicide research in naturalistic clinical settings. *Journal of Clinical Psychology, 65*, 382–395.

Jobes, D. A., Casey, J. O., Berman, A. L., & Wright, D. G. (1991). Empirical criteria for the determination of suicide manner of death. *Journal of Forensic Sciences, 36*, 244–256.

Jobes, D. A., Comtois, K., Brenner, L., & Gutierrez, P. (2011). Clinical trial feasibility studies of the Collaborative Assessment and Management of Suicidality (CAMS). In R. C. O'Connor, S. Platt, & J. Gordon (Eds.), *International handbook of suicide prevention: Research, policy, and practice* (pp. 383–400). West Sussex, UK: Wiley-Blackwell.

Jobes, D. A., Comtois, K. A., Brenner, L. A., Gutierrez, P. M., & O'Connor, S. S. (2016). Lessons learned from clinical trials of the Collaborative Assessment and Management of Suicidality (CAMS). In R. C. O'Connor & J. Pirkis (Eds.), *International handbook of suicide prevention* (2nd ed., pp. 431–449). West Sussex, UK: Wiley-Blackwell.

Jobes, D. A., Comtois, K. A., Brown, G. K., & Sung, J. (2015, April). *Evidence-based practice for suicidal risk: Rhetoric vs. reality.* Panel presentation at the annual conference of the American Association of Suicidology, Atlanta, GA.

Jobes, D. A., & Drozd, J. F. (2004). The CAMS approach to working with suicidal patients. *Journal of Contemporary Psychotherapy, 34,* 73–85.

Jobes, D. A., Eyman, J. R., & Yufit, R. I. (1995). How clinicians assess suicide risk in adolescents and adults. *Crisis Intervention and Time-Limited Treatment, 2,* 1–12.

Jobes, D. A., & Flemming, E. P. (2004, August). *Qualitative SSF assessments of suicidality and treatment outcome.* Paper presented at the 10th European Symposium on Suicide and Suicide Behaviors, Copenhagen, Denmark.

Jobes, D. A., Jacoby, A. M., Cimbolic, P., & Hustead, L. A. T. (1997). Assessment and treatment of suicidal clients in a university counseling center. *Journal of Counseling Psychology, 44,* 368–377.

Jobes, D. A., & Jennings, K. W. (2011). The collaborative assessment and management of suicidality (CAMS) with college students. In D. Lamis & D. Lester (Eds.), *Understanding and preventing college student suicide* (pp. 236–254). Springfield, IL: Charles C Thomas.

Jobes, D. A., Kahn-Greene, E., Greene, J., & Goeke-Morey, M. (2009). Clinical improvements of suicidal outpatients: Examining suicide status form responses as predictors and moderators. *Archives of Suicide Research, 13,* 147–159.

Jobes, D. A., & Karmel, M. P. (1996). Case consultation with a suicidal adolescent. In A. Leenaars & D. Lester (Eds.), *Suicide and the unconscious* (pp. 175–193). Northvale, NJ: Aronson.

Jobes, D. A., Luoma, J. B., Hustead, L. A. T., & Mann, R. (2000). In the wake of suicide: Survivorship and postvention. In R. Maris (Ed.), *Textbook of suicidology and suicide prevention* (pp. 536–561). New York: Guilford Press.

Jobes, D. A., Luoma, J. B., Jacoby, A. M., & Mann, R. E. (1998). *Manual for the collaborative assessment and management of suicidality (CAMS).* Unpublished manuscript, The Catholic University of America, Washington, DC.

Jobes, D. A., & Maltsberger, J. T. (1995). The hazards of treating suicidal patients. In M. B. Sussman (Ed.), *A perilous calling: The hazards of psychotherapy practice* (pp. 200–214). New York: Wiley.

Jobes, D. A., & Mann, R. E. (1999). Reasons for living versus reasons for dying: Examining the internal debate of suicide. *Suicide and Life-Threatening Behavior, 29,* 97–104.

Jobes, D. A., & Mann, R. E. (2000). Letters to the editor—Reply. *Suicide and Life-Threatening Behavior, 30,* 182.

Jobes, D. A., & Nelson, K. N. (2006). Shneidman's contributions to the understanding of suicidal thinking. In T. E. Ellis (Ed.), *Cognition and suicide: Theory, research, and therapy* (pp. 29–49). Washington, DC: American Psychological Association.

Jobes, D. A., Nelson, K. N., Peterson, E. M., Pentiuc, D., Downing, V., Francini, K., et al. (2004). Describing suicidality: An investigation of qualitative SSF responses. *Suicide and Life-Threatening Behavior, 34,* 99–112.

Jobes, D. A., & O'Connor, S. (2009). The duty to protect: Suicide assessment and intervention. In J. Werth, E. Welfel, & G. Benjamin (Eds.), *The duty to protect: Ethical, legal, and professional considerations in risk assessment and intervention* (pp. 163–180). Washington, DC: American Psychological Association.

Jobes, D. A., Rudd, M. D., Overholser, J. C., & Joiner, T. E. (2008). Ethical and competent care of suicidal patients: Contemporary challenges, new developments, and considerations for clinical practice. *Professional Psychology: Research and Practice, 39,* 405–413.

Jobes, D. A., Stone, G., Wagner, B., Conrad, A., & Lineberry, T. (2010, September). *Suicide facilitating and preventive aspects of self vs. relational orientations.* Paper presented at the 13th European Symposium of Suicide and Suicidal Behavior, Rome, Italy.

Jobes, D. A., Wong, S. A., Conrad, A., Drozd, J. F., & Neal-Walden, T. (2005). The collaborative assessment and management of suicidality vs. treatment as usual: A retrospective study with suicidal outpatients. *Suicide and Life-Threatening Behavior, 35,* 483–497.

Johnson, L. (2012, June). *Group therapy for individuals with increased risk for suicide: Provider and veteran perspectives.* Poster presented at the Annual DOD/VA Suicide Prevention Conference, Washington, DC.

Johnson, L. L., O'Connor, S. S., Kaminer, B., Jobes, D. A., & Gutierrez, P. M. (2014). Suicide-focused group therapy for veterans. *Military Behavioral Health, 2,* 327–336.

Joiner, T. E. (2005). *Why people die by suicide.* Cambridge, MA: Harvard University Press.

Joiner, T. E. (2015, May). *Optimizing screening and risk assessment for suicide risk in the US military.* Presentation at Suicide Prevention Research Interim Progress Report meeting, Military Operational Medicine Research Program, Ft. Detrick, MD.

Joiner, T. E., Conwell, Y., Fitzpatrick, K. K., Witte, T. K., Schmidt, N. B., Berlim, M. T., et al. (2005). Four studies on how past and current suicidality relate even when "everything but the kitchen sink" is covaried. *Journal of Abnormal Psychology, 114,* 291–303.

Joiner, T. E., Steer, R. A., Brown, G., Beck, A. T., Pettit, J. W., & Rudd, M. D. (2003). Worst-point suicidal plans: A dimension of suicidality predictive of past suicide attempts and eventual death by suicide. *Behaviour Research and Therapy, 41,* 1469–1480.

Joiner, T. E., Walker, R. L., Rudd, M. D., & Jobes, D. A. (1999). Scientizing and routinizing the assessment of suicidality in outpatient practice. *Professional Psychology: Research and Practice, 30,* 447–453.

The Joint Commission. (2010). A follow-up report on preventing suicide: Focus on medical/surgical units and the emergency department. *Sentinel Event Alert, 46,* 1–4.

The Joint Commission. (2013). Sentinel event data: Root causes by event type 2004–June 2013. Retrieved March 20, 2015, from *www.jointcommission.org/assets/1/18/Root_Causes_by_Event_Type_2004-2Q2013.pdf.*

The Joint Commission. (2016). Detecting and treating suicidal ideation in all settings. *Sentinel Event Alert, 56,* 1–7.

Joubert, L., Petrakis, M., & Cementon, E. (2012). Suicide attempt presentations at the emergency department: Outcomes from a pilot study examining precipitating factors in deliberate self-harm and issues in primary care physician management. *Social Work in Health Care, 51,* 66–76.

Judd, S., Jobes, D. A., Arnkoff, D. B., & Fenton, W. (1999). *Negative countertransference and suicide: An empirical evaluation.* Unpublished manuscript, The Catholic University of America, Washington, DC.

Kahl, K. G., Winter, L., & Schweiger, U. (2012). The third wave of cognitive behavioural therapies: What is new and what is effective? *Current Opinion in Psychiatry, 25,* 522–528.

Karlin, B. E., Ruzek, J. I., Chard, K. M., Eftekhari, A., Monson, C. M., Hembree, E. A., et al. (2010). Dissemination of evidence-based psychological treatments for posttraumatic stress disorder in the Veterans Health Administration. *Journal of Traumatic Stress, 23,* 663–673.

Kayser, S., Bewernick, B. H., Grubert, C., Hadrysiewicz, B. L., Axmacher, N., & Schlaepfer, T. E. (2011). Antidepressant effects, of magnetic seizure therapy and electroconvulsive therapy, in treatment-resistant depression. *Journal of Psychiatric Research, 45,* 569–576.

Kinsler, P. J., & Saxman, A. (2007). Traumatized offenders: Don't look now, but your jail's also your mental health center. *Journal of Trauma and Dissociation, 8,* 81–95

Klonsky, E. D., & May, A. (2010). Rethinking impulsivity in suicide. *Suicide and Life-Threatening Behavior, 40,* 612–619.

Klonsky, E. D., & May, A. (2015). The three-step theory (3ST): A new theory of suicide rooted in the "ideation-to-action" framework. *International Journal of Cognitive Therapy, 8,* 114–129.

Knox, K. L., Stanley, B., Currier, G. W., Brenner, L., Ghahramanlou-Holloway, M., & Brown, B. (2012). An emergency department-based brief intervention for veterans at risk for suicide (SAFE VET). *American Journal of Public Health, 102,* 33–37.

Kohen, D. (2004). Diabetes mellitus and schizophrenia: Historical perspective. *British Journal of Psychiatry, 184,* s64–s66.

Kopta, S. M., & Lowry, J. L. (2002). Psychometric evaluation of the Behavioral Health Questionnaire–20: A brief instrument for assessing global mental health and the three phases of psychotherapy outcome. *Society for Psychotherapy Research, 12,* 413–426.

Kopta, S. M., Petrik, M., Saunders, S., Mond, M., Hirsch, G., Kadison, R., et al. (2014). The utility of an efficient outcomes assessment system at university counseling centers. *Journal of College Student Psychotherapy, 28,* 97–116.

Kovacs, M., & Beck, A. T. (1977). The wish to die and the wish to live in attempted suicides. *Journal of Clinical Psychology, 33,* 361–365.

Kraft, T. L., Jobes, D. A., Lineberry, T. L., & Conrad, A. K. (2010). Brief report: Why suicide? Perceptions of suicidal inpatients and reflections of clinical researchers. *Archives of Suicide Research, 14,* 375–382.

Kulish, A., Jobes, D. A., & Lineberry, T. (2012, April). Development of a reliable coding system for the SSF "one thing" response. Poster presented at the annual conference of the American Association of Suicidology, Baltimore, MD.

Lahti, A., Keränen, S., Hakko, H., Riala, K., & Räsänen, P. (2014). Northern excess in adolescent male firearm suicides: A register-based regional study from Finland, 1972–2009. *European Child and Adolescent Psychiatry, 23,* 45–52.

Lambert, M. J., Burlingame, G., Umphress, V., Hansen, N., Vermeersch, D., Clouse, G., et al. (1996). The reliability and validity of the Outcome Questionnaire. *Clinical Psychology and Psychotherapy, 3,* 106–116.

Lambert, M. J., Hansen, N. B, Umphress, V., Lunnen, K., Okiishi, J., Burlingame, G., et al. (1996). *Administration and scoring manual for the Outcome Questionnaire (OQ 45.2).* Wilmington, DE: American Professional Credentialing Services.

Lambert, M. J., & Shimokawa, K. (2011). Collecting client feedback. *Psychotherapy, 48,* 72–79.

Lebensohn, Z. M. (1999). The history of electroconvulsive therapy in the United States and its place in American psychiatry: A personal memoir. *Comprehensive Psychiatry, 40,* 173–181.

Leenaars, A. A. (2004). *Psychotherapy with suicidal people: A person-centered approach.* New York: Wiley.

Lento, R. M., Ellis, T. E., Hinnant, B. J., & Jobes, D. A. (2013). Using the suicide index score to predict treatment outcomes among psychiatric inpatients. *Suicide and Life-Threatening Behavior, 43,* 547–561.

Lento, R. M., Ellis, T. E., & Jobes, D. A. (2013, April). *Self vs. relational suicidal orientation: Implications for treatment course and outcome.* Paper session presented at the 46th annual conference of the American Association of Suicidology, Austin, TX.

Lewis, L. M. (2007). No-harm contracts: A review of what we know. *Suicide and Life-Threatening Behavior, 37,* 50–57.

Lineberry, T. W., Brancu, M., Varghese, R., Jobes, D. A., Jacoby, A. M., Conrad, A. K., et al. (2006, March). *Clinical use of the suicide status form on a psychiatric inpatient unit.* Poster presented at the Fourth Aeschi Conference, Aeschi, Switzerland.

Linehan, M. M. (1993a). *Cognitive-behavioral treatment of borderline personality disorder.* New York: Guilford Press.

Linehan, M. M. (1993b). *Skills training manual for treating borderline personality disorder.* New York: Guilford Press.

Linehan, M. M. (1998, April). *Is anything effective for reducing suicidal behavior?* Paper presented at the annual conference of the American Association of Suicidology, Bethesda, MD.

Linehan, M. M. (2005, August). *Latest research on suicide and DBT*. Paper presented at the annual convention of the American Psychological Association, Washington, DC.

Linehan, M. M. (2014). *DBT skills training manual* (2nd ed.). New York: Guilford Press.

Linehan, M. M. (2015, February). Effective suicide care: Evidence-based treatments. Suicide Prevention Resource Center, Zero Suicide webinar presentation. Recording link available at *http://edc.adobeconnect.com/p3b5v78vwue..*

Linehan, M. M., Armstrong, H. E., Suarez, A., Allmon, D., & Heard, H. L. (1991). Cognitive-behavioral treatment of chronically parasuicidal borderline patients. *Archives of General Psychiatry, 48,* 1060–1064.

Linehan, M. M., Comtois, K. A., Murray, A M., Brown, M. Z. Gallop, R. J., Heard, H. L., et al. (2006). Two year randomized controlled trial and follow up of dialectical behavioral therapy vs. therapy by experts for suicidal behaviors and borderline personality disorder. *Archives of General Psychiatry, 63,* 757–766.

Linehan, M. M., Goodstein, J. L., Nielsen, S. L., & Chiles, J. A. (1983). Reasons for staying alive when you are thinking of killing yourself: The reasons for living inventory. *Journal of Consulting and Clinical Psychology, 51,* 276–286.

Linehan, M. M., Korslund, K. E., Harned, M. S., Gallop, R. J., Lungu, A., Neacsiu, A. D., et al. (2015). Dialectical behavior therapy for high suicide risk in individuals with borderline personality disorder: A randomized clinical trial and component analysis. *JAMA Psychiatry, 72,* 475–482.

Linehan, M. M., Schmidt, H., Dimeff, L., Craft, J. C., Kanter, J., & Comtois, K. A. (1999). Dialectical behavioral therapy for patients with borderline personality disorder and drug dependence. *American Journal on Addictions, 8,* 279–292.

Longcamp, M., Boucard, C., Gilhodes, J. C., Anton, J., Roth, M., Nazarian, B., et al. (2008). Learning through hand- or typewriting influences visual recognition of new graphic shapes: Behavioral and functional imaging evidence. *Journal of Cognitive Neuroscience, 20,* 802–815.

Longcamp, M., Boucard, C., Gilhodes, J. C., & Velay, J. L. (2006). Remembering the orientation of newly learned characters depends on the associated writing knowledge: A comparison between handwriting and typing. *Human Movement Science, 25,* 646–656.

Luoma, J. B. (1999). *Students' perceptions of items on the Suicide Status Form.* Unpublished manuscript, The Catholic University of American, Washington, DC.

Luoma, J. B., Martin, K. E., & Pearson, J. L. (2002). Contact with mental health and primary care providers before suicide: A review of the evidence. *American Journal of Psychiatry, 159,* 909–916.

Luoma, J. B., & Villatte, J. L. (2012). Mindfulness in treatment of suicidal individuals. *Cognitive and Behavioral Practice, 19,* 265–276.

Luxton, D. D., June, J. D., & Comtois, K. A. (2013). Can post-discharge follow-up contacts prevent suicide and suicidal behavior?: A review of the evidence. *Crisis, 34,* 32–41.

Maltsberger, J. T. (1994). Calculated risk-taking in the treatment of suicidal patients: Ethical and legal problems. In A. Leenaars, J. Maltsberger, & R. Neimeyer (Eds.), *Treatment of suicidal people* (pp. 195–205). Washington, DC: Taylor & Francis.

Maltsberger, J. T., & Buie, E. H. (1974). Countertransference hate in the treatment of suicidal patients. *Archives of General Psychiatry, 30,* 625–633.

Mann, J. J., Apter, A., Bertolote, J., Beautrais, A., Currier, D., Haas, A., et al. (2005). Suicide prevention strategies: A systematic review. *Journal of the American Medical Association, 294,* 2064–2074.

Mann, R. (2002). *Reasons for living vs. reasons for dying: The development of suicidal typologies for predicting treatment outcomes.* Unpublished dissertation, The Catholic University of America, Washington, DC.

Maris, R. W., Berman, A. L., & Maltsberger, J. T. (1992). Summary and conclusions: What have we learned about suicide assessment and prediction? In R. W. Maris, A. L. Maris, J. T. Maltsberger, & R. I. Yufit (Eds.), *Assessment and prediction of suicide* (pp. 640–668). New York: Guilford Press.

Maris, R. W., Berman, A, L., & Silverman, M. M. (2000). *Comprehensive textbook of suicidology.* New York: Guilford Press.

Mark, T. L. (2010). For what diagnoses are psychotropic medications being prescribed? *CNS Drugs, 24*, 319–326.

Marshall, E., York, J., Magruder, K., Yeager, D., Knapp, R., De Santis, M., et al. (2014). Implementation of online suicide-specific training for VA providers. *Academic Psychiatry, 38*, 566–574.

Martell, C. R., Dimidjian, S., & Herman-Dunn, R. (2013). *Behavioral activation for depression: A clinician's guide.* New York: Guilford Press.

Mashour, G. A., Walker, E. E., & Martuza, R. L. (2005). Psychosurgery: Past, present, and future. *Brain Research Reviews, 48*, 409–419.

Matulis, S., Resick, P. A., Rosner, R., & Steil, R. (2014). Developmentally adapted cognitive processing therapy for adolescents suffering from posttraumatic stress disorder after childhood sexual or physical abuse: A pilot study. *Clinical Child and Family Psychology Review, 17*, 173–190.

McHugh, R. K., & Barlow, D. H. (2010). The dissemination and implementation of evidence-based psychological treatments: A review of current efforts. *American Psychologist, 65*, 73–84.

McLaren, S., & Challis, C. (2009). Resilience among men farmers: The protective roles of social support and sense of belonging in the depression-suicidal ideation relation. *Death Studies, 33*, 262–276.

McWilliams, N. (2011). *Psychoanalytic diagnosis: Understanding personality structure in the clinical process* (2nd ed.). New York: Guilford Press.

Meehan, J., Kapur, N., Hunt, I. M., Turnbull, P., Robinson, J., Bickley, H., et al. (2006). Suicide in mental health in-patients and within 3 months of discharge: National clinical survey. *British Journal of Psychiatry, 188*, 129–134.

Meehl, P. E. (1997). Credentialed persons, credentialed knowledge. *Clinical Psychology: Science and Practice, 4*, 91–98.

Melonas, J. M. (2011). Patients at risk for suicide: Risk management and patient safety considerations to protect the patient and the physician. *Innovations in Clinical Neuroscience, 8*, 45–49.

Meltzer, H. Y., Alphs, L., Green, A. I., Altamura, A. C., Anand, R., Bertoldi, A., et al. (2003). Clozapine treatment for suicidality in schizophrenia: International suicide prevention trial (InterSePT). *Archives of General Psychiatry, 60*, 82–91.

Michaelsen, K., & Shankar, C. (2014). Suicide: Who is to blame? *Journal of the American Academy of Psychiatry and the Law, 42*, 109–111.

Michel, K., & Gysin-Maillart, A. (2015). *ASSIP: Attempted suicide short intervention program: A manual for clinicians.* Boston: Hogrefe.

Michel, K., & Jobes, D. A. (2010). *Building a therapeutic alliance with the suicidal patient.* Washington, DC: American Psychological Association Press.

Michel, K., Maltsberger, J. T., Jobes, D. A., Leenaars, A., Orbach, I., Young, R., et al. (2002). Discovering the truth in attempted suicide. *American Journal of Psychotherapy, 56*, 424–437.

Michel, K., Valach, L., & Waeber, V. (1994). Understanding deliberate self-harm: The patient's view. *Crisis, 15*, 172–178.

Millon, T. (2004). *Masters of the mind: Exploring the story of mental illness from ancient times to the new millennium.* Hoboken, NJ: Wiley.

Mills, P. D., Watts, B. V., Miller, S., Kemp, J., Knox, K., DeRosier, J. M., et al. (2010). A checklist to identify inpatient suicide hazards in veterans affairs hospitals. *Joint Commission Journal on Quality and Patient Safety, 36*, 87–93.

Mishara, B. L., Chagnon, F., Daigle, M., Bogdan, B., Raymond, S., Marcous, I., et al. (2005, April). *Practical implications for crisis centers of the AAS-Hopeline Silent Monitoring Evaluation Study.* Paper presented at the annual conference of the American Association of Suicidology, Denver, CO.

Monahan, M., Saghafi, S., Holmes, J., Cardeli, E., & Jobes, D. (2014, April). *"Manipulative" vs. "genuine" suicidal risk: An examination of juvenile offenders.* Paper presented at the 47th annual conference of the American Association of Suicidology, Los Angeles, CA.

Motto, J. A. (1976). Suicide prevention for high-risk persons who refuse treatment. *Suicide and Life-Threatening Behavior, 6*, 223–230.

Motto, J. A., & Bostrom, A. G. (2001). A randomized controlled trial of postcrisis suicide prevention. *Psychiatric Services, 52*, 828–833.

Murray, H. A. (1938). *Explorations in personality.* New York: Oxford University Press.

Nademin, E., Jobes, D. A., Downing, V., & Mann, R. (2005). *Reasons for living among college students: A comparison between suicidal and non-suicidal samples.* Unpublished manuscript, The Catholic University of America, Washington, DC.

Najavits, L. M. (2002). *Seeking safety: A treatment manual for PTSD and substance abuse.* New York: Guilford Press.

National Action Alliance: Clinical Care and Intervention Task Force. (2011). Suicide care in systems framework. Available at *http://actionallianceforsuicideprevention.org.*

National Alliance for the Mentally Ill. (2000, November 17). *Outpatient services experience big decline in availability according to new study* [Press release]. Available at *www.nami.org.*

National Alliance on Mental Illness (NAMI). (2014). Psychiatric hospitalization. Retrieved from *www.nami.org/Template.cfm?Section=About_Treatments_and_Supports&Template=/ContentManagement/ContentDisplay.cfm&ContentID=150789.*

Neacsiu, A. D., Rizvi, S. L., & Linehan, M. M. (2010). Dialectical behavior therapy skills use as a mediator and outcome of treatment for borderline personality disorder. *Behaviour Research and Therapy, 48*, 832–839.

Nestoriuc, Y., Martin, A., Rief, W., & Andrasik, F. (2008). Biofeedback treatment for headache disorders: A comprehensive efficacy review. *Applied Psychophysiology and Biofeedback, 33*, 125–140.

Nielsen, A. C., Alberdi, F., & Rosenbaum, B. (2011). Collaborative assessment and management of suicidality method shows effect. *Danish Medical Bulletin, 58*, A4300.

Nock, M. K., & Dinakar, K. (2015, April). *Using advances in technology and computing to improve the understanding, prediction, and prevention of suicidal behavior.* Plenary presentation at the annual conference of the American Association of Suicidology, Atlanta, GA.

Nock, M. K., Hwang, I., Sampson, N., Kessler, R. C., Angermeyer, M., Beautrais, A., et al. (2009). Cross-national analysis of the associations among mental disorders and suicidal behavior: Findings from the WHO World Mental Health Surveys. *PLoS Medicine, 6*, e1000123.

Nock, M. K., Park, J. M., Finn, C. T., Deliberto, T. L., Dour, H. J., & Banaji, M. R. (2010). Measuring the suicidal mind implicit cognition predicts suicidal behavior. *Psychological Science, 21*, 511–517.

Nock, M. K., & Prinstein, M. J. (2004). A functional approach to the assessment of self-mutilative behavior. *Journal of Consulting and Clinical Psychology, 72*, 885–890.

O'Connor, R. C. (2011). Towards and Integrated Motivational-Volitional Model of Suicidal Behaviour. In R. C. O'Connor, S. Platt, & J. Gordon (Eds.), *International handbook of suicide prevention: Research, policy and practice* (pp. 181–198). Chichester, UK: Wiley-Blackwell.

O'Connor, R. C., O'Connor, D. B., O'Connor, S. M., Smallwood, J., & Miles, J. (2004). Hopelessness, stress, perfectionism: The moderating effects of future thinking. *Cognitions and Emotions, 18*, 1099–1120.

O'Connor, R. C., Smyth, R., Ferguson, E., Ryan, C., & Williams, J. M. G. (2013). Psychological processes and repeat suicidal behavior: A four-year prospective study. *Journal of Consulting and Clinical Psychology, 81*, 1137–1143.

O'Connor, R. C., Smyth, R., & Williams, J. M. G. (2014). Intrapersonal positive future thinking predicts repeat suicide attempts in hospital-treated suicide attempters. *Journal of Consulting and Clinical Psychology, 83*, 169–176.

O'Connor, S. S., Beebe, T. J., Jobes, D. A., Lineberry, T. W., & Conrad, A. K. (2012). The association between the K10 and suicidality: A cross-sectional analysis. *Comprehensive Psychiatry, 53*, 48–53.

O'Connor, S. S., Brausch, A., Anderson, A. R., & Jobes, D. A. (2014). Applying the collaborative assessment and management of suicidality (CAMS) to suicidal adolescents. *International Journal of Behavioral Consultation and Therapy, 9*, 53–58.

O'Connor, S. S., Comtois, K. A., Wang, J., Russo, J., Peterson, R., Lapping-Carr, L., et al. (2015).

The development and implementation of a brief intervention for medically admitted suicide attempt survivors. *General Hospital Psychiatry, 37,* 427–433.

O'Connor, S. S., Jobes, D. A., Comtois, K. A., Atkins, D. C., Janis, K., Chessen, C. E., et al. (2012). Identifying entrenched suicidal ideation following hospital discharge. *Suicide and Life-Threatening Behavior, 42,* 173–184.

O'Connor, S., Jobes, D. A., Lineberry, T., & Bostwick, J. M. (2010). An investigation of emotional upset in suicidal inpatients. *Archives of Suicide Research, 14,* 35–43.

O'Connor, S. S., Jobes, D. A., Yeargin, M. K., Fitzgerald, M., Rodriguez, V., Conrad, A. K., et al. (2012). A cross-sectional investigation of the suicidal spectrum: Typologies of suicidality based upon ambivalence about living and dying. *Comprehensive Psychiatry, 53,* 461–467.

Ogrodniczuk, J. S., Joyce, A. S., & Piper, W. E. (2005). Strategies for reducing patient-initiated premature termination of psychotherapy. *Harvard Review of Psychiatry, 13,* 57–70.

Olfson, M., Gameroff, M. J., Marcus, S. C., Greenberg, T., & Shaffer, D. (2005). National trends in hospitalization of youth with intentional self-inflicted injuries. *American Journal of Psychiatry, 162,* 1328–1335.

Oordt, M., Jobes, D. A., Fonseca, V. P., & Schmidt, S. M. (2009). Training mental health professionals to assess and manage suicidal behavior: Can provider confidence and practice behaviors be altered? *Suicide and Life-Threatening Behavior, 39,* 21–32.

Oordt, M., Jobes, D., Rudd, M., Fonseca, V., Russ, C., Stea, J., et al. (2005). Development of a clinical guide to enhance care for suicidal patients. *Professional Psychology: Research and Practice, 36,* 208–218.

Orbach, I. (2001). Therapeutic empathy with the suicidal wish. *American Journal of Psychotherapy, 55,* 166–184.

Overholser, J. C. (2005). Contemporary psychotherapy: Promoting personal responsibility for therapeutic change. *Journal of Contemporary Psychotherapy, 35,* 369–376.

Owens, P. L., Mutter, R., & Stocks, C. (2010, July). Healthcare Cost and Utilization Project (HCUP) statistical brief #92: Mental health and substance abuse-related emergency department visits among adults, 2007. Retrieved from *www.hcup-us.ahrq.gov/reports/statbriefs/sb92.pdf.*

Patient Protection and Affordable Care Act (Public Law No: 111–148). (2010, March 23).

Patterson, D. R., & Jensen, M. P. (2003). Hypnosis and clinical pain. *Psychological Bulletin, 129,* 495–521.

Pennebaker, J. W., Chung, C. K., Ireland, M., Gonzales, A., & Booth, R. J. (2007). *The development and psychometric properties of LIWC2007.* Austin, TX: LIWC.net.

Peterson, E. M. (2003). *Assessing suicide risk and predicting treatment outcomes: The role of suicide history, suicide status form qualitative responses, and response style.* Unpublished doctoral dissertation, The Catholic University of America, Washington, DC.

Peterson, E. M., Luoma, J. B., & Dunne, E. (2002). Suicide survivors' perceptions of the treating clinician. *Suicide and Life-Threatening Behavior, 32,* 158–166.

Piet, J., & Hougaard, E. (2011). The effect of mindfulness-based cognitive therapy for prevention of relapse in recurrent major depressive disorder: A systematic review and meta-analysis. *Clinical Psychology Review, 31,* 1032–1040.

Pigeon, W. R., Britton, P. C., Ilgen, M. A., Chapman, B., & Conner, K. R. (2012). Sleep disturbance preceding suicide among veterans. *American Journal of Public Health, 102,* S93–S97.

Pigeon, W. R., Pinquart, M., & Conner, K. (2012). Meta-analysis of sleep disturbance and suicidal thoughts and behaviors. *Journal of Clinical Psychiatry, 73,* 1160–1167.

Pisani, A. R., Cross, W. F., & Gould, M. S. (2011). The assessment and management of suicide risk: State of workshop education. *Suicide and Life-Threatening Behavior, 41,* 255–276.

Pistorello, J., & Jobes, D. (2014, September). *Feasibility of adaptive treatments for suicidal college students: A SMART design.* Paper presented at the Dialectical Behavior Therapy Strategic Planning Meeting sponsored by University of Washington, Seattle.

Pompili, M., Innamorati, M., Szanto, K., Di Vittorio, C., Conwell, Y., Lester, D., et al. (2011). Life events as precipitants of suicide attempts among first-time suicide attempters, repeaters, and non-attempters. *Psychiatry Research, 186*(2), 300–305.

Pope, K. S., & Tabachnik, B. G. (1993). Therapists' anger, fear, and sexual feelings: National survey of therapist responses, client characteristics, critical, formal complaints, and training. *Professional Psychology: Research and Practice, 24,* 142–152.

Posner, K., Brown, G. K., Stanley, B., Brent, D. A., Yershova, K. V., Oquendo, M. A., et al. (2011). The Columbia–Suicide Severity Rating Scale: Initial validity and internal consistency findings from three multisite studies with adolescents and adults. *American Journal of Psychiatry, 168,* 1266–1277.

Poston, J. M., & Hanson, W. E. (2010). Meta-analysis of psychological assessment as a therapeutic intervention. *Psychological Assessment, 22,* 203–212.

Poulin, C., Shiner, B., Thompson, P., Vepstas, L. Young-Xu, Y., Goertzel, B., et al. (2014). Predicting the risk of suicide by analyzing the text of clinical notes. *PLoS ONE, 9,* e85733.

Powers, M. B., Halpern, J. M., Ferenschak, M. P., Gillihan, S. J., & Foa, E. B. (2010). A meta-analytic review of prolonged exposure for posttraumatic stress disorder. *Clinical Psychology Review, 30,* 635–641.

Price, R. B., Nock, M. K., Charney, D. S., & Mathew, S. J. (2009). Effects of intravenous ketamine on explicit and implicit measures of suicidality in treatment-resistant depression. *Biological Psychiatry, 66,* 522–526.

Qin, P., & Nordentoft, M. (2005). Suicide risk in relation to psychiatric hospitalization: Evidence based on longitudinal registers. *Archives of General Psychiatry, 62,* 427–432.

Randall, J. R., Rowe, B. H., Dong, K. A., Nock, M. K., & Colman, I. (2013). Assessment of self-harm risk using implicit thoughts. *Psychological Assessment, 25,* 714–721.

Range, L. M., & Penton, S. R. (1994). Hope, hopelessness, and suicidality in college students. *Psychological Reports, 75,* 456–458.

Resick, P. A., & Schnicke, M. K. (1992). Cognitive processing therapy for sexual assault victims. *Journal of Consulting and Clinical Psychology, 60,* 748–756.

Ribeiro, J. D., Bender, T. W., Selby, E. A., Hames, J. L., & Joiner, T. E. (2011). Development and validation of a brief self-report measure of agitation: The brief agitation measure. *Journal of Personality Assessment, 93,* 597–604.

Rice, R. E. (2002). *Assessing agentic and communal traits in suicidal outpatients: A potential model for predicting typologies, severity, and treatment outcome.* Unpublished doctoral dissertation, The Catholic University of America, Washington, DC.

Roberts, A. R., Monferrari, I., & Yeager, K. R. (2008). Avoiding malpractice lawsuits by following risk assessment and suicide prevention guidelines. *Brief Treatment and Crisis Intervention, 8,* 5–14.

Roemer, L., & Orsillo, S. M. (2009). *Mindfulness- and acceptance-based behavioral therapies in practice.* New York: Guilford Press.

Rogers, C. R. (1957). The necessary and sufficient conditions of therapeutic personality change. *Journal of Consulting Psychology, 21,* 95–103.

Romanowicz, M., O'Connor, S. S., Schak, K. M., Swintak, C. C., & Lineberry, T. W. (2013). Use of the Suicide Status Form-II to investigate correlates of suicide risk factors in psychiatrically hospitalized children and adolescents. *Journal of Affective Disorders, 151,* 467–473.

Rosenberg, M., Davidson, L., Smith, J., Berman, A., Buzbe, H., Gantner, G., et al. (1988). Operational criteria for the determination of suicide. *Journal of Forensic Sciences, 33,* 1445–1456.

Rotter, J. B., & Rafferty, J. E. (1950). *Manual for the Rotter Incomplete Sentence Blank, college form.* New York: Psychological Corporation.

Rowe, J. L., Conwell, Y., Schulberg, H. C., & Bruce, M. L. (2006). Social support and suicidal ideation in older adults using home healthcare services. *American Journal of Geriatric Psychiatry, 14,* 758–766.

Rudd, M. D. (2008). Suicide warning signs in clinical practice. *Current Psychiatry Reports, 10,* 87–90.

Rudd, M. D., Berman, A. L., Joiner, T. E., Nock, M. K., Silverman, M. M., Mandrusiak, M., et al.

(2006). Warning signs for suicide: Theory, research, and clinical applications. *Suicide and Life-Threatening Behavior, 36,* 255–262.

Rudd, M. D., Bryan, C. J., Wertenberger, E. G., Peterson, A. L., Young-McCaughan, S., Mintz, J., et al. (2015). Brief cognitive-behavioral therapy effects on post-treatment suicide attempts in a military sample: Results of a randomized clinical trial with 2-year follow-up. *American Journal of Psychiatry, 172,* 441–449.

Rudd, M., & Joiner, T. (1998). Relationships among suicide ideators, attempters, and multiples attempters in a young adult sample. *Journal of Abnormal Psychology, 105,* 541–550.

Rudd, M. D., Joiner, T., Brown, G. K., Cukrowicz, K., Jobes, D. A., Silverman, M. M., et al. (2009). Informed consent with suicidal patients: Rethinking risks in (and out of) treatment. *Psychotherapy Theory, Research, Practice, Training, 46,* 459–468.

Rudd, M. D., Joiner, T., Jobes, D. A., & King, C. A. (1999). Practice guidelines in the outpatient treatment of suicidality: An integration of science and a recognition of its limitations. *Professional Psychology: Research and Practice, 30,* 437–446.

Rudd, M. D., Joiner, T., & Rajab, M. H. (2001). *Treating suicidal behavior: An effective, time-limited approach.* New York: Guilford Press.

Rudd, M. D., Mandrusiak, M., & Joiner, T. (2006). The case against no-suicide contracts: The commitment to treatment statement as a practice alternative. *Journal of Clinical Psychology, 62,* 243–251.

Saghafi, S., Monahan, M. F., Holmes, J., Cardeli, E., & Jobes, D. A. (2014, April). *The subjective experience of suicide among youth: A comparison between suicidal college students and incarcerated juvenile offenders.* Paper presented at the 47th annual conference of the American Association of Suicidology, Los Angeles, CA.

Sakel, M. (1935). Schizopheniebehandlung mittels insulin-hypoglykämie sowie hypoglykämischer schock. *Weiner Medizinische Wochenschrift, 84,* 1211–1215.

Sanna, L., Stuart, A. L., Pasco, J. A., Kotowicz, M. A., Berk, M., Girardi, P., et al. (2014). Suicidal ideation and physical illness: Does the link lie with depression? *Journal of Affective Disorders, 152,* 422–426.

Schembari, B. C., & Jobes, D. A. (2015, June). *The cross-cultural applicability of American-based theories of suicide.* Paper presented at the Congress of the International Association for Suicide Prevention, Montreal, Quebec, Canada.

Schembari, B. C., Jobes, D. A., & Horgan, R. (2016). Successful treatment of suicidal risk: What helped and what was internalized? *Crisis: Journal of Crisis Intervention and Suicide Prevention* [Epub ahead of print].

Schilling, N., Harbauer, G., Andreae, A., & Haas, S. (2006, March). *Suicide risk assessment in inpatient crisis intervention.* Poster presented at the Fourth Aeschi Conference, Aeschi, Switzerland.

Schuberg, K., Jobes, D. A., Ballard, E., Kraft, T. L., Kerr, N. A., Hyland, C. A., et al. (2009, April). *Pre/post/post evaluations of CAMS-trained VA clinicians.* Poster presented at the annual meeting of the American Association of Suicidology, San Francisco, CA.

Schwartz, A. J. (2011). Rate, relative risk, and method of suicide by students at 4-year colleges and universities in the United States, 2004–2005 through 2008–2009. *Suicide and Life-Threatening Behavior, 41,* 353–371.

Segal, Z. V., Williams, J. M. G., & Teasdale, J. D. (2012). *Mindfulness-based cognitive therapy for depression* (2nd ed.). New York: Guilford Press.

Selaman, Z. M. H., Chartrand, H. K., Bolton, J. M., & Sareen, J. (2014). Which symptoms of post-traumatic stress disorder are associated with suicide attempts? *Journal of Anxiety Disorders, 28,* 246–251.

Shafran, R., Clark, D. M., Fairburn, C. G., Arntz, A., Barlow, D. H., Ehlers, A., et al. (2009). Mind the gap: Improving the dissemination of CBT. *Behaviour Research and Therapy, 47,* 902–909.

Shapiro, F. (1996). Eye movement desensitization and reprocessing (EMDR): Evaluation of controlled PTSD research. *Journal of Behavior Therapy and Experimental Psychiatry, 27,* 209–218.

Shea, S. C. (1999). *The practical art of suicide assessment: A guide for mental health professionals and substance abuse counselors.* New York: Wiley.

Sher, L. (2015). Suicide medical malpractice: An educational overview. *International Journal of Adolescent Medicine and Health, 27,* 203–206.

Shneidman, E. S. (1985). *The definition of suicide.* New York: Wiley.

Shneidman, E. S. (1987). A psychological approach to suicide. In G. R. Vanden Box & B. K. Bryant (Eds.), *Cataclysms, crises, and catastrophies: Psychology in action* (pp. 147–183). Washington, DC: American Psychological Association.

Shneidman, E. S. (1988). Some reflections of a founder. *Suicide and Life-Threatening Behavior, 18,* 1–12.

Shneidman, E. (1993). *Suicide as psychache: A clinical approach to self-destructive behavior.* Northvale, NJ: Aronson.

Shneidman, E. S. (1998). *The suicidal mind.* Northfield, NJ: Aronson.

Siepmann, M., Aykac, V., Unterdörfer, J., Petrowski, K., & Mueck-Weymann, M. (2008). A pilot study on the effects of heart rate variability biofeedback in patients with depression and in healthy subjects. *Applied Psychophysiology and Biofeedback, 33,* 195–201.

Simon, G. E., Rutter, C. M., Peterson, D., Oliver, M., Whiteside, U., Operskalski, B., et al. (2013). Does response on the PHQ-9 depression questionnaire predict subsequent suicide attempt or suicide death? *Psychiatric Services, 64,* 1195–1202

Simon, T. R., & Crosby, A. E. (2000). Suicide planning among high school students who report attempting suicide. *Suicide and Life-Threatening Behavior, 30,* 213–221.

Simon, T. R., Swann, A. C., Powell, K. E., Potter, L. B., Kresnow, M. J., & O'Carroll, P. W. (2002). Characteristics of impulsive suicide attempts and attempters. *Suicide and Life-Threatening Behavior, 32,* 49–59.

Simpson, S., & Stacy, M. (2004). Avoiding the malpractice snare: Documenting suicide risk assessment. *Journal of Psychiatric Practice, 10,* 1–5.

Slotema, C. W., Blom, D. J., Hoek, H. W., & Sommer, I. E. (2010). Should we expand the toolbox of psychiatric treatment methods to include repetitive transcranial magnetic stimulation (rTMS)?: A meta-analysis of the efficacy of rTMS in psychiatric disorders. *Journal of Clinical Psychiatry, 71,* 873–884.

Smith, A. R., Witte, T. K., Teale, N. E., King, S. L., Bender, T. W., & Joiner, T. E. (2008). Revisiting impulsivity in suicide: implications for civil liability of third parties. *Behavioral Sciences and the Law, 26,* 779–797.

Smith, M. T., Edwards, R. R., Robinson, R. C., & Dworkin, R. H. (2004). Suicidal ideation, plans, and attempts in chronic pain patients: Factors associated with increased risk. *Pain, 111,* 201–208.

Stack, S., & Scourfield, J. (2015). Recency of divorce, depression, and suicide risk. *Journal of Family Issues, 36,* 695–715.

Stanley, B., & Brown, G. K. (2012). Safety planning intervention: A brief intervention to mitigate suicide risk. *Cognitive and Behavioral Practice, 19,* 256–264.

Stefan, S. (2016). *Rational suicide, irrational laws.* New York: Oxford University Press.

Stefansson, J., Nordström, P., & Jokinen, J. (2012). Suicide Intent Scale in the prediction of suicide. *Journal of Affective Disorders, 136,* 167–171.

Stensland, M. D., Zhu, B., Ascher Svanum, H., & Ball, D. E. (2010). Costs associated with attempted suicide among individuals with bipolar disorder. *Journal of Mental Health Policy and Economics, 13,* 87–92.

Stoffers, J. M., Völlm, B. A., Rücker, G., Timmer, A., Huband, N., & Lieb, K. (2012). Psychological therapies for people with borderline personality disorder. *Cochrane Database of Systematic Reviews, CD005652*(8), 1–186.

Stranges, E., Levit, K., Stocks, C., & Santora, P. (2011, June). Healthcare Cost and Utilization Project (HCUP) statistical brief #117: State variation in inpatient hospitalizations for mental health and substance abuse conditions, 2002–2008. Retrieved from *www.hcup-us.ahrq.gov/reports/statbriefs/sb117.pdf.*

Street, R. L., Makoul, G., Arora, N. K., & Epstein, R. M. (2009). How does communication heal?: Pathways linking clinician–patient communication to health outcomes. *Patient Education and Counseling, 74,* 295–301.

Stroebe, W. (2013). Firearm possession and violent death: A critical review. *Aggression and Violent Behavior, 18,* 709–721.

Suarez-Balcazar, Y., Balcazar, F., Taylor-Ritzler, T., Portillo, N., Rodakowsk, J., Garcia-Ramirez, M., et al. (2011). Development and validation of the cultural competence assessment instrument: A factorial analysis. *Journal of Rehabilitation, 77,* 1–11.

Sublette, M. E., Galfalvy, H. C., Fuchs, D., Lapidus, M., Grunebaum, M. F., Oquendo, M. A., et al. (2011). Plasma kynurenine levels are elevated in suicide attempters with major depressive disorder. *Brain, Behavior, and Immunity, 25,* 1272–1278.

Sveticic, J., & De Leo, D. (2012). The hypothesis of a continuum in suicidality: A discussion on its validity and practical implications. *Mental Illness, 4,* 73–78.

Tang, J., Wu, S., & Miao, D. (2013). Experimental test of escape theory: Accessibility to implicit suicidal mind. *Suicide and Life-Threatening Behavior, 43,* 347–355.

Tarescavage, A. M., & Ben-Porath, Y. S. (2014). Psychotherapeutic outcomes measures: A critical review for practitioners. *Journal of Clinical Psychology, 70,* 808–830.

Tohen, M., Waternaux, C., & Oepen, G. (1994). One hundred years of schizophrenia: A meta-analysis of the outcome literature. *American Journal of Psychiatry, 151,* 1409–1416.

Tondo, L., Hennen, J., & Baldessarini, R. J. (2001). Lower suicide risk with long-term lithium treatment in major affective illness: A meta-analysis. *Acta Psychiatrica Scandinavica, 104,* 163–172.

Tucker, R. P., Crowley, K. J., Davidson, C. L., & Gutierrez, P. M. (2015). Risk factors, warning signs, and drivers of suicide: What are they, how do they differ, and why does it matter? *Suicide and Life-Threatening Behavior* [Epub ahead of print].

Unsworth, G., Cowie, H., & Green, A. (2011). Therapist' and clients' perceptions of routine outcome measurement in the NHS: A qualitative study. *Counselling and Psychotherapy Research, 12,* 71–80.

U.S. Department of Health and Human Services. (n.d.). Does depression increase the risk for suicide? Retrieved from *http://answers.hhs.gov/questions/3200.*

U.S. Department of Health and Human Services. (1996). Health Insurance Portability and Accountability Act of 1996 (Public Law 104-191, 104th Congress). Retrieved March 25, 2015, from *www.hhs.gov/ocr/privacy/index.html.*

Valenstein, E. S. (1986). *Great and desperate cures: The rise and decline of psychosurgery and other radical treatments for mental illness.* New York: Basic Books.

Valenstein, M., Eisenberg, D., McCarthy, J. F., Austin, K. L., Ganoczy, D., Kim, H. M., et al. (2009). Service implications of providing intensive monitoring during high-risk periods for suicide among VA patients with depression. *Psychiatric Services, 60,* 439–444.

Wagner, B. M., Wong, S. A., & Jobes, D. A. (2002). Mental health professionals' determinations of adolescent suicide attempts. *Suicide and Life-Threatening Behavior, 32,* 284–300.

Walsh, B. W. (2014). *Treating self-injury: A practical guide* (2nd ed.). New York: Guilford Press.

Weinstein, M. J. (2002). *Psychotherapy progress of suicidal students at the Johns Hopkins University Counseling and Student Development Center.* Unpublished doctoral dissertation, Chicago School of Professional Psychology, Chicago, IL.

Wenzel, A., Brown, G. K., & Beck, A. T. (2009). *Cognitive therapy for suicidal patients: Scientific and clinical applications.* Washington, DC: American Psychological Association.

Wilcox, H. C., Conner, K. R., & Caine, E. D. (2004). Association of alcohol and drug use disorders and completed suicide: An empirical review of cohort studies. *Drug and Alcohol Dependence, 76,* S11–S19.

Williams, M. (2001). *Suicide and attempted suicide.* London: Penguin.

Wingate, L. R., Joiner, T. E., Walker, R. L., Rudd, M. D., & Jobes, D. A. (2004). Empirically informed approaches to topics in suicide risk assessment. *Behavioral Science and Law, 22,* 1–15.

Winsper, C., & Tang, N. K. Y. (2014). Linkages between insomnia and suicidality: Prospective associations, high-risk subgroups and possible psychological mechanisms. *International Review of Psychiatry, 26,* 189–204.

Wise, T. L., Jobes, D. A., Simpson, S., & Berman, A. L. (2005, April). *Suicidal client and clinician: Approach or avoidance.* Panel presentation at the annual conference of the American Association of Suicidology, Denver, CO.

World Health Organization. (1992). *International classification of diseases, 10th revision (ICD-10).* Geneva: Author.

Yanez, D. C. (2015, February). *Effective suicide care: Evidence-based treatments.* Suicide Prevention Resource Center, Zero Suicide webinar presentation. Retrieved from *http://edc.adobeconnect.com/p3b5v78vwue.*

Yang, B., & Lester, D. (2007). Recalculating the economic cost of suicide. *Death Studies, 31,* 351–361.

Younes, N., Melchior, M., Turbelin, C., Blanchon, T., Hanslik, T., & Chee, C. C. (2015). Attempted and completed suicide in primary care: Not what we expected? *Journal of Affective Disorders, 170,* 150–154.

Zimbardo, P. G., & Boyd, J. N. (1999). Putting time in perspective: A valid, reliable individual-differences metric. *Journal of Personality and Social Psychology, 77,* 1271–1288.

Zisook, S., Lesser, I. M., Lebowitz, B., Rush, A., Kallenberg, G., Wisniewski, S. R., et al. (2011). Effect of antidepressant medication treatment on suicidal ideation and behavior in a randomized trial: An exploratory report from the Combining Medications to Enhance Depression Outcomes Study. *Journal of Clinical Psychiatry, 72,* 1322–1332.

Index

Page numbers followed by *f* indicate figure, *t* indicate table